GENDER IDENTITY DISORDER AND PSYCHOSEXUAL PROBLEMS IN CHILDREN AND ADOLESCENTS

Gender Identity Disorder and Psychosexual Problems in Children and Adolescents

KENNETH J. ZUCKER, Ph.D.
SUSAN J. BRADLEY, M.D.

THE GUILFORD PRESS
New York   London

Published by The Guilford Press
A Division of Guilford Publications, Inc.
72 Spring Street, New York, NY 10012

Printed in the United States of America

This book is printed on acid-free paper.

Last digit is print number: 9   8   7   6   5   4   3   2   1

Library of Congress Cataloging-in-Publication Data

Zucker, Kenneth J.
    Gender identity disorder and psychosexual problems in children and
adolescents / Kenneth J. Zucker, Susan J. Bradley.
        p.   cm.
    Includes bibliographical references and index.
    ISBN 0-89862-266-2
    1. Gender identity disorders in children.   2. Gender identity
disorders in adolescence.   3. Psychosexual disorders in adolescence.
I. Bradley, Susan J.   II. Title.
    [DNLM: 1. Gender Identity—in infancy and childhood.   2. Gender
Identity—in adolescence.   3. Psychosexual Development—in
adolescence.   4. Psychosexual Development—in infancy & childhood.
WS 105.5.P3 Z94g 1995]
RJ506.G35Z83   1995
618.92'8583—dc20
DNLM/DLC
for Library of Congress   95-2174
                                                              CIP

Preface

In the mid-1970s, Kenneth J. Zucker was a graduate student in developmental psychology at the University of Toronto. Susan J. Bradley, a child psychiatrist, was on staff at the Child and Adolescent Service (now the Child and Family Studies Centre) at the Clarke Institute of Psychiatry, a government-funded psychiatric research institute and one of the primary teaching hospitals of the University of Toronto Medical School. Zucker's awe of the imposing Clarke Institute edifice inspired him to meet with the then chief of psychology, Dr. Kingsley Ferguson. He learned from Ferguson that Bradley had recently assembled a working group to assess children and adolescents with gender identity problems. Having read Green's (1974) volume, *Sexual Identity Conflict in Children and Adults,* Zucker, who had recently received his master's degree in clinical psychology and completed a thesis on normative gender development in children, was intrigued and arranged to meet Bradley. Thus began a collaboration that has continued to the present.

The Clarke Institute of Psychiatry was established in 1966. Over the years, it has supported many new investigators and topics. In 1968, Dr. Betty W. Steiner, an adult psychiatrist, was asked to establish a gender identity clinic for adults (Steiner, 1985a; Steiner, Zajac, & Mohr, 1974), which continues today under the leadership of Dr. Robert Dickey, a psychiatrist, and Dr. Ray Blanchard, a psychologist. The Adult Gender Identity Clinic is authorized by the Ontario provincial health insurance program to evaluate adults with gender dysphoria and to recommend, when appropriate, hormonal and surgical sex reassignment, which are then fully covered by the Ontario provincial health care plan.

By the mid-1970s, children were also being referred to the adult clinic. Dr. Steiner then asked the chief of the Child and Adolescent Service, Dr. Gordon Warme, whether anyone would be interested in evaluating these youngsters. Bradley's multidisciplinary team expressed an interest in doing so. This resulted in the establishment of what has since become a very busy Child and Adolescent Gender Identity Clinic (Bradley et al., 1978), which Zucker heads. Over the years, our work has been supported by many colleagues, including Drs. Freda Martin, Joseph H. Beitchman, Fred Lowy, Vivian Rakoff, Paul Garfinkel, Christopher Webster, and H. Bruce Ferguson. We are grateful to them for their collegiality.

We would like to thank a number of colleagues in the field who, through their professional work and more informal conversations, have greatly enriched our understanding of psychosexual differentiation and its disorders. In alphabetical order, they are J. Michael Bailey, Michael J. Baum, Ray Blanchard, Susan Coates, Anke A. Ehrhardt, Beverly I. Fagot, Kurt Freund, Richard C. Friedman, Brian A. Gladue, Louis J. G. Gooren, Richard Green, Melissa Hines, Stephen B. Levine, Heino F. L. Meyer-Bahlburg, John Money, Robert J. Stoller (deceased), and Kim Wallen. Of course, they should not be held accountable for the content of this work, but we hope that their contributions, both direct and indirect, are recognized. We would also like to thank Professor Meyer-Bahlburg for reviewing this volume in its entirety and providing his usual trenchant commentary.

We would also like to extend our gratitude to local colleagues in Toronto for their help in formulating ideas in this book and for agreeing to work therapeutically with many of the children and their families: Claire B. Lowry Sullivan (a close collaborator for several years), Marino Battigelli, Maria Becker, Alan Beitel, Andrea Birkenfeld-Adams, Miriam Byrne, Claudia Koshinsky Clipsham, Robert W. Doering, Jo-Anne K. Finegan, Cynthia Gertsmann, Joey Gladding, Jeremy Harman, Sam Izenberg, Myra Kuksis, Jodi A. Lozinski, Sally Manning, Klaus Minde, Faye Mishna, Janet N. Mitchell, Arnold H. Rubenstein, H. David Sackin, Stephen J. Sibalis, Ruth Stirtzinger, Costas Tirovolas, and Rod Wachsmuth. Lastly, thanks to Cathy Spegg for her computer wizardry, Lori Bothner for her data reduction skills, Pierro Fazzini for his artistry with Harvard graphics, and Wilma Aranha for assistance in typing portions of the manuscript.

In preparing this volume, Zucker wrote the first drafts for Chapters 1–7 and 9–10, and Bradley wrote the first drafts for Chapters 8 and 11–13.

Some of our research reported in this volume was supported by grants from the Sonor Foundation, the Laidlaw Foundation, the Dean's Fund (University of Toronto), and the Clarke Institute of Psychiatry's Research Fund.

KENNETH J. ZUCKER
SUSAN J. BRADLEY

Contents

GENDER IDENTITY DISORDER AND PSYCHOSEXUAL PROBLEMS IN CHILDREN AND ADOLESCENTS

CHAPTER I

An Overview

This volume is about gender identity disorder and psychosexual problems in children and adolescents. It can be divided into two parts: The first part concerns gender identity problems in children; the second part concerns gender identity and psychosexual problems in adolescents. Broadly stated, our goal is to provide the reader with an overview of the clinical and research literature in this field.

The study of psychosexual development and its attendant problems requires a strong interdisciplinary focus. It will become apparent that advances in our knowledge have come from many disciplines that cut across the biological and social sciences. An understanding of the clinical phenomena we explore in this volume will be facilitated by knowledge about normative psychosexual development (cf. Hines, 1982). Hence, we strongly endorse what has become an established axiom in developmental psychiatry and psychology: namely, that the growing knowledge bases about normative and atypical development are mutually enhancing enterprises—they are, so to speak, two sides of the same coin (Cicchetti, 1984, 1993; Sroufe & Rutter, 1984). Of course, this is not a particularly new idea, but one that has guided biomedical and psychological research for a long time. Regarding sexological matters in particular, we might recall a remark made by Freud (1905/1953) regarding the origins of homosexuality: "Psycho-analytic research is most decidedly opposed to any attempt at separating off homosexuals from the rest of mankind. . . . from the point of view of psycho-analysis the exclusive sexual interest felt by men for women *is also a problem that needs elucidating and is not a self-evident fact*" (pp. 145–146, italics added).[1]

In this introductory chapter, we provide the reader with a brief re-

1

view of some key terminology, a short historical overview of the field, and the aims of this volume.

TERMINOLOGY

The study of psychosexual development and its attendant problems requires, first of all, some familiarity with basic terminology. For professionals who work in clinical sexology or study normative psychosexual development, this will be quite familiar; for professionals with other primary interests, however, it will provide at least a rudimentary framework for conceptualizing the varied components of psychosexual differentiation.

Sex

In contemporary sexology, the term *sex* refers to attributes that collectively, and usually harmoniously, characterize biological maleness and femaleness. In humans, the best-known attributes that constitute biological sex include the sex-determining genes, the sex chromosomes, the H-Y sex-determining antigen, the gonads, the sex hormones, the internal reproductive structures, and the external genitalia (Money & Ehrhardt, 1972; Olsen, 1992). Humans with various types of physical intersex conditions (also referred to as *true hermaphroditism* and *pseudohermaphroditism*) show at least one type of anomaly with regard to these biological parameters (see, e.g., Imperato-McGinley, 1983; Money, 1994a; Money & Ehrhardt, 1972; Shearman, 1982).

Gender Identity, Gender Role, and Sexual Orientation

Although there continues to be healthy disagreement among scholars regarding the precise behavioral and phenomenological markers of psychosexuality, many contemporary researchers accept, at minimum, a tripartite model whose components are identified by the terms *gender identity, gender role,* and *sexual orientation.*

Researchers and clinicians used these terms with increasing frequency in the 1960s (see Money, 1973, 1994b). Initially, however, all three components of the tripartite model had been subsumed under the single term *gender role,* introduced by Money (1955) and defined as "all those things that a person says or does to disclose himself or herself as having the status of boy or man, girl or woman, respectively. It includes, but is not restricted to, sexuality in the sense of eroticism" (p. 254).

In the 1960s and 1970s, *gender role* was decomposed into the three conceptually distinct components noted above (see, e.g., Fagot & Leinbach, 1985; Money, 1985; Rosen & Rekers, 1980). *Gender identity* was distinguished from *gender role* by several scholars. Stoller (1964a, 1964b, 1965, 1968a), for example, used the slightly different term *core gender identity* to describe a young child's developing "fundamental sense of belonging to one sex" (1964a, p. 453). Cognitive-developmental psychologists (e.g., Kohlberg, 1966) began to use the term *gender identity* to indicate primarily that a child could accurately discriminate males from females and identify his or her own gender status correctly—a task considered by some to be the first "stage" in "gender constancy" development, whose end state is the knowledge of gender invariance (see, e.g., Eaton & Von Bargen, 1981; Kohlberg, 1966).

A child's acquisition of gender identity is, however, more than a cognitive milestone; it is also surrounded by affective significance. Many youngsters take the knowledge that they are male or female quite seriously. In our experience of administering gender constancy tasks (e.g., Slaby & Frey, 1975) to "normal" preschoolers, we have observed that some find it quite hilarious to be asked whether they are members of the opposite sex. Others seem offended and irritated! Yet, as noted by Fagot and Leinbach (1989), the role of affect in early gender identity formation has been relatively neglected by developmentalists. For clinicians, however, affect has always been a cornerstone in their thinking about this subject. For example, the term *gender dysphoria* was used with increasing regularity to describe patients, particularly adults, who felt so unhappy about their biological status as males or females that they sought surgical sex reassignment (Fisk, 1973). Clinicians working with children also noted the importance of affect that surrounded early gender identity development (e.g., Green, 1974; Money, 1968; Stoller, 1965, 1968b).

The term *gender role* is now defined more narrowly than Money (1955) defined it originally. Many scholars, particularly developmental psychologists, have used the term to refer to behaviors, attitudes, and personality traits that a society, in a given culture and historical period, designates as masculine or feminine—that is, as more "appropriate" to or typical of the male or female social role (Huston, 1983). In young children, the measurement of gender role behavior includes several easily observable phenomena, including affiliative preference for same-sex versus opposite-sex peers, fantasy roles, toy interests, dress-up play, and interest in rough-and-tumble play. In older children, gender role has also been measured using personality attributes with stereotypic masculine or feminine connotations (e.g., Absi-Semaan, Crombie, & Freeman, 1993; Alpert-Gillis & Connell, 1989; Hall & Halberstadt, 1980).

Defining gender roles in this way assumes that they are completely arbitrary and social in origin—a view not universally shared by researchers in the field. The notion of complete arbitrariness is particularly apparent among scholars who cede *sex* to biology and *gender* to the social sciences. (For critiques of this division, see Maccoby, 1988, Money, 1985, and Unger, 1979; for a recent exchange on this point, see Deaux, 1993, Gentile, 1993, and Unger & Crawford, 1993.) In lower animals, certain "gender role" behaviors that, on average, show quantitative sex differences (e.g., rough-and-tumble play) are influenced by biological variables, such as prenatal sex hormones (e.g., Gerall, Moltz, & Ward, 1992; Reinisch, Rosenblum, & Sanders, 1987). Given the phenotypic similarity of these behaviors to some human gender role behaviors, this might argue against a purely social analysis of their origins (Kenrick, 1987; Money, 1987a, 1988). As a result, some researchers who study humans employ such terms as *sex-typical, sex-dimorphic,* and *sex-typed* to characterize sex differences in behavior, since terms of this kind are descriptively more neutral with regard to putative etiology. The use of these terms, however, runs some risk of including behaviors relatively unrelated to how the term *gender role* is used in psychology, sociology, and anthropology. For example, art activities seem to be sex-preferred by female preschoolers (Fagot, 1977, 1978), yet it is not clear that the culture at large considers such behavior to be "feminine."

One further nuance regarding the term *gender role* requires consideration. Some developmental psychologists differentiate between children's expressed or observed gender role preferences and their knowledge (or stereotypes) concerning gender roles. Indeed, there is some merit in this distinction. For example, there is evidence that as children grow older, they become more flexible regarding behaviors considered appropriate for the male or female social role; thus, older children are more willing to concede that both boys and girls can engage in certain activities or are able to work in certain occupational roles (e.g., doctor and nurse). Yet children's actual gender role preferences remain considerably more sex-dimorphic over time. There appear to be distinct influences that account for this split between cognition and affect (e.g., Katz & Boswell, 1986; Liben & Signorella, 1987; Serbin, Powlishta, & Gulko, 1993).

Lastly, the term *sexual orientation* is defined by a person's responsiveness to sexual stimuli. The most salient dimension of sexual orientation is probably the sex of one's partner. This stimulus class is obviously how one defines a person's sexual orientation as heterosexual, bisexual, or homosexual. In contemporary sexology, sexual orientation is often assessed by psychophysiological techniques such as penile plethysmography and vaginal photoplethysmography (e.g., Freund, 1963, 1977; Langevin, 1983; Rosen & Beck, 1988), although structured interview schedules have become increasingly common, particularly when respondents do not have a compelling reason to conceal their sexual orientation.

It is important to uncouple the concept of *sexual orientation* from the concept of *sexual identity*. A person may, for example, be predominantly aroused by homosexual stimuli, yet may not regard himself or herself as "a homosexual," for whatever reason. Sociologists (particularly those of the "social scripting" and "social constructionist" schools) have articulated this notion most forcefully, arguing that the incorporation of sexual orientation into one's sense of identity is a relatively recent phenomenon, is culturally variable, and is the result of a complex interplay of sociohistorical events (e.g., Boswell, 1982–1983, 1990; Chauncey, 1994; Epstein, 1987, 1991; Escoffier, 1985; Gagnon, 1990; Gagnon & Simon, 1973; Greenberg, 1989; Interdisciplinary Centre for the Study of Science, Society, and Religion, 1989; McIntosh, 1968; Weeks, 1985, 1991). For example, several historians have pointed out that the word *homosexual* was first used as a noun only in the middle of the 19th century; it was coined by a German man known as Karl Maria Kertbeny (born Karl Maria Benkert) in 1869 (Bullough, 1990; Herzer, 1985). Anthropologists such as Herdt (1980, 1981, 1984, 1990a), who have described ritualized, age-structured homosexual behavior in non-Western cultures, note that such behavior is not at all tied to a homosexual sexual identity, but rather is a rite of passage to mature adult heterosexuality. In contemporary Western culture, there are many individuals (e.g., married men) who are primarily or exclusively sexually responsive to same-sex persons, yet do not adopt a homosexual or "gay" identity (see, e.g., Ross, 1983).[2] There are also individuals who engage in extensive homosexual behavior but who are not predominantly aroused by homosexual stimuli or do not consider themselves to "be" homosexual (e.g., male adolescents who have sex with men for money).

The *paraphilias* (*para:* akin to, faulty, abnormal; *philia:* abnormal appetite or liking for) also need to be considered in relation to the concept of sexual orientation (see Money, 1984, 1986a). For example, the stimulus class of age is of importance in determining whether a person's sexual orientation is complicated by an age-atypical sexual preference, as in the cases of pedophilia (a preference for prepubertal children) and hebephilia (a preference for pubescent children, usually about 11–14 years of age), regardless of whether the superordinate sexual orientation is heterosexual or homosexual (e.g., Freund, Watson, & Rienzo, 1989). In this volume, we consider one specific paraphilia, transvestic fetishism, as we observe it *in statu nascendi* during adolescence.

The literal meaning of the term *transvestism* is wearing the clothing of the opposite sex (Hirschfeld, 1910). In the older clinical literature on adults, the term *transvestism* was used by clinicians in diverse ways (see, e.g., Housden, 1965; Lukianowicz, 1959, 1962; Randell, 1959); without studying the actual case material, one could never be certain whether the patient was, in "modern" terminology, a *transsexual* (a person who experiences himself or herself as a member of the opposite sex, who wishes to be perceived that way by others, and who seeks out hormonal and surgical sex reassignment when it is available), a *transvestite* (a person who cross-dresses, in part, for the purpose of sexual arousal), or a homosexual cross-dresser or "drag queen" (Person & Ovesey, 1984). The term *transvestism* has also been used as a label characterizing the behavior of young children who show patterns of marked cross-gender behavior that signal a strong identification with the opposite sex, including the desire to change sex, even though the cross-dressing itself is not accompanied by sexual arousal (e.g., Bakwin, 1960). In contemporary sexology, the accepted clinical use of the term *transvestism* is limited to describing biological males who cross-dress because doing so is accompanied by sexual arousal (e.g., Blanchard, 1991; Ovesey & Person, 1976; Person & Ovesey, 1978; Stoller, 1971), and that is how the term is used in this volume.[3]

HISTORICAL BACKGROUND

Although the bulk of the early European literature in sexology pertained to adult homosexuality, the paraphilias, and alleged problems of sexual function (e.g., masturbation), there were several accounts of adults who struggled with a sense of profound discomfort about what we now term their gender identity.[4]

Both Hoenig (1982, 1985a) and Bullough (1987b) have summarized some of the landmark reports. Frankel (1853) is credited with describing the first case of a transsexual. He was followed by Westphal (1869), who coined the term *Konträre Sexualempfindung* (contrary sexual self-awareness); this term was meant in some instances to capture the phenomenology of an inverted gender identity, although more generally it referred to homosexual attractions (Moll, 1891). Ferenczi (1914/1980), one of Freud's close colleagues, employed another descriptor, *subject homoerotics*, to describe men who felt and behaved like women. Case examples of transsexuals subsequently appeared in such major texts as those by Krafft-Ebing (1886), Hirschfeld (1910), and Ellis (1910/1936).

Hirschfeld (1923) introduced the term *transsexual,* which Cauldwell (1949) transformed into *psychopathia transsexualis.* Hirschfeld's term was popularized by Benjamin (1954, 1966), an endocrinologist who played a pivotal role in humanizing the modern clinical care of adults with gender dysphoria ("Memorial for Harry Benjamin," 1988). Hoenig (1982) noted that the *Cumulative Index Medicus* introduced the term *transsexualism* as a subject heading only in 1969.

A turning point in the recognition of transsexualism as a clinical phenomenon was the publication of the Christine Jorgensen case by the Danish endocrinologist Hamburger (1953; Hamburger, Sturup, & Dahl-Iverson, 1953). Although there had been other personal and scientific reports along the same lines (e.g., Benjamin, 1954), including accounts of the first patient who received sex reassignment surgery (Abraham, 1931; Hoyer, 1933; Mühsam, 1921), the Jorgensen case helped crystallize the notion that adults' discontent with their gender identity might impel them to seek radical physical transformations.

Since the 1950s, the study of adults with gender identity disorder has been the focus of considerable clinical and scientific effort, including the publication of many books (Benjamin, 1966; Blanchard & Steiner, 1990; Bolin, 1987; Devor, 1989; Green & Money, 1969; Kando, 1973; King, 1993; Koranyi, 1980; Lothstein, 1983; Pfäfflin & Junge, 1992; Steiner, 1985b; Stoller, 1975; Tully, 1992; Walinder, 1967; Walters & Ross, 1986); the establishment of specialized adult gender identity clinics and standards of care (Pauly & Edgerton, 1986; "Standards of Care," 1985); and the entry of transsexualism into the psychiatric nomenclature (American Psychiatric Association, 1980).

From a historical point of view, several summary accounts have made the case that the wish to become a member of the opposite sex is not a novelty of 20th-century social life in the West (see, e.g., Bullough, 1974, 1975, 1987b; Bullough & Bullough, 1993; De Savitsch, 1958; Green, 1969, 1974; Lothstein, 1983; Nanda, 1990; Sweet & Zwilling, 1993)—a modern-day "social construction," as has been charged by some critics (e.g., Billings & Urban, 1982; Birrell & Cole, 1990; Garber, 1989; Irvine, 1990; King, 1984; Raymond, 1979; Risman, 1982; Sulcov, 1973; Yudkin, 1978). Perhaps the novelty lies in the availability of hormonal and surgical techniques for transforming aspects of biological sex to conform to the felt psychological state (Hausman, 1992). Indeed, the historical record on the phenomenon of gender dysphoria has deepened in recent years (e.g., Bullough & Bullough, 1993; Dekker & van de Pol, 1989; Herdt, 1994; Perry, 1987; Sullivan, 1990). Moreover, the evidence is increasingly compelling that gender dysphoria (and, more broadly, cross-gender identity) in adults occurs in many non-Western cultures (e.g., Blackwood, 1984; Hauser, 1990; Herdt, 1994; Roscoe, 1991; Ruan & Bullough, 1988; Ruan, Bullough, & Tsai, 1989; Stevenson, 1977; Weinrich, 1976; Whitehead, 1981; Wikan, 1977; Williams, 1986), although it may not be conceptualized and managed in the same way—by the individual or by his or her society—that this is done by mental health professionals in Western cultures.[5]

The relevance of the adult syndrome of transsexualism to the study of children became apparent from life history interviews, which indicated that the patient's gender dysphoria or discontent often originated in childhood. Such data were also hinted at in the anecdotal reports on psychosexual "inversion" (*inversion* was another forerunner of the term *transsexualism*) in the writings of the early sexologists (see, e.g., Hirschfeld, 1910/1991, Chap. 12).

But it was only 35 years ago that Green and Money (1960) published a series of five cases of young boys with marked cross-gender behavior, which they called "incongruous gender role," in the *Journal of Nervous and Mental Disease*. Although there had been previous reports on such youngsters (e.g., Bakwin & Bakwin, 1953; Bender & Paster, 1941; Friend, Schiddel, Klein, & Dunaeff, 1954; MacDonald, 1938), Green and Money (1960) were the first authors to begin to characterize this childhood behavioral pattern within the taxonomic framework that used the forerunners of the modern terms *gender identity, gender role,* and *sexual orientation* (see also Bakwin, 1960; Green & Money, 1961a, 1961b). By the late 1960s, the study of youngsters with marked cross-gender behavior was recommended as one strategy for understanding the development of gender identity disorder or transsexualism *in statu nascendi* (Green, 1968; Stoller, 1968b).

When these case reports first appeared, however, childhood cross-gender behavior was linked more closely to sexual orientation (homosexuality) than to transsexualism (cf. Brown, 1957, 1958).[6] The reason for this may have been that much more had been written about homosexuality than about transsexualism. Moreover, as will be noted in Chapter 3, homosexuality is much more common than transsexualism. If we return again to the writings of the early sexologists, there is evidence that the relation between childhood sex-typed behavior and later sexual orientation was no surprise. Moll (1907/1919), for example, wrote that

> the characteristics of effemination [male homosexuality] and of viraginity [female homosexuality] are displayed in early childhood. We are told that a boy with these tendencies prefers the society of little girls to that of boys, that he likes to play with dolls, and to help

his mother in her housework. He takes naturally to cooking, sewing, and darning; he becomes clever in the selection of feminine dress, so that he can help his sisters in the choice of their clothes. Contrariwise, the girl who is destined in later life to display the characteristics of viraginity will be found frequenting the playground of the boys. Such a girl will have nothing to do with dolls, but exhibits a passion for the rocking horse, and for playing at soldiers and robbers. (p. 126)

It is possible that in the modern era the relation of childhood sex-typed behavior to sexual orientation took a back seat to the relation of such behavior to transsexualism, because the latter was receiving so much clinical attention by the late 1960s. In addition, the imperial hold of psychoanalysis on clinical discourse pertaining to homosexuality through the 1960s may have resulted in a neglect of the nonerotic, developmental aspects of sexual orientation, given its focus on putative psychodynamics and family influences (see, e.g., Abelove, 1986; Friedman, 1988; Lewes, 1988). But, as we indicate throughout this volume, the connection between childhood sex-typed behavior and later sexual orientation and transsexualism has received considerable scrutiny over the past two decades.

AIMS OF THIS VOLUME

Two landmark books by Green (1974, 1987) have previously summarized our understanding of gender identity conflicts in children, particularly boys. In this volume, we wish to provide the reader with a comprehensive analysis of the clinical and research literature on children and adolescents with gender identity disorder and other psychosexual problems. The section on children (Chapters 2–10) provides a detailed analysis of gender identity disorder in both boys and girls that includes information on its core phenomenology, epidemiology, diagnosis and assessment, associated psychopathology, biological and psychosocial etiology, clinical formulation, treatment, and long-term follow-up. The section on adolescents (Chapters 11–13) provides information about gender identity disorder, transvestic fetishism, and homosexuality. Both sections include a great deal of material from our own work and attempt to integrate it with the extant literature that has accumulated, particularly over the past three decades. We hope that this volume will encourage other researchers and clinicians to continue to expand the understanding of psychosexual development in all people.

NOTES

1. Given this remark by Freud, it is astonishing that Chodorow (1992) recently claimed that psychoanalysis takes "as given a psychosexuality of normal hetero-sexual development" (p. 268) that does not require explanation.
2. In recent years, some activists in the homophile political subculture have even characterized their sexual identity as "queer," thus transforming a pernicious slur into a positive attribute (Duggan, 1992).
3. Stoller (1982) described three cases of possible transvestic fetishism in biological females: one reported by Gutheil (1930), another who corresponded with Stoller, and a third who had been seen in psychotherapy.
4. Although a discussion of the subject would go beyond the scope of this brief synopsis, we should mention that there is considerable current interest in the more general history of sexology or sexual science (e.g., Birken, 1988; Bullough, 1987a, 1994; Chauncey, 1982–1983; Faderman, 1992; Haeberle, 1982; Hansen, 1989; Hoenig, 1977a, 1977b; Hutter, 1993; Johnson, 1973; Martin, 1993; Matlock, 1993; Minton, 1986, 1988; Money, 1976a; Nye, 1989a, 1989b, 1991, 1993; Salessi, 1994). This interest is embedded in a much broader endeavor—an interdisciplinary examination of the history of sexuality, by scholars in social history and the humanities (e.g., Abelove, Barale, & Halperin, 1993; Bullough, 1976; Burnham, 1972; Fout, 1990; Halperin, 1989; Padgug, 1979).
5. Of course, the same can be said for what we would consider psychiatric phenomena in general, as psychiatrists and anthropologists interested in the interface between culture and psychopathology have long pointed out (e.g., Fabrega, 1975, 1994; Stein, 1993).
6. Some of the early clinical reports also made reference to transvestism. For example, Bakwin's (1960) clinical essay was entitled "Transvestism in Children." His case material was about children with marked cross-gender behavior, and not about the type of cross-dressing associated with sexual arousal. Bakwin may have meant to use the term *transvestism* to signify what we now term *transsexualism*, but this is not clear. From a modern perspective, therefore, Bakwin's use of the term *transvestism* was confusing but typical of this period. Green and Money (1961a) also wrote about the relation between childhood cross-gender behavior and "adult effeminacy, including homosexuality and transvestism" (p. 286), but did not specifically mention transsexualism. It is not clear whether their use of the term *transvestism* was meant to signify what we now mean by transsexualism. The ambiguous use of the term *transvestism* is apparently still quite common in psychoanalytic circles (see, e.g., Karush, 1993, p. 60).

CHAPTER 2

Phenomenology

Boys and girls diagnosed with gender identity disorder, as described in the fourth edition of the *Diagnostic and Statistical Manual of Mental Disorders* (DSM-IV; American Psychiatric Association, 1994), display an array of sex-typed behavior signaling a strong psychological identification with the opposite sex. These behaviors include (1) identity statements, (2) dress-up play, (3) toy play, (4) role play, (5) peer relations, (6) motoric and speech characteristics, (7) statements about sexual anatomy, and (8) involvement in rough-and-tumble play. In general, there is a strong preference for sex-typed behaviors more characteristic of the opposite sex, and a rejection or avoidance of sex-typed behaviors more characteristic of one's own sex. There are also signs of distress and discomfort about one's status as a boy or a girl. The behaviors that characterize gender identity disorder in children occur in concert, not in isolation. It is this behavioral patterning that is of clinical significance, and recognition of the patterning is extremely important in conducting a diagnostic assessment (see Chapter 4).

The onset of most of the behaviors occurs during the preschool years (2–4 years). At times, however, some of the behaviors, particularly cross-dressing (especially in boys), are observed even prior to the age of 2 years. Some boys develop what their parents describe as "an obsession" with their mothers' shoes or apparel prior to the age of 1 year—a process that is sometimes documented with photographs or with videotapes. Clinical referral often occurs when parents begin to feel that a pattern of behavior is no longer a "phase" (a common initial parental appraisal) that their child will "grow out of" (Stoller, 1967). From a developmental perspective, the onset occurs during the same period that more typical sex-dimorphic behaviors can be observed in young children (Fagot, 1985a; Huston, 1983).

The following two vignettes[1] are typical of children referred for clinical assessment.

CASE EXAMPLE 2.1

Max, a 5-year-old boy with an IQ of 124, was referred at the request of a psychiatric social worker whom the parents had consulted. Max lived with his parents, who had a middle-class socioeconomic background, and a younger sister. The parents had noted signs of cross-gender behavior since Max was 2 years old. When he was 3, they consulted their family physician, who apparently was not overly concerned. He presented as a thin and pale-looking, though cute, youngster with straight blonde hair that covered his forehead.

Max preferred girls as playmates but would shy away from them if they became too boisterous. Since age 2 Max had enjoyed cross-dressing, and currently he engaged in it both at home and at nursery school. His father commented that he was "creative" in his cross-dressing. Max had stereotypical feminine toy preferences, including female dolls, purses, and jewelry. His parents reported that he sometimes "carried" himself in a feminine way and spoke in a high-pitched voice when playing house. Max avoided rough-and-tumble activity and refused to participate in T-ball, a form of baseball for young children. Since age 3, Max had "sporadically" expressed the wish to be a girl. He sat to urinate and on occasion tried to hide his penis by covering it with his scrotum. He had said to his parents that he wished his penis would "fly away"; however, the parents also noted that he was "proud" when he experienced penile erection.

In addition to manifesting extensive cross-gender identification, Max was an extremely anxious, tense, and inhibited youngster. The parents recalled that as an infant Max had disliked vigorous play and loud noises, and had had extremely negative reactions to strangers. He had always been a poor sleeper and had often insisted on layering himself with clothing before bedtime (e.g., with several pairs of socks). Currently Max experienced marked anxiety in novel situations, such as going to school or encountering new peers. During the assessment, Max refused to separate from his parents for an individual interview. He was extremely closed when questions were posed to him; for example, he acknowledged "scary" dreams but could not provide information about their content. When seen for psychological testing, Max initially clung to his mother with tremendous intensity and cried. Once alone with the female examiner, he settled; nevertheless, he required a lot of checking in with his mother during the day.

CASE EXAMPLE 2.2

Sally, a 6-year-old girl with an IQ of 125, was referred at her mother's request. The parents were of a working-class socioeconomic background. The mother had had concerns about Sally's gender identity development for at least 2 years, but the family pediatrician did not agree with her. Finally, Sally's mother asked for help from her own physician, who referred her to our clinic. Although Sally's father attended the assessment, he expressed less concern about her behavior than did her mother, believing that it was only a phase in her development.

At the initial assessment, Sally wore black sweatpants and a black sweatshirt. For the first hour of the interview, she concealed her head behind the hood of the sweatshirt, so that her face could not be seen. Later, she took the hood down, lay on the floor, and bit her nails continuously. When she removed the hood, it was noted that her hair was short and styled in a fashion more culturally typical of boys than of girls. From the style of her hair and her clothing, a naive observer would have judged her to be a boy.

Sally's mother noted that at about the age of 3 she had developed a strong aversion to wearing culturally typical feminine apparel, such as dresses. Sally would have intense temper tantrums when asked to wear a dress, and insisted—relentlessly, in her parents' view—on having her hair cut in the fashion of a boy.

At the time of clinical assessment, Sally preferred boys as playmates; played only with stereotypical masculine toys; always took the male role in fantasy play; and was preoccupied with aggressive, culturally stereotypic masculine activities, such as hockey. At times her motoric style had an exaggerated masculine quality, although this was not observed in speech characteristics, such as pitch. Sally was preoccupied with the desire to be a boy. She had informed her mother that her male peers had told her about a "machine" that could change one's sex, and she demanded to be turned into a boy. She stated that if her parents refused this request, she would have "an operation" when she turned "25."

Apart from Sally's marked cross-gender identification, she presented as a tense, inhibited, and anxious youngster. She was described by her teacher as an anxious youngster who rarely spoke spontaneously. During the clinical interview, it was noted that from about the age of 3 Sally had been extremely jealous of her older brother, age 10. The parents stated that they lived in a neighborhood with few other children of her age and that there had been chronic conflict between Sally and her older brother, who did not want her to join him in his play with his male friends. During the individual clinical interview, Sally indicated that she wanted to be strong, and in doll-play interaction with the examiner she took great pleasure in throwing the brother doll off a cliff. Although largely mute, she indicated with affirmative head nods that she often felt scared and that she believed becoming a boy would make her stronger.

During the family interview, Sally did not seem particularly close to either of her parents. She did not look at her mother very often, and she never approached her mother for contact. By the end of the interview, she sat on her father's lap in a rather quiet, frozen way. Both parents noted that at home Sally tended to ignore typical parental requests, although they did not feel that she was grossly oppositional.

We now describe these clinical features in more detail (for other accounts, see Coates, 1985; Green, 1974, 1987, 1994a; Stoller, 1968b; Zucker & Green, 1993; Zuger, 1966).

IDENTITY STATEMENTS

Prior to school age, a few children rigidly maintain that they are in fact members of the opposite sex. Despite attempts at correction, they hold steadfastly to this belief. Clinically, it is not always clear whether these youngsters have made a literal error in gender self-labeling or whether these are defensive remarks. Other children, a larger number, are aware of their status as boys or girls but want to become members of the opposite sex. The repetitively expressed desire to be a member of the opposite sex is a common reason for clinical referral. Still other children do not voice cross-sex desires, but their sex-typed behavior nevertheless points to a marked cross-gender identification, as in this case.

CASE EXAMPLE 2.3

Matthew was an 8-year-old boy with an IQ of 98. He was referred for assessment because of maternal concern regarding his gender identity development. His parents, who were of a middle-class socioeconomic background, had been separated for 5 years.

At the time of assessment, Matthew displayed the following behaviors: He preferred to play with girls and was frightened of boys; his favorite toys were female dolls, such as Barbie and Cabbage Patch Kids; he loved to play with dolls' hair and his mother's hair, and indicated that he would be a hairdresser when he grew up; he liked to cross-dress and wear barrettes in his hair in public; he took only female roles in fantasy play, and his favorite heroine was Wonder Woman, whose transformational powers fascinated him; he displayed effeminate motoric movements; he dreaded rough-and-tumble play and group sports; he occasionally sat to urinate; and he had said on at least one occasion that he would like to be rid of his genitals. Matthew did not verbalize a current desire to be a girl, or indicate that he had such a desire but was afraid to tell anyone. He did state, however, that he had previously wanted this very much: "When I was 4 . . . I wanted to be a girl every day." Despite Matthew's failure to verbalize a current desire to be a girl, it seemed obvious that he manifested a significant cross-gender identification. There was little in his behavior or in his fantasy that connoted a masculine identification or satisfaction in being a boy.

By middle childhood, it is not unusual for the open wish to be of the opposite sex to dissipate—a diagnostic issue discussed in detail in Chapter 4. Among severely gender-dysphoric children, however, the wish remains open, and some of these children begin to wonder about how they could change sex.

CROSS-DRESSING

Cross-dressing is one of the more dramatic signs of marked cross-gender identification. In early childhood, the use of their mothers' clothes by boys is very common, including high-heeled shoes, dresses, jewelry, and makeup. In Green's (1976) study, for example, the modal time of onset of cross-dressing was between age 2 and 3, and 94% of the boys were cross-dressing by age 6. In many boys, cross-dressing has an obligatory quality (e.g., insistence on cross-dressing outside the home) and is not restricted to play situations. A common precipitant for referral is extensive cross-dressing by a boy in preschool or kindergarten. The driven quality of the cross-dressing is sometimes manifested by the boy's need to sleep in female clothing or by his agitation when female clothing is unavailable. Some parents report that when their son comes home from school, he manifests a frantic need to change into women's clothing. Even among parents who have a generally ambivalent or supportive reaction to their sons' cross-gender identification (see Chapter 7), there is an emerging unease with the chronic display of cross-dressing, and by school age such parents have usually attempted to set limits on the behavior. Some boys therefore resort to veiled maneuvers, such as creating costumes, using towels, or simply cross-dressing when no one is around. By late childhood, the interest in cross-dressing may be transformed into a preoccupation with the appearance of female movie stars or other popular figures.

Although most of these boys wear conventional masculine clothing in social settings, they often prefer colors that are stereotypically feminine, such as pink or purple (Picariello, Greenberg, & Pillemer, 1990). Some boys adamantly refuse to wear sweatshirts or other items of clothing that represent masculinity, such as those with male insignia (Batman, Teenage Mutant Ninja Turtles, Power Rangers, etc.). Some parents report that their youngsters are extremely picky about clothing, so that they have to be quite careful in their shopping; otherwise, there is intense conflict around dressing.

In girls, the marked rejection of stereotypical feminine clothing results in a great deal of conflict with their parents, particularly their mothers. The preference of these girls for a masculine style of dress does not result from a desire for more comfortable clothing (e.g., slacks or sweatpants, which many girls wear in social settings for this reason); it results from marked distress about being a girl. Some parents report that asking their daughters to wear stereotypical feminine clothing on special occasions (e.g., to church) gives rise to intense temper tantrums. Many of the girls also demand that their hair be cut extremely short, which results in a phenotypic appearance as male. As a result, a number of these girls are perceived by others as boys. For example, one 4-year-old girl seen in our clinic was presumed by her kindergarten teacher to be a boy because of her physical appearance. This girl was from an Asian country and did not yet speak English, and her Caucasian teacher was unable to infer her sex from her given name. The teacher presumed that the parents had simply erred in identifying her as a girl on the registration form. Despite parental assurance, the teacher was unconvinced and took the girl to the washroom "to check."

TOY AND ROLE PLAY

Many boys role-play female figures, including their mothers, their sisters, or characters from films or books. The toy interests and activities of these boys are also stereotypically feminine, with a particular interest in female dolls, such as Barbie or any other figure that is popular among girls (e.g., Kimberly and Trini from the *Mighty Morphin Power Rangers,* the latest television show that has captured the imagination of North American children). They show very little interest in toys and roles that are stereotypically masculine.

Clinically, we have been impressed with two major forms of this play, one or the other of which usually predominates. One form involves identification in fantasy with benevolent, idealized females, such as the Little Mermaid or Snow White. Boys preoccupied with Barbie (or her variants) spend inordinate amounts of time brushing her hair and dressing and undressing her. However, we have noticed very little nurturant play, such as parenting baby dolls. Although we have not studied this matter formally, our impression is that these boys are considerably less interested than girls are in nurturant, maternal role play. Such play is, for example, rarely observed during individual psychotherapy. The other form involves a preoccupation and identification with "evil" females, such as the Wicked Witch of the West (from *The Wizard of Oz*), Cruella DeVille (from *101 Dalmatians*), and Ursula

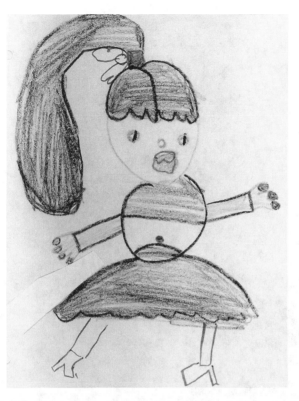

FIGURE 2.1. Drawing of a girl by an 8-year-old boy with gender identity disorder. Note the emphasis on detail (e.g., nail polish on fingernails), the oversized ponytail, the high-heeled shoes, and so on.

(from *The Little Mermaid*). Figures 2.1 and 2.2 display drawings by two boys that reflect these two types of female representations.

Many girls role-play male figures, including their fathers, their brothers, or characters from films or books. Their toy interests and activities are also stereotypically masculine. They are often preoccupied with violent and aggressive fantasy play, although they rarely act this out, unlike children with the disruptive behavior disorders. In this play, they often take on the role of protector. They show very little interest in toys and roles that are stereotypically feminine, including nurturant play. Figure 2.3 displays a drawing by one girl that reflects her preoccupation with the strength and power she associated with the male social role, and her own specific desire to become a weightlifter.

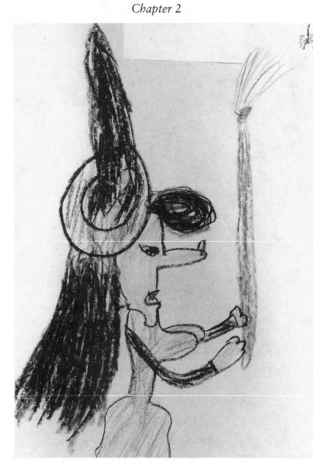

FIGURE 2.2. Spontaneous drawing of a witch by a 9-year-old boy with gender identity disorder, as he spoke about his mother during an individual interview.

PEER RELATIONS

The vast majority of these boys show a strong affiliation with girls as playmates. This preference remains in older boys, but they tend to become socially isolated (see, e.g., Green, 1976) as boys and girls develop stronger patterns of peer group "sex segregation" (La Freniere, Strayer, & Gauthier, 1984; Leaper, 1994; Maccoby & Jacklin, 1987). A minority of the boys have chronically poor peer relations and no close friends of either sex.

The quality of peer relations with girls varies. Some of the boys have genuinely close friendships with girls. Others seem to feel that

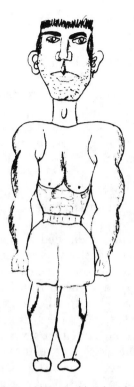

FIGURE 2.3. Drawing of a man by an 11-year-old girl with gender identity disorder, who wanted to be a weightlifter so that she could be strong enough to protect her mother from potential rapists.

they can be more "in control" with girls or younger children, and several clinicians have described these relationships as "bossy" (e.g., Bakwin, 1968; Zuger, 1966). Coates, Friedman, and Wolfe (1991) characterized as "omnipotent" or extremely egocentric some boys who "insist on their own rules in games . . . and when they do not get their way, they either withdraw or have temper tantrums" (p. 483). In general, the boys appear to experience less teasing from girls than from other boys regarding their feminine interests and activities, at least during early childhood.

There is usually a strong avoidance of boys as playmates. Some of the boys worry a great deal about bodily injury that they anticipate will occur during rough-and-tumble play. They appear to have trouble distinguishing between rough-and-tumble play and intent to hurt (cf. Costabile et al., 1991; Pellegrini, 1989; Smith & Boulton, 1990). Teasing by other boys becomes particularly prominent by middle childhood. One 6-year-old boy seen in our clinic appeared to deal with the teasing at school by announcing to his classmates that he really was a girl; however, he was rejected by both boys and girls. It is well known that boys form stable dominance hierarchies more commonly than do girls (e.g., Edelman & Omark, 1973). One boy seen in our clinic was subsequently placed in a day treatment milieu because of several co-oc-current behavioral difficulties. Serendipitously, he was a participant in a research study that focused on dominance hierarchies within the peer group. He was judged to be lowest in rank (M. M. Konstantareas, personal communication, August 19, 1993; Konstantareas & Homatidis, 1985).

The vast majority of the girls show a strong affiliation with boys as playmates. Although the girls appear to be less ostracized for their cross-gender interests than do the boys, it has been our impression that the markedly cross-gender-identified girls are disliked. For example, a 6-year-old girl who had transformed her female given name into a male given name (the pronunciation of the two names was identical) was rejected by both the boys and the girls in her class, who complained to the teacher that they were confused as to whether she was in fact a boy or a girl. Like the boys, some of the girls have chronically poor peer relations and no close friends of either sex.

The quality of the girls' peer relations with boys varies. Some of the girls have genuinely close friendships with boys that revolve around shared interests. Some of the school-age girls seem to have a strong need to compete with boys, but they tend to be excluded from the male peer group, which results in a sense of alienation. These girls usually reject other girls as playmates, in part because of the perception that girls do not share any of their interests.

MANNERISMS AND VOICE

Some boys display stereotypical feminine or "effeminate" body movements, such as flexing the elbow and letting the wrist go limp (see, e.g., Rekers, Amaro-Plotkin, & Low, 1977; Rekers & Morey, 1989a; Zucker, 1992a). Some of these boys speak in a high-pitched voice that parents and others perceive as girlish. The father of a 7-year-old boy (IQ = 115) described these behaviors as follows:

> "He at times becomes very effeminate in his mannerisms and his voice, particularly when he's under stress . . . he's under stress typically because he's either shy or . . . reacting to something, he gets very effeminate. . . . It's short-lived . . . but it's a, it's a very effeminate reac-

tion. . . . In terms of his hands or . . . the way he'll, he'll, I don't know if he actually flips his hand or whether he, or whether he sort of goes like, like this and he rolls his eyes, just strange little quirks, you know."

Some girls display stereotypical masculine body movements, in that they walk in an exaggerated manner (e.g., large strides) and lower their pitch to sound more like a boy. These characteristics do not, however, occur as routinely as do some of the other behavioral traits.

ANATOMIC DYSPHORIA

Expressions of dislike about sexual anatomy have not as yet been assessed in formal empirical studies. Because many children develop the same inhibitions about sexuality that adults do, inquiry about attitudes toward the genitalia meets with variable success (cf. Balk, Dreyfus, & Harris, 1982; Fraley, Nelson, Wolf, & Lozoff, 1991).

Clinical assessment reveals that some of these boys prefer to sit to urinate, which seems to fuel a fantasy that they have female genitalia. These boys often refuse to stand to urinate. Some boys attempt to hide or tuck the penis between the thighs, and then announce that they are girls. Other signs of anatomic dysphoria include efforts to simulate breasts and remarks that they hate their genitalia. Lothstein (1992) described several examples of "genital dysphoria" in young boys. For instance, one 5-year-old commented, "When my penis goes up, I get mad and angry. I hate it when it goes up. I want to shoot it off with a gun. I want to get rid of it. I want to shoot myself and die" (p. 95). On one occasion, this boy tried to cut off his penis; on another occasion, he tried to use his father's gun to shoot his penis. Card IV of the Rorschach inkblot test, which has a rather obvious "phallic" connotation, occasionally elicits unique responses. One 5-year-old boy seen in our clinic commented that he saw a "giant monster" (D7), and then pointed to a portion of the blot (D1) and said, "They have a big thing like that, going down. Know what? It's a dick. . . . It's not a nice thing to say. It's sort of rude. It's okay if you say 'dick' [said softly] but not if you say it like this—DICK [said loudly]." Later, he commented that the monster was wearing high heels (D2) and that "they should make the dick smaller." Other boys refuse to comment on D1 (the "phallic" protrusion) and appear to become quite anxious, turning the card, looking away, or handing it back to the examiner.

Anatomic dysphoria in girls often centers on a preoccupation with acquiring a penis. One girl slept with Magic Markers (felt pens) inserted in her underwear. Another girl walked around her house with a hot dog protruding from the zipper on her pants. A third stated that when she was older she would "murder" a man and cut off his penis.[2] A fourth was referred by her parents, in part because she had been making efforts to cut off her brother's penis with scissors and was very distressed when told by them that she could not do this. A fifth would draw pictures with "hundreds of penises" and pray to God at night for one. A sixth was persistent in claiming that she had male genitalia "hidden inside," despite her parents' efforts to dissuade her of this notion. If hit in the stomach with a hockey puck, she would clutch herself and exclaim, "Oh, my balls!" Information from interviews and psychological testing indicated that she was aware of her status as a girl but was struggling with intense desires that this not be so. For example, she stated that she knew she didn't really have a penis and testicles hidden inside her, but that she said she did so "just to be like a boy."

Some of the older girls become very distressed when they learn about the physical changes associated with puberty. By late childhood, they often refuse to wear bathing suits and wear several layers of T-shirts so that early breast development cannot be observed by others.

ROUGH-AND-TUMBLE PLAY

The boys generally dislike intensely rough-and-tumble activity, competitive group sports, and aggression, all of which often cause them to experience marked anxiety. Although some clinicians have observed that these boys are motorically clumsy (e.g., Bates, Skilbeck, Smith, & Bentler, 1974), we have noted that many of them are competent at individual athletic activities, such as swimming. Some of them have a phobic-like reaction to aggressive language and refuse to swear. They often complain about children who utter obscenities, and they are quite uneasy if they happen to have a teacher who yells a lot.

In contrast, some of the girls are quite involved in rough-and-tumble activity and, as noted earlier, are preoccupied with aggressive fantasy.

NOTES

1. Throughout this volume, we have followed Clifft's (1986) guidelines for confidentiality in reporting clinical material.
2. Fantasy sometimes becomes reality. An adolescent gender-dysphoric female was evaluated in our forensic division after being charged with homicide. This

youngster was passing socially as a male and was involved in a love relationship with a teenage girl. Her partner's father became suspicious about her true sex and demanded "proof" that she was in fact a male. The patient lured a taxicab driver into her apartment, murdered him, removed his penis and testicles, and attached them to her body with Krazy Glue. She was found not guilty by reason of insanity. This case, which received a great deal of attention in the local press, was likely the stimulus for the fictional character Paulie in the critically acclaimed novel *The Wives of Bath*, by Susan Swan (1993). Better fantasy than reality.

CHAPTER 3

Epidemiology

PREVALENCE

The prevalence of gender identity disorder in children has not been formally studied by epidemiological methods. Nevertheless, Meyer-Bahlburg's (1985) characterization of gender identity disorder as a "rare phenomenon" is not unreasonable. Gender identity disorder is an uncommon child psychiatric condition (like, say, autistic disorder), and can in no way compete in a prevalence race with such conditions as the disruptive behavior disorders.

If one relies on prevalence estimates of gender identity disorder (transsexualism) in adults, then one summary account suggested an occurrence of 1 in 24,000–37,000 men and 1 in 103,000–150,000 women (Meyer-Bahlburg, 1985). More recently, Bakker, van Kesteren, Gooren, and Bezemer (1993) inferred the prevalence of transsexualism in the Netherlands from the number of persons receiving "cross-gender" hormonal treatment at the main adult gender identity clinic in that country—1 in 11,000 men and 1 in 30,400 women.

This approach suffers, however, from at least three limitations. First, it relies on the number of persons who attend specialty clinics serving as gateways for surgical and hormonal sex reassignment; such clinics may not see all gender-dysphoric adults. Second, the assumption that gender identity disorder in children will in fact persist into adulthood is not necessarily true (see Chapter 10). Nevertheless, prevalence estimates of gender identity disorder derived from data on adult transsexualism support the notion of its rarity. Lastly, unlike adult females with gender dysphoria, who are invariably attracted sexually to biological females, adult males with gender dysphoria are about equally likely to be attracted sexually to biological males or females (e.g., Blanchard, 1985a, 1988, 1989; Blanchard, Clemmensen, & Steiner, 1987).[1] A childhood history of gender identity disorder, or its subclinical manifestation, occurs largely among gender-dysphoric adults with a homosexual orientation. Estimates of the prevalence of childhood gender identity disorder inferred from the prevalence of adult transsexualism in males should take this into account.

As will be discussed in detail in Chapter 10, gender identity disorder in childhood is strongly associated with subsequent homosexuality. Accordingly, the prevalence of gender identity disorder might also be derived from the literature on the epidemiology of homosexuality. Determining the prevalence of homosexuality is, however, no simple task and has been beset by a host of methodological and interpretive problems. For example, it is fairly well recognized that homosexual experiences are not equivalent to a homosexual orientation. Thus, the oft-cited finding by Kinsey, Pomeroy, and Martin (1948, p. 623) that 37% of the adult males they surveyed in the United States had had at least one postpubertal homosexual experience leading to orgasm is not of particular value in establishing the prevalence of a bona fide homosexual orientation (cf. Diamond, 1993a).

Estimates of the prevalence of a homosexual orientation based on other aspects of the Kinsey et al. (1948) data set differ considerably. Voeller (1990) recently concluded that "an average of 10% of the population [men and women combined] could be designated as Gay [homosexual]" (p. 33, italics omitted). Other scholars who have reworked the Kinsey et al. terrain suggest much lower prevalence rates, typically between 2% and 6% for men and about 2% for women (e.g., Diamond, 1993a; Fay, Turner, Klassen, & Gagnon, 1989; Gebhard, 1972; Rogers & Turner, 1991; Whitam & Mathy, 1986). Even lower estimates for men and women have emerged from studies pertaining to the AIDS epidemic (Billy, Tanfer, Grady, & Klepinger, 1993; Laumann, Gagnon, Michael, & Michaels, 1994; Leigh, Temple, & Trocki, 1993; Spira, Bajos, & the ACSF Group, 1994; Wellings, Field, Johnson, & Wadsworth, 1994).

Although these recent sex surveys constitute an improvement over Kinsey et al.'s work, they are far from satisfactory with regard to the actual prevalence of a homosexual orientation. Important distinctions between current and lifetime sexual experiences have not always been made. Operational definitions of homosexual behavior have varied from survey to survey. Interpersonal sexual behavior has been the main focus of assessment, with less attention given to fantasy (e.g., masturbation imagery). Assessment of sexual orientation in fantasy is important, since some adults with a homosexual preference may not engage in overt homosexual behavior for a variety of reasons. The issue of nonrespondents also remains a vexatious problem (cf. Fay et al., 1989; Wiederman, 1993). And none of these surveys have attempted to correct for the loss of people with a homosexual orientation to the AIDS epidemic. All of these factors may have resulted in underestimates of a homosexual orientation.

Remafedi, Resnick, Blum, and Harris (1992) conducted a unique study of sexual orientation among 36,741 adolescents (mean age = 15 years; range = 12–18 years; response rate = 69%). As part of the Minnesota Adolescent Health Survey, several questions were asked pertaining to sexual orientation: (1) sexual fantasy (males, females, both); (2) sexual experience of any kind with males and females; (3) sexual orientation self-labeling (from exclusively homosexual to exclusively heterosexual, or "unsure"); (4) sexual attraction; and (5) sexual interest.

Regarding sexual fantasy, 2.2% of males and 3.1% of females reported bisexual or homosexual fantasy. With respect to sexual attraction, 4.5% of males and 5.7% of females reported bisexual or homosexual feelings. With regard to self-labeling, however, only 1.1% of the participants described themselves as bisexual or homosexual. From these data, it appears that adolescents are more likely to report bisexual or homosexual feelings/attractions than to identify themselves as "bisexual" or "homosexual"—a pattern that has been observed by others (e.g., Meyer-Bahlburg et al., 1992).

The percentage of participants who did not respond to each of these questions ranged from 3.6% to 7.4%. The percentage of participants who were "unsure" of their sexual orientation was strongly related to age. For example, 25.9% of 12-year-olds were unsure, in contrast to only 5.0% of 17-year-olds.

Unfortunately, it is difficult to give a definitive interpretation of the absence of answers to these questions. Regarding fantasy or attraction, for example, the failure to respond could mean a reluctance to report atypical feelings or a failure to experience sexual fantasy or attraction. The questions may have been left unanswered because the option "no sexual fantasy or attraction" was not available. Moreover, because of the nature of the survey, we do not know how accurately the participants interpreted the questions. To ensure an accurate interpretation, a much more detailed psychosexual interview would be required. Lastly, we do not know whether the 31% who did not answer the questionnaire were disproportionately represented in one of the sexual orientation classifications.

The use of prevalence data on homosexuality to determine the prevalence of childhood gender identity disorder is based on retrospective studies that have shown a substantial proportion of homosexual men and women to recall greater rates of childhood cross-gender behavior than those of their heterosexual counterparts (e.g., Bell, Weinberg, & Hammersmith, 1981). To provide a more formal quantitative analysis of the retrospective literature pertaining to childhood sex-typed behavior and later sexual orientation, Bailey and Zucker (1995) conducted a meta-analysis based on 48 independent effect sizes from 41 different citations—32 effect sizes for heterosexual versus homosexual men, and 16 effect sizes for heterosexual versus homosexual women. The mean effect sizes for the within-sex sexual orientation comparisons were "large" by Cohen's (1988) criteria: 1.31 for men and 0.96 for women, respectively. Figures 3.1 and 3.2 display the frequency distributions of the pooled samples of men and women, respectively. The male distribution indicated that 89% of homosexual men exceeded the heterosexual median and that only 2% of heterosexual men exceed-

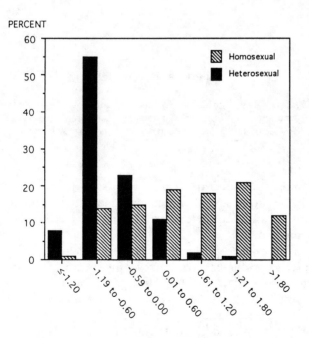

Recalled Sex-typed Behavior (Z)

FIGURE 3.1. Frequency distributions for recalled childhood sex-typed behavior for composite distributions of homosexual and heterosexual men. From Bailey and Zucker (1995, p. 48), Copyright 1995 by the American Psychological Association. Reprinted by permission.

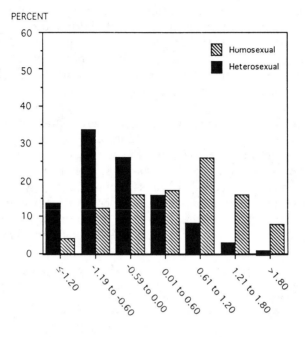

Recalled Sex-typed Behavior (Z)

FIGURE 3.2. Frequency distributions for recalled childhood sex-typed behavior for composite distributions of homosexual and heterosexual women. From Bailey and Zucker (1995, p. 48), Copyright 1995 by the American Psychological Association. Reprinted by permission.

ed the homosexual median. There was slightly more overlap for women: 81% of homosexual women exceeded the heterosexual female median, and only 12% of heterosexual women exceeded the homosexual female median.

From a prevalence perspective, however, these studies pose their own interpretive problems. For example, the specific behaviors assessed varied from one study to the next. How one should determine whether or not an individual was cross-gendered versus not cross-gendered ("caseness") is rarely specified; moreover, as noted by Friedman (1988), among others, individuals classified as cross-gendered would not necessarily meet the complete diagnostic criteria for gender identity disorder. A formal retrospective diagnostic study on the occurrence of gender identity disorder during childhood among homosexual men and women (compared to heterosexual men and women) remains to be done.

More liberal estimates of prevalence of gender identity disorder might be derived from studies of children in whom specific cross-gender behaviors were assessed (see, e.g., Zucker, 1985, pp. 87–95). For example, Fagot (1977) made an attempt at statistical identification of preschool children with "moderate" levels of cross-gender behavior. Such children were defined as obtaining preference scores for opposite-sex activities that were at least 1 SD above the mean of the opposite sex and preference scores for same-sex activities that were at least 1 SD below the mean of their own sex. According to these criteria, 7 (6.6%) of 106 boys and 5 (4.9%) of 101 girls displayed moderate cross-gender preferences.

Another source of information, based on a broader age range of children, comes from the widely used Child Behavior Checklist (CBCL; Achenbach & Edelbrock, 1981), a parent-report behavior problem questionnaire with excellent psychometric properties. It includes 2 items (out of 118) that pertain to cross-gender identification: "Behaves like opposite sex" and "Wishes to be of opposite sex." In the standardization study (see Table 3.1), endorsement of both items was more common for girls than for boys, regardless of age and clinical status (referred vs. nonreferred). Among referred boys, the desire to be of the opposite sex was quite high for the 4- to 5-year-olds (15.5%), but dropped off sharply thereafter for older children. Among referred girls, the desire to be of the opposite sex was more stable (ranging from 4.2% to 8.3%), and was consistently higher than that of the nonreferred girls.

Although both items significantly differentiated the clinic from the nonclinic samples, they did so quite poorly. In fact, they were among the five smallest differences in the entire questionnaire; hence, they were deemed nonsignificant after correction for the number of simultaneous comparisons (Achenbach & Edelbrock, 1981, p. 36). Similar results were obtained from a newly developed parent-report questionnaire, the ACQ Behavior Checklist (Achenbach, Howell, Quay, & Conners, 1991), which contains 3 items pertaining to cross-gender identification out of a total of 215 (two from the original CBCL and a third, "Dresses like or plays at being opposite sex"). If anything, endorsement of these items appeared to be less common on the new questionnaire than on the original CBCL, which supports the general point that extreme cross-gender behavior is relatively uncommon.

The main problem with such data is that they do not identify adequately patterns of cross-gender behavior that would be of use in determining "caseness." Thus, such data may be best viewed as screening devices for more intensive evaluation (cf. Pleak, Meyer-Bahlburg, O'Brien, Bowen, & Morganstein, 1989; Pleak, Sandberg, Hirsch, &

TABLE 3.1. Percentage of Children Whose Mothers Endorsed CBCL Items Relevant to Cross-Gender Identification

Group	Age grouping				
	4–5	6–7	8–9	10–11	12–13
Behaves like opposite sex (item 5)					
Boys					
Referred	16.3	11.2	9.5	10.7	2.7
Nonreferred	6.0	5.9	2.7	4.9	0.7
Girls					
Referred	18.6	9.1	14.5	13.1	16.5
Nonreferred	11.8	9.6	11.0	12.5	12.9
Wishes to be of opposite sex (item 110)					
Boys					
Referred	15.5	2.7	5.1	1.1	2.4
Nonreferred	1.3	0.0	0.0	2.3	0.0
Girls					
Referred	6.5	5.8	8.3	7.4	4.2
Nonreferred	5.0	2.6	2.7	1.9	2.7

Note. Data from Achenbach and Edelbrock (1981). Exact percentages from Achenbach (personal communication, December 7, 1982). $n = 100$ per cell. Percentages are not exact in some cases because of missing data.

Anderson, 1991; Sandberg, Meyer-Bahlburg, Ehrhardt, & Yager, 1993). Unfortunately, extant child psychiatric diagnostic interview schedules have not included an adequate number of items pertaining to gender identity disorder (Orvaschel, 1989). According to D. Shaffer (personal communication, August 4, 1994), however, such items will be considered for inclusion in the epidemiological field trials of the revised edition of the Diagnostic Interview Schedule for Children (Shaffer et al., 1993), so new information on prevalence rates can be expected to become available.

INCIDENCE

On the basis of clinical experience, Lothstein (1983) speculated that parents who had been influenced by the cultural *Zeitgeist* to use "non-sexist" socialization techniques may have inadvertently induced gender identity conflict in their children. There are, however, no systematic data regarding changes (or the lack thereof) in the incidence of gender identity disorder over the past several decades.

Figure 3.3 shows the number of referrals of children to our clinic from 1978 to 1994 (and to the adult clinic from 1975 to 1977, before the child clinic was opened). It can be seen that the referral rate increased somewhat from 1987 to 1994, but it is obviously impossible to know whether this has any bearing on incidence, which can only be studied epidemiologically. At present, the increased referral rate may simply reflect changes in "local conditions." It is possible, for example, that our clinic has more visibility, although we have never actively solicited referrals. It has been our impression that general practitioners, pediatricians, and school psychologists have become more sensitive to gender identity issues in children, in part because gender identity disorder now has "official" standing in the DSM. Parents may also have become more sensitive to gender identity issues, given that so much more is now being written about these matters in the popular press, magazines for parents, and so on. Although issues pertaining to long-term psychosexual outcome (transsexualism, homosexuality) have always been raised by many of the parents we see (as we discuss in more detail in Chapter 4), these matters may have become even more salient in

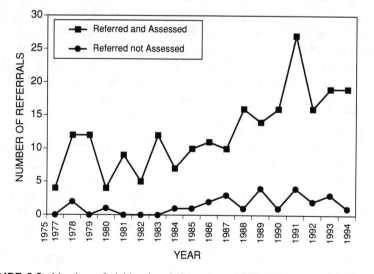

FIGURE 3.3. Number of child referrals by year in 1975–1977 to the Adult Gender Identity Clinic, Clarke Institute of Psychiatry, Toronto, Ontario, and in 1978–1994 to the Child and Adolescent Gender Identity Clinic, Child and Family Studies Centre, Clarke Institute of Psychiatry.

light of the AIDS epidemic. But these are only speculations and we have not attempted to test any of these ideas empirically.

SEX DIFFERENCES IN REFERRAL RATES

Consistently, it has been observed that boys are referred more often than girls for concerns regarding gender identity. This has been reflected in both research studies and case reports of treatment. Since its inception in 1978, our clinic has had a referral ratio of 6.3:1 ($n = 249$) of boys to girls.

How might this disparity be best understood? It may be that the true prevalence of psychosexual disorders is greater in males, perhaps because of a greater biological vulnerability. For example, it has been noted that among mammals, development along male lines is dependent on the production of androgen during early fetal development. If appropriate androgen secretion does not occur, or if cell receptors do not respond to circulating androgen, then fetal development proceeds along female lines, despite the presence of XY sex chromosomes. The androgen insensitivity (testicular feminization) syndrome (see, e.g., Pérez-Palacios, Chávez, Méndez, Imperato-McGinley, & Ulloa-Aguirre, 1987) in genetic males is the most poignant illustration of this possibility. Accordingly, it has been suggested that male fetal development is more "complex" than female fetal development, and thus more susceptible to errors that may affect postnatal psychosexual differentiation (e.g., Gadpaille, 1972; Money & Ehrhardt, 1972; Stoller, 1972).

Whatever the contribution of biological events, social factors appear to play a role in accounting for the disparity in referral rates. For example, the peer group is less tolerant of cross-gender behavior in boys than in girls (reviewed by Zucker, 1985), which might influence the likelihood of clinical referral.

Zucker, Wilson, Kurita, and Stern (1995) evaluated children's appraisals of clinically relevant cross-gender behaviors in boys and girls— that is, an array of behavior characteristics of children who would meet diagnostic criteria for gender identity disorder. Five stories were constructed that varied the ratio of same-gender to cross-gender behaviors: 4:0, 3:1, 2:2, 1:3, and 0:4. Children in Grades 3–6 read each story and then used a 5-point multiple-choice format to answer several questions, including one that asked whether they would like to be friends with the target child. Figures 3.4 and 3.5 display the results. For the experiment in which the target child was a boy (Figure 3.4), the boy raters liked most the boy who engaged in four same-gender behaviors. With each addition of a cross-gender behavior (and subtraction of a same-gender

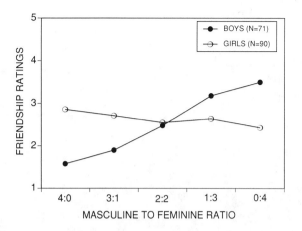

FIGURE 3.4. Peer ratings of friendship as a function of story content and rater's sex (male target child). Data from Zucker, Wilson, Kurita, and Stern (1995).

behavior), the target boy was preferred as a friend less and less. The girls' ratings indicated a general indifference toward being friends with the target boy, though there was some tendency for the boy to be liked as the number of his feminine behaviors increased. For the experiment in which the target child was a girl, the effects were much less pronounced (Figure 3.5).

More direct clinical evidence for the differential reaction to cross-gender behavior in boys versus girls comes from Green's studies of feminine boys and masculine girls. Green (1976) and Green, Williams, and Harper (1980) obtained parental assessments of the male peer group relations of 55 feminine and 45 control boys (all of whom proved conventionally masculine). The former had been referred by various professionals for participation in a research study (see Green, 1970). Green, Williams, and Goodman (1982) also obtained parental assessments of the female peer group relations of 50 masculine ("tomboy") girls and 49 feminine ("nontomboy") girls, who were solicited through newspaper advertisements.

Maternal ratings of same-sex peer group relations for these four groups of children are shown in Table 3.2. It can be seen that the masculine boys were more likely to have good same-sex peer group relations than were the feminine boys, especially as judged by the "good mixer" category. (As an aside, raw data provided by Green and analyzed elsewhere [Zucker et al., 1995] showed that the "rejected" feminine boys were significantly older than the feminine boys in the other three categories.)

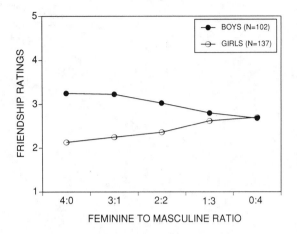

FIGURE 3.5. Peer ratings of friendship as a function of story content and rater's sex (female target child). Data from Zucker, Wilson, Kurita, and Stern (1995).

The masculine girls tended to do less well than the feminine girls with female peers, although this trend was not confirmed in the analysis of paternal ratings (Green et al., 1982). It is apparent from Table 3.2, however, that the masculine girls were less likely to be rejected by same-sex peers than were the feminine boys, and were more likely to be regarded as leaders or good mixers. One caveat in interpreting these

TABLE 3.2. Maternal Judgments of Same-Sex Peer Group Relations of Masculine and Feminine Boys and Masculine and Feminine Girls

Group	Same-sex peer group relations (%)			
	Leader	Good mixer	Voluntary loner	Rejected
Masculine boys (n = 45)	19	70	3	8
Feminine boys (n = 55)	14	29	38	18
Masculine girls (n = 50)	32	44	24	0
Feminine girls (n = 49)	27	63	8	2

Note. Data from Green (1976, Table 20) and Green, Williams, and Goodman (1982, Table 22).

differences is to recall that the masculine girls, unlike the feminine boys, were not referred through clinical channels.

Adults (e.g., parents, teachers) are also less tolerant of cross- gender behavior in boys than in girls (e.g., Fagot, 1977, 1985b; Langlois & Downs, 1980). Weisz and Weiss (1991) devised a "referability index" (RI), which reflected the frequency with which a child problem, adjusted for its prevalence in the general population, resulted in a clinic referral. All 118 items from the CBCL were analyzed in a comparison of clinic-referred and nonreferred children. Among parents in the United States, the 20 most referable problems (e.g., vandalism, poor schoolwork, attacks people) appeared to be relatively serious. In contrast, the 20 least referable problems (e.g., bragging, teases a lot, likes to be alone) appeared less so. B. Weiss (personal communication, March 4, 1992) indicated that for boys, the CBCL item "Wishes to be of opposite sex" had an RI of 91/118 (i.e., in the upper quartile), and "Behaves like opposite sex" had an RI of 80/118. For girls, the RI was lower: 55/118 for "Wishes to be of opposite sex" and 14/118 for "Behaves like opposite sex." In addition to their immediate differential reactions to cross-gender behavior in boys and girls, adults are more likely to predict long-term atypical outcomes (e.g., homosexuality) in feminine boys than in masculine girls (Antill, 1987; Martin, 1990).

These studies, particularly that of Weisz and Weiss (1991), led us to predict that girls would be required to display more extreme cross-gender behavior than boys before parents sought out a clinical assessment. Figure 3.6 shows that the mothers of gender-referred girls seen in our clinic were significantly more likely than the mothers of gender-referred boys to rate the two items pertaining to gender development on the CBCL as a "2" ("very true or often true" on a scale from 0 to 2). This was not, however, the case for ratings by fathers (Figure 3.6). Although mother–father ratings for the two CBCL ratings were significantly correlated, r (128) = .56, $p < .001$, it can also be seen in Figure 3.6 that the mothers were more likely than were the fathers to rate both items as a "2" for both the boys and the girls, χ^2 (1) = 5.11, $p < .05$, and χ^2 (1) = 3.18, $p < .10$, respectively.

If one assumes that mothers on average are more likely than fathers to initiate a clinical referral (a phenomenon we certainly have noted in our experience), there may well be a sex-related threshold difference associated with this process. This raises the question of whether boys are overreferred (i.e., the threshold is too low) or girls are underreferred (i.e., the threshold is too high). This question could be examined by testing for sex differences in the percentage of false-positive referrals. We will address this question further in Chapter 4.

Chapter 3

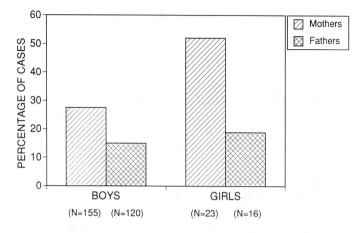

FIGURE 3.6. Percentage of mothers and fathers who rated the two CBCL items pertaining to gender identity (item 5, "Behaves like opposite sex"; item 110, "Wishes to be of opposite sex") as a "2" on a rating scale from 0 to 2.

A final possibility regarding the sex difference in referral rates is that the base rate of cross-gender behavior differs for boys and girls in the general population. The developmental literature is inconsistent on this point, but, if anything, girls are more likely to display masculine behavior than boys are to display feminine behavior (e.g., Brown, 1956; Cole, Zucker, & Bradley, 1982; Sandberg et al., 1993; Serbin et al., 1993). Thus, from a comparative standpoint, one would predict that girls need to show more cross-gender behavior than boys in order to be perceived as notably different from same-sex peers. To test this possibility, we compared our CBCL data with the normative data from the standardization sample (Achenbach & Edelbrock, 1983). We calculated the percentage of nonreferred boys and girls, aged 4–11 years, who received a rating of "2" on both CBCL items pertaining to gender development.[2] Of 398 boys, none were given ratings of a "2" on both items; of 398 girls, only 2 were rated in this way. Thus, it appears that the CBCL sex difference in our sample of gender-referred children does not seem to be accounted for by a sex difference in the way these items are rated for nonreferred children.

NOTES

1. Recent case studies have, however, identified a small number of biological females with gender dysphoria who report a sexual attraction to biological males

with a homosexual orientation (e.g., Blanchard, 1990a; Blanchard et al., 1987; Clare & Tully, 1989; Coleman, Bockting, & Gooren, 1993; Devor, 1993a, 1993b; Dickey & Stephens, 1995; Stoller, 1982, Case 2).

2. The CBCL raw data were provided on diskette by T. M. Achenbach.

CHAPTER 4

Diagnosis and Assessment

The diagnosis of gender identity disorder of childhood appeared in the psychiatric nomenclature for the first time in the DSM-III (American Psychiatric Association, 1980). Prior to this, at least 23 other descriptors were used by different writers to label the cluster of characteristics suggestive of marked cross-gender identification (listed in Zucker, 1992b, p. 309). Eventually, the DSM-III Advisory Committee on Psychosexual Disorders settled on Green's (1971) term, *gender identity disorder*, to represent the phenomenology described in the literature before 1980.

There were revisions to the criteria, particularly for girls, in the DSM-III-R (American Psychiatric Association, 1987); the Subcommittee on Gender Identity Disorders (hereafter, the DSM-IV Subcommittee; Bradley et al., 1991) recommended further revisions for the DSM-IV (American Psychiatric Association, 1994). In the first part of this chapter, we review some of the central diagnostic issues pertaining to the DSM-IV criteria for gender identity disorder.[1] Detailed analyses of the DSM-III and DSM-III-R diagnostic criteria for gender identity disorder of childhood can be found elsewhere (Zucker, 1982, 1992b; Zucker, Bradley, & Lowry Sullivan, 1992). In the second part of the chapter, we discuss issues pertaining to assessment.

DIAGNOSTIC ISSUES

Placement in the Nomenclature

Within the DSM, the section placement of gender identity disorder of childhood has had an interesting history. In the DSM-III it had somewhat of an "outlaw" status, as it was the only disorder for children not located in the section entitled "Disorders Usually First Evident in Infancy, Childhood, or Adolescence." Instead, it was included in the section entitled "Psychosexual Disorders," along with other new sexological diagnoses such as transsexualism. Perhaps because of this separation, several texts devoted exclusively to child psychiatric diagnosis did not include a chapter on gender identity disorder (e.g., Frame & Matson, 1987; Ollendick & Hersen, 1983). In the DSM-III-R, gender identity disorder of childhood was moved to the child section of the manual, which may have resulted in its inclusion in several new texts on child psychiatric diagnosis (e.g., Garfinkel, Carlson, & Weller, 1990; Hooper, Hynd, & Mattison, 1992; Kestenbaum & Williams, 1988; Last & Hersen, 1989).

For better or worse, the situation changed yet again in the DSM-IV. Because the largely adult diagnosis of transsexualism (and its variants, such as gender identity disorder of adolescence or adulthood, nontranssexual type) had also been moved to the child section in the DSM-III-R (the section "Psychosexual Disorders" was eliminated and replaced with "Sexual Disorders"), clinicians working with adults were not particularly pleased with this state of affairs (Bradley et al., 1991; Pauly, 1992). In addition, the DSM-IV Subcommittee took the position that gender identity disorder of childhood, transsexualism, and gender identity disorder of adolescence or adulthood, nontranssexual type, were not qualitatively distinct disorders; rather, they reflected differences in both developmental and severity parameters. As a result, the DSM-IV Subcommittee recommended one overarching diagnosis, gender identity disorder, that could be used with appropriate variations in criteria across the life cycle (Bradley et al., 1991). Accordingly, it was suggested that gender identity disorders be assigned to a distinct section that would have the same status as, for example, "Anxiety Disorders" and "Mood Disorders." The framers of the DSM-IV eventually settled on a section termed "Sexual and Gender Identity Disorders," which is perhaps a more descriptively accurate heading than the original DSM-III section title, "Psychosexual Disorders."

DSM-IV Diagnostic Criteria:
Changes from DSM-III-R

Table 4.1 shows the criteria for the DSM-III-R diagnosis of gender identity disorder of childhood, and Table 4.2 shows the DSM-IV criteria for gender identity disorder for use with children (see Chapter 11 for the criteria for use with adolescents and adults). It can be seen that

TABLE 4.1. DSM-III-R Diagnostic Criteria for Gender Identity Disorder of Childhood

For Females:
A. Persistent and intense distress about being a girl, and a stated desire to be a boy (not merely a desire for any perceived cultural advantages from being a boy), or insistence that she is a boy.

B. Either (1) or (2):
    (1) persistent marked aversion to normative feminine clothing and insistence on wearing stereotypical masculine clothing, e.g., boys' underwear and other accessories
    (2) persistent repudiation of female anatomic structures, as evidenced by at least one of the following:
        (a) an assertion that she has, or will grow, a penis
        (b) rejection of urinating in a sitting position
        (c) assertion that she does not want to grow breasts or menstruate

C. The girl has not yet reached puberty.

For Males:
A. Persistent and intense distress about being a boy and an intense desire to be a girl or, more rarely, insistence that he is a girl.

B. Either (1) or (2):
    (1) preoccupation with female stereotypical activities, as shown by a preference for either cross-dressing or simulating female attire, or by an intense desire to participate in the games and pastimes of girls and rejection of male stereotypical toys, games, and activities
    (2) persistent repudiation of male anatomic structures, as indicated by at least one of the following repeated assertions:
        (a) that he will grow up to become a woman (not merely in role)
        (b) that his penis or testes are disgusting or will disappear
        (c) that it would be better not to have a penis or testes

C. The boy has not yet reached puberty.

Note. Reprinted with permission from the *Diagnostic and Statistical Manual of Mental Disorders,* Third Edition, Revised (pp. 73–74). Copyright 1987 by the American Psychiatric Association.

three criteria (A, B, and D) are required for the diagnosis and that C is an exclusion criterion.

Compared to the DSM-III and DSM-III-R, there have been five main changes in the DSM-IV criteria for use with children:

1. Criterion A reflects the child's cross-gender identification, indexed by a total of five behavioral characteristics, of which at least four must be manifested. Previously, these characteristics were listed in either Criterion A or Criterion B in the DSM-III-R. In addition, they are more distinct in the DSM-IV.

TABLE 4.2. DSM-IV Diagnostic Criteria for Gender Identity Disorder (Child Criteria)

A. A strong and persistent cross-gender identification (not merely a desire for any perceived cultural advantages of being the other sex).

   In children, the disturbance is manifested by four (or more) of the following:

   (1) repeatedly stated desire to be, or insistence that he or she is, the other sex
   (2) in boys, preference for cross-dressing or simulating female attire; in girls, insistence on wearing only stereotypical masculine clothing
   (3) strong and persistent preferences for cross-sex roles in make-believe play or persistent fantasies of being the other sex
   (4) intense desire to participate in the stereotypical games and pastimes of the other sex
   (5) strong preference for playmates of the other sex

B. Persistent discomfort with his or her sex or sense of inappropriateness in the gender role of that sex.

   In children, the disturbance is manifested by any of the following: in boys, assertion that his penis or testes are disgusting or will disappear or assertion that it would be better not to have a penis, or aversion toward rough-and-tumble play and rejection of male stereotypical toys, games, and activities; in girls, rejection of urinating in a sitting position, assertion that she has or will grow a penis, or assertion that she does not want to grow breasts or menstruate, or marked aversion toward normative feminine clothing.

C. The disturbance is not concurrent with a physical intersex condition.

D. The disturbance causes clinically significant distress or impairment in social, occupational, or other important areas of functioning.

Note. Reprinted with permission from the *Diagnostic and Statistical Manual of Mental Disorders,* Fourth Edition (pp. 537–538). Copyright 1994 by the American Psychiatric Association.

2. Criterion B reflects the child's rejection of his or her own anatomic status and/or rejection of same-sex stereotypical activities. In the DSM-III-R, Criterion B also included some of the behavioral signs of cross-gender identification, which are now restricted to Criterion A.

3. The criteria for boys and girls are more similar than they were in the DSM-III-R. For example, in the DSM-III-R girls had to have a "stated" desire to be a boy, whereas boys had to have an "intense" desire to be a girl. Zucker (1992b) noted that the basis for this distinction was unclear and was particularly confusing, inasmuch as the phraseology had been identical for the two sexes in the DSM-III: "strongly and persistently *stated* desire to be a boy [girl]" (American Psychiatric Association, 1980, p. 265; italics added). Moreover, the passage for girls in the DSM-III-R contained no reference to intensity or chronicity. In the DSM-IV, both boys and girls must manifest a "repeatedly stated" desire

to be of the other sex. In addition, the other behavioral characteristics required for the diagnosis are more similar for boys and girls than they were in the DSM-III-R.

4. In the DSM-III-R, a girl's wish to be of the other sex could not be "merely a desire for any perceived cultural advantages from being a boy," whereas this proviso was not included for boys. In the DSM-IV, this proviso applies to both boys and girls.

5. In the DSM-III-R, Criterion A specified that a child must show "persistent and intense distress" about being a boy or a girl. This phrase had not appeared in the DSM-III criteria, and in the DSM-III-R it was not specified how a clinician should assess such distress or in what ways it might be distinct from other operationalized components in the criteria. This phrase has been deleted in the DSM-IV Criterion A, but Criterion D asserts that the child must experience "clinically significant distress or impairment in social, occupational, or other important areas of functioning."

Appraisal of the DSM-IV Criteria

Reliability and Validity

Can the DSM-IV diagnosis of gender identity disorder be made reliably? Because the criteria have been changed and because no field trials were conducted, this question cannot yet be answered. We conducted one study pertaining to the reliability of the earlier DSM-III criteria (Zucker, Finegan, Doering, & Bradley, 1984), which involved 36 consecutive referrals to our clinic. Kappas of .89 and .80 were obtained for Criteria A and B, respectively (both p's < .001).

In the Zucker, Finegan, et al. (1984) study, the validity of the DSM-III criteria was also assessed by comparing the children who met the complete criteria with those children who did not meet the complete criteria on a number of demographic variables and sex-typed behaviors. It should be noted that, by and large, the children who did not meet the complete DSM-III criteria showed at least some characteristics of cross-gender-identification and were not necessarily inappropriate referrals.

Tables 4.3 and 4.4 provide an update of these initial analyses, based on a considerably larger sample size. In Table 4.3, it can be seen that the children who met the complete criteria for gender identity disorder of childhood were significantly younger, were more likely to be of a higher social class background, and were more likely to come from intact, two-parent families than the children who did not meet the com-

TABLE 4.3. Demographic Characteristics as a Function of Diagnostic Status for Gender Identity Disorder of Childhood

Variables	Diagnostic status	
	DSM-III (n = 113)	Non-DSM-III (n = 80)
Sex of child		
Male (n)	95	72
Female (n)	18	8
p	n.s.	
Age (in years)		
M	6.1	8.7
SD	1.9	2.5
n	113	80
p	.000	
Full Scale IQ		
M	109.4	105.7
SD	16.3	18.0
n	110	79
p	n.s.	
Social class[a]		
M	44.3	38.0
SD	14.9	15.4
n	111	79
p	.005	
Family status		
Both parents (n)	86	44
Mother only/reconstituted (n)	27	36
p	.003	

[a]Hollingshead's (1975) Four-Factor Index of Social Status (absolute range = 8–66).

plete criteria. The two subgroups did not differ significantly with regard to sex and IQ. Correlational analyses indicated that the variables of age, IQ, parents' social class, and parents' marital status were all significantly correlated with one another (absolute r's ranged from .32 to .50). Sex of child was unrelated to any of the other demographic variables.

To test which variables, if any, contributed to the correct classification of the subjects in the two diagnostic groups, we performed a discriminant-function analysis. Age, sex, IQ, and parents' marital status contributed to the discriminant function, with age showing the greatest power. In the DSM-III group, 82.6% were correctly classified, and in the non-DSM-III group, 68.8% were correctly classified.

We next compared the two diagnostic subgroups on several measures of sex-typed behavior (Table 4.4). We performed t tests, with age,

TABLE 4.4. Measures of Gender Identity and Gender Role Behavior as a Function of Diagnostic Status for Gender Identity Disorder of Childhood

Measures	Diagnostic status				
	DSM-III		Non-DSM-III		
	M	*SD*	*M*	*SD*	p^a
Parent measures					
Revised Gender Behavior Inventory for Boys[b]					
Factor 1 (Masculinity)	2.7	0.5	2.8	0.6	.047
Factor 2 (Femininity I)	3.0	0.8	2.3	0.7	.000
Factor 3 (Femininity II)	3.2	1.1	2.3	1.0	.001
Factor 4 (Mother's boy)	3.7	0.9	3.6	0.9	.021
Play and Games Questionnaire[b]					
Scale 1 (Feminine/Preschool)	18.9	4.7	17.0	5.6	n.s.
Scale 2 (Masculine, Nonathletic)	9.1	3.5	10.7	4.3	.065
Scale 3 (Masculine, Athletic)	3.1	2.1	5.3	3.2	.001
Enjoyment (Scale 1)	4.0	0.5	3.9	0.6	n.s.
Enjoyment (Scale 2)	3.5	0.7	3.7	0.6	.009
Enjoyment (Scale 3)	3.0	1.1	3.2	1.1	.008
Activity Level/Extraversion[c]	3.1	0.5	3.0	0.6	n.s.
Gender Identity Questionnaire[d]	2.7	0.5	3.2	0.5	.000
Child measures					
Draw-a-Person test[e]					
Percentage opposite-sex persons drawn first[f]	1.7	0.4	1.3	0.5	.000
Height of same-sex person – height of opposite-sex person (in centimeters)[g]	−0.6	3.6	0.1	2.8	n.s.
Rorschach test					
Number of same-sex responses – number of cross-sex responses[h]	−1.3	4.2	−0.3	4.5	n.s.
Free-play task					
Percentage of same-sex play – cross-sex play[i]	−0.4	0.5	0.3	0.6	.000
Gender Identity Interview					
Factor 1 (Affective Gender Confusion)[j]	1.0	0.6	0.3	0.3	.000
Factor 2 (Cognitive Gender Confusion)[j]	0.3	0.6	0.04	0.2	n.s.

Note. The *n*'s in footnotes *b–d* and *f–j* indicate the number of children in the DSM-III and non-DSM-III subgroups, respectively. For the four factors of the Gender Behavior Inventory,

(continued on next page)

social class, and marital status covaried. The DSM-III subgroup showed significantly more cross-gender behavior or less same-gender behavior than the non-DSM-III subgroup on 11 of 18 measures; thus, there seemed to be at least some behavioral differences between the two diagnostic subgroups in the degree of same-sex-typed or cross-sex-typed behavior, even after the demographic variables that also differed between the two subgroups were controlled.

Empirical Analyses

In general, the DSM-IV work groups were encouraged to use extant or new databases to support recommended changes in diagnostic criteria (e.g., Widiger, Frances, Pincus, & Davis, 1990).

Initially, the DSM-IV Subcommittee had recommended that the DSM-III-R Criteria A and B for children be collapsed into one criterion. In part, this was because the two criteria appeared conceptually and empirically related (e.g., Bentler, Rekers, & Rosen, 1979; Rosen, Rekers, & Friar, 1977). Moreover, research utilizing the DSM-III and DSM-III-R criteria found that younger children (mean age = 6.4 years, $n = 54$) were significantly more likely to receive the diagnosis than were older children (mean age = 9.0 years, $n = 54$) (Zucker, 1992b; Zucker, Finegan, et al., 1984). This seemed mainly attributable to the fact that older children did not meet Criterion A. Despite marked clinical evidence of cross-gender identification, these children did not frequently voice the desire to be of the opposite sex. In part, this seemed a function of social desirability and fear of stigma (cf. Bentler, 1976).

If, in fact, the stated desire to be of the opposite sex is simply one of a series of behavioral markers suggestive of gender identity disorder, then a factor analysis of these markers should yield one common factor. The DSM-IV Subcommittee tested this hypothesis in a reanalysis of parent reports and clinician ratings of cross-gender behavior in Green's (1987) sample of feminine and control boys (Zucker et al., in press). A principal axis factor analysis with varimax rotation yielded one strong

---

the absolute ranges were 1.00–5.75, 1.00–5.80, 1.00–6.84, and 1.00–5.75. For the three scales on the Play and Games Questionnaire, the absolute ranges were 0–29, 0–22, and 0–14. For the Enjoyment ratings, the Activity Level factor, and the Gender Identity Questionnaire, absolute ranges were 1–5. For the Gender Identity Interview, absolute range was 0–2.

[a] p value is based on t tests with age and parents' social class and marital status covaried.

[b] $n = 91/65$. [c] $n = 92/64$. [d] $n = 74/49$.

[e] Dummy variables were used, where 1 = same-sex person and 2 = opposite-sex person. Actual percentages of opposite-sex persons drawn first were 72.5% and 30.4%, respectively.

[f] $n = 110/78$. [g] $n = 108/78$. [h] $n = 105/73$. [i] $n = 106/60$. [j] $n = 64/43$.

factor, accounting for 51.2% of the variance (Table 4.5). The variable "Son states wish to be a girl" was one of 15 cross-gender behaviors that loaded on this factor (all factor loadings ≥ .40). Thus, there was some empirical support for the hypothesis.

As noted earlier, clinical experience and some research data (Bates et al., 1974; Zucker, Finegan, et al., 1984) suggested that the wish to change sex is negatively related to age; that is, older children may be less likely to voice this wish, perhaps because of social desirability factors. Green's (1987) data were reanalyzed to explore the relation between age and the wish to be of the opposite sex. Given the age effects suggested by other analyses (Zucker, 1992b), Green's data were analyzed by comparing children 3–9 years of age to children 9–12 years of age. Of the 47 boys in the younger age grouping, 43 (91.5%) were reported by their mothers to occasionally or frequently state the wish to be a girl, compared to 9 (69.2%) of 13 boys in the older age grouping (Fisher's exact test, p = .0588, one-tailed). Frequency of the wish to be of the opposite sex was not associated with several other demographic variables.

Given the changes that the DSM-IV Subcommittee was considering making in Criterion A (see Table 4.2), we (Zucker et al., in press)

TABLE 4.5. Factor Analysis of Green's (1987) Data

Behavioral variables	Factor 1
1. Female role playing	.840
2. Sex-typed role playing (male vs. female)	.826
3. Role when playing house (female)	.772
4. Sex-typed pictures drawn	.757
5. Wears girls' clothes	.732
6. Frequency of cross-dressing	.690
7. Doll playing	.684
8. Composition of peer group	.661
9. Masculine behavior	−.659
10. Relates best to (women)	.650
11. Son states wish to be a girl	.611
12. Doll play	.607
13. Wishes to grow up like dad	−.544
14. Interest in women's clothing	.471
15. Interest in play acting	.437

Note. Data derived from Green (1987) and reported in Zucker et al. (in press). Only factor loadings ≥ .40 are reported. Where not explicit, a positive loading reflects a higher feminine/female rating. Items 1, 3, 5, 6, 8, 10–13, and 15 were maternal ratings; items 2, 4, 7, 9, and 14 were interviewer global ratings.

then re-examined the symptom ratings from parent interview data regarding a cohort of 54 children who did not meet the DSM-III criteria for gender identity disorder (Zucker, 1992b). In this analysis, we assessed whether children would meet the proposed DSM-IV Criterion A for gender identity disorder. Because these children did not repeatedly state the desire to be of the opposite sex, we coded as present or absent four remaining traits: cross-dressing, cross-sex roles in fantasy play, cross-sex activity/toy interests, and cross-sex peer preference. If all four traits were present, these children would meet the proposed cutoff for the new Criterion A. (We chose not to reanalyze the data on the 54 other children who met the DSM-III criteria for gender identity disorder of childhood, since it was our impression that there would not be any substantive change, given that these children had already verbalized the wish to be of the opposite sex and had displayed marked cross- gender role behaviors.)

Of the 54 children, the mean number of symptoms rated as present was 2.36 (SD = 1.33, range = 0–4). Only 7 children did not have any symptoms rated as present. Of the 54 children, 16 (29.6%) had all four symptoms, thus meeting the new Criterion A.

The subgroup that met Criterion A was also compared with the subgroup that did not with regard to the demographic variables of age, IQ, parents' social class, and parents' marital status. There was a trend for the children who met Criterion A to be younger than the children who did not (8.0 vs. 9.4 years), t (52) = 1.74, p = .087 (two-tailed). Thus, age continued to be a correlate of diagnostic status, but the correlation appeared to be weaker than that found in our earlier research (Zucker, Finegan, et al., 1984). None of the other demographic variables distinguished the two subgroups. These reanalyses suggest that the revisions to the diagnostic criteria in the DSM-IV may result in a modest increase in the number of cases that will meet the complete criteria.

After these reanalyses were completed, the DSM-IV Subcommittee, with feedback from the DSM-IV main office, developed the new Criterion B (see Table 4.2); this should, if anything, make the diagnosis even harder to meet. Unfortunately, the reanalyses just described did not focus explicitly on this criterion, so this conjecture will require additional empirical analysis.

Cultural Influences

We have noted earlier that in the DSM-IV the simple perception of cultural advantage of being the other sex is deemed inadequate for Criterion A. A difference from the DSM-III and DSM-III-R is that this exclusion requirement no longer applies only to girls.

Interestingly, the DSM-IV Subcommittee had initially recommended that this proviso be deleted, since it was argued that although the motivational basis for the desire to be the other sex may have relevance for such parameters as natural history and response to treatment, it was not clear why it should be used diagnostically (Bradley et al., 1991). For example, it could be argued that boys who wish to be girls perceive similar, albeit inverted, cultural advantages (e.g., "Girls can wear dresses *and* pants," "Girls don't have to play rough, boys do") (cf. Coates, 1985; Green, 1974; J. W. Thompson, personal communication to J. E. Mezzich, June 22, 1993; K. J. Zucker, personal communication to J. E. Mezzich, August 10, 1993). Before the DSM-IV went into print, there was a compromise in the deliberations between the DSM-IV Subcommittee and the DSM-IV Task Force on this matter. Empirical research will have to resolve the question of whether including this proviso has any clinical utility or validity.

Judgments of Persistence

Judgments of behavioral persistence are required by the DSM-IV in both Criteria A and B. For example, Criterion A requires a clinical judgment in determining what qualifies as a "repeatedly stated desire to be . . . the other sex." What criteria should clinicians utilize in deciding whether the desire to change sex is persistent? To some extent, the answer to this question hinges on what is known about the prevalence and intensity of cross-sex wishes in the general population. As we have noted in Chapter 3 on epidemiology, it is likely that the persistent desire to change sex is relatively uncommon, but there is really no "gold standard" for the clinician to use. Of course, this is a problem not unique to diagnosing gender identity disorder. For example, to diagnose attention-deficit/hyperactivity disorder, one has to decide whether a child "often leaves seat in classroom . . ." (American Psychiatric Association, 1994, p. 84). The DSM-IV does not provide explicit guidelines for these matters.

Differential Diagnosis

We have identified four differential diagnostic issues that need to be considered in evaluating children. First, although this has not been described formally in the literature, youngsters are occasionally encountered who display an acute onset of symptoms of gender identity disorder, but whose symptoms usually prove to be transient. In our experience, such an acute onset can usually be understood as a stress response to a specific life event. For example, some youngsters with a newborn sibling of the opposite sex may display delimited cross-gender behaviors (e.g., cross-dressing, "penis envy" in girls), which can be understood as related to feelings of displacement or jealousy. Such behaviors can be easily distinguished from the chronic feelings of jealousy that are sometimes observed among children with the full-blown disorder. Transient symptoms may also be manifested by youngsters who, after having experienced temporary setbacks in same-sex peer groups, may voice unhappiness about their status as boys or girls. Once the stress has been removed or the focal conflict reduced, the symptoms rapidly dissipate.

Moreover, in the clinical psychoanalytic literature on toddlers and preschool children, it is not uncommon to encounter case reports of youngsters who show signs of gender dysphoria (e.g., "penis envy" in girls) that are understood to arise in the context of specific developmental crises (e.g., becoming more aware of the anatomic differences between the sexes). Our reading of this literature suggests that these symptoms are not pervasive and remit over time without much in the way of formal intervention (see, e.g., Fast, 1984; Frenkel, 1993; Linday, 1994; Renik, Spielman, & Afterman, 1978; Roiphe & Galenson, 1981; Roiphe & Spira, 1991).

A second differential diagnostic issue involves a type of cross-dressing in boys that appears to be qualitatively different from the type of cross-dressing that characterizes gender identity disorder. In the latter, cross-dressing typically involves outerwear (e.g., dresses, shoes, and jewelry) that helps enhance the fantasy of being like the opposite sex. In the former, cross-dressing involves the use of undergarments, such as panties and nylons (Scharfman, 1976; Stoller, 1985a). Clinical data show that such cross-dressing is not accompanied by other signs of cross-gender identification; in fact, the appearance and behavior of boys who engage in it are conventionally masculine. Clinical experience also suggests that this type of cross-dressing is associated with self-soothing or reduction of anxiety. Many male adolescents and adults who display transvestic fetishism (American Psychiatric Association, 1994) recall having engaged in this type of cross-dressing during childhood (Bradley & Zucker, 1990; see also Chapter 12). It should be noted, however, that prospective study has not verified the assumption that such cross-dressing is fully contiguous with later transvestism.

The following case vignette illustrates this type of cross-dressing.

CASE EXAMPLE 4.1

Jimmy was a 5-year-old boy with an IQ of 108. He was referred because of his mother's concern about his stealing, hiding, and wearing her clothes, and also because of his encopresis. His parents, who were from a lower-middle-class socioeconomic background, were separated; Jimmy lived with his mother, but his father participated in the assessment.

At age 3, Jimmy had begun cross-dressing in his mother's nightgown, swimsuit, and underwear. He would wear these under his own clothes when he had to be away from his mother (e.g., when he went to nursery school). Jimmy also took underwear from his father's girlfriend. In addition, he tended to "disappear" into the women's lingerie section whenever he was in a department store.

Jimmy's soiling had also concerned his parents for the past 2 years. This soiling consisted of staining his underwear and sometimes of defecating on the carpet. His parents reported that the frequencies of the cross-dressing and the soiling were inversely related.

Jimmy preferred boys as playmates, liked stereotypically masculine toys, and enjoyed rough-and-tumble play. He never voiced a dislike of his sexual anatomy or displayed feminine mannerisms. On one occasion, after his mother tried to persuade him to stop cross-dressing, he told her that he would like to be a girl, "so that I can wear your clothes." Clinically, however, there was little evidence that Jimmy had a pervasive wish to become a girl.

When all the clinical signs of gender identity disorder are present, it is not difficult to make the diagnosis (cf. Zucker, Finegan, et al., 1984). But the clinician who accepts the notion that there is a spectrum of cross-gender identification must be prepared to identify what Meyer-Bahlburg (1985) has described as the "zone of transition between clinically significant cross-gender behavior and mere statistical deviations from the gender norm" (p. 682). Clinical experience suggests that boys who fall into this ambiguous zone do poorly in male peer groups, avoid rough-and-tumble play, are disinclined toward athletics and other conventionally masculine activities, and feel somewhat uncomfortable about being male; however, these boys do not wish to be girls and do not show an intense preoccupation with femininity. Friedman (1988) coined the term *juvenile unmasculinity* to describe such boys, who, he argued, suffer from a "persistent, profound feeling of masculine inadequacy which leads to negative valuing of the self" (p. 199). (Although this was not discussed by Friedman and has not been well studied clinically, one might speculate that an analogous phenomenon, *juvenile unfemininity*, is manifested among girls.) It is not clear, however, whether this putative behavior pattern constitutes a distinct syndrome, which

Friedman (personal communication to S. J. Bradley, June 16, 1989) has subsequently labeled *juvenile phase atypical gender identity disorder,* or is simply below the clinical threshold for gender identity disorder; in any case, the residual diagnosis of gender identity disorder not otherwise specified (American Psychiatric Association, 1994) could be employed in such cases.

In girls, the primary differential diagnostic issue concerns the distinction between gender identity disorder and "tomboyism." The study of a community sample of tomboys by Green et al. (1982) showed that these girls shared a number of the cross-gender traits observed in clinic-referred gender-disturbed girls (Zucker, 1982). In part, the DSM-III-R criteria for gender identity disorder in girls were modified in the hope of better differentiating these two groups of girls (Zucker, 1992b). At least three characteristics may be most useful in making the differential diagnosis: (1) By definition, girls with gender identity disorder indicate an intense unhappiness with their status as females, whereas this should not be the case for tomboys; (2) girls with gender identity disorder display an intense aversion to the wearing of culturally defined feminine clothing under any circumstances, whereas tomboys do not manifest this reaction with the same intensity, though they may prefer to wear casual clothing (e.g., jeans); and (3) girls with gender identity disorder, unlike tomboys, manifest a verbalized or acted-out discomfort with sexual anatomy.

The final differential diagnostic issue concerns children with physical intersex (hermaphroditic) conditions. In the DSM-III (American Psychiatric Association, 1980), an intersex condition was an exclusion criterion for the adult diagnosis of transsexualism; however, it was not an exclusion criterion for gender identity disorder of childhood, although the DSM-III noted that "physical abnormalities of the sex organs are rarely associated with gender identity disorder" (American Psychiatric Association, 1980, p. 256). In the DSM-III-R (American Psychiatric Association, 1987), this exclusion criterion was eliminated for transsexualism.

Given that some children with intersex conditions have been observed to experience severe gender identity conflict, the DSM-IV Subcommittee considered the relevant diagnostic issues. As noted by Meyer-Bahlburg (1994), neither the DSM-III nor the DSM-III-R contained substantive information regarding the conceptual issues. The DSM-III-R did not explicitly address the question of whether children who displayed significant cross-gender identification and had an intersex condition should be given the diagnosis of gender identity disorder.

Meyer-Bahlburg (1994) has recently pointed out that the intersex case report literature has rarely attempted to utilize DSM criteria in describing patients with gender identity and gender role conflicts (cf. Zucker, Bradley, & Hughes, 1987). Thus, it is not possible to specify what percentage of intersex patients with gender identity problems would meet the formal criteria for gender identity disorder. Meyer-Bahlburg (1994) has also argued that it is unclear whether the phenomenology surrounding gender identity concerns is the same as that observed in nonintersex persons with gender identity problems (see also Bradley et al., 1991); however, the DSM-IV Subcommittee did not reach a consensus on this issue.

Even if the phenomenology of intersex and nonintersex youngsters is similar, there appear to be substantial differences between them in other variables, including associated features, prevalence, sex ratio, and age of onset (Meyer-Bahlburg, 1994); these suggest an etiology at least somewhat different from that involved in nonintersex youngsters with gender identity disorder. For example, gender dysphoria seems to be experienced more frequently by intersex youngsters assigned to the female sex than by intersex youngsters assigned to the male sex, which is the opposite of what is observed among nonintersex youngsters with gender identity disorder (at least as inferred from referral rates).

The very real possibility of distinct etiological influences in intersex youngsters raises the question of whether there may be a risk in applying the same diagnosis to them that is applied to physically normal children (e.g., offering the same type of therapeutic intervention that is used with the latter). On the other hand, the risk is reduced if it is recognized that a particular diagnosis does not dictate identical treatment across cases. From an etiological standpoint, the use of Axis III for physical disorders or conditions would be important in noting the role of the physical anomaly, but this would not preclude using the gender identity disorder diagnosis if it seemed to be clinically justified (for further discussion, see Bradley et al., 1991; Meyer-Bahlburg, 1994).

Following additional consultation with the DSM-IV Task Force, it was decided to allow inclusion of intersex persons with gender identity conflicts under the residual diagnosis of gender identity disorder not otherwise specified.

Is Gender Identity Disorder Really a "Disorder"?

So far in this chapter, we have considered diagnostic issues within the relatively narrow confines of nosological matters and conventional questions that are important with regard to the reliability and validity of psychiatric diagnosis. It would be remiss on our part, however, not to comment on the more controversial issues that have surrounded the gender identity disorder diagnosis.

Critics of psychiatric diagnosis have long mused about how behavioral phenomena come to be viewed as "disorders." Szasz's (1961) seminal critique of the concept of *mental illness* probably represents the best-known intellectual springboard for discourse on this matter. Interestingly, the debate in the 1970s regarding the pathological status of homosexuality, and the subsequent dropping of homosexuality from the DSM, played a major role in the DSM framers' conceptualization of the boundaries of mental disorder (see, e.g., Bayer, 1981; Bayer & Spitzer, 1982; Kirk & Kutchins, 1992, pp. 81–90; Spitzer, 1981).

What is the basis, then, for considering gender identity disorder a disorder? As noted earlier, homosexuality is the most common postpubertal psychosexual outcome for children followed prospectively with gender identity disorder (Green, 1987): The vast majority of the children followed so far have not requested sex reassignment surgery, nor do they appear to meet the pre-DSM-IV criteria for transsexualism. Some authors have, in fact, argued that the cross-gendered behavioral pattern observable during childhood is nothing more than the immature expression of homosexuality proper (e.g., Harry, 1982; Zuger, 1988). Isay (1989) even claims that the very early adoption of feminine gender role traits by boys is a way of "[sexually] attracting the father's love and attention" (p. 30). Other authors have wondered why children who appear to be primarily "prehomosexual" should deserve a psychiatric diagnosis at one phase in the life cycle (childhood), but not at a later phase (adulthood) (see, e.g., Bem, 1993, pp. 106–111; Fagot, 1992; McConaghy & Silove, 1991; Neisen, 1992; Sedgwick, 1991; Thorne, 1986, 1993). Thorne (1986, p. 31), for example, has asked, "Who has the problem, one wishes the literature more vigorously inquired, the labelled or the labellers?" There are, then, two distinct questions that need to be addressed: (1) Is gender identity disorder of childhood really nothing more than homosexuality? (2) What constitutes a disorder?

On both conceptual and empirical grounds, we do not agree with the argument that the behavioral patterns corresponding to gender identity disorder and postpubertal homoeroticism are isomorphic phenomena (cf. Coates et al., 1991, p. 518; Friedman, 1988). (This does not, however, deny their intimate statistical association, which, as noted in Chapter 3, is strong. See Bailey & Zucker, 1995.) If, for example, gender identity and sexual orientation are not viewed as distinct variables, how does one explain the phenomenon of transsexualism in, say, a man who wishes for sex reassignment and is erotically attracted to other men? From an empirical point of view, neither prospective nor retrospective studies support the view that a complete concordance exists between gender identity disorder and later homosexuality. Prospectively, a small minority of children with gender identity disorder become "transsexual," and a minority appear to develop a heterosexual orientation (Green, 1987; Zucker, 1985, 1990a). Retrospectively, not all homosexual men and women recall a childhood behavioral pattern consistent with gender identity disorder or lesser forms of cross-gender identification (e.g., Bailey & Zucker, 1995; Friedman, 1988). Second, we are not persuaded that the evidence supports Isay's (1989) "inversion" of the relation between gender identity and eroticism (for further discussion on this point, see Zucker, 1990a).

But even if it can be agreed that gender identity disorder should be conceptually and empirically distinguished from a homosexual sexual orientation, one still needs to make the case that the behavioral pattern itself is a "disorder" and not just a cluster of behaviors that go together. What is the basis, then, for arguing that the cluster is in fact a disorder? On this point, one must acknowledge the absence of intellectual consensus regarding the definition of *mental disorder* (see, e.g., Scott, 1958; Spitzer & Endicott, 1978; Wakefield, 1992a, 1992b). Given this state of affairs, we will comment on whether gender identity disorder is consistent with the DSM's definition of disorder—in other words, with the "rules of the game."

Spitzer and Endicott (1978) argued that *distress, disability,* and *disadvantage* should be present for a behavioral syndrome to qualify as a disorder. Spitzer and Endicott contended that the concept of disorder presupposes "negative consequences of the condition, an inferred or identified organismic dysfunction, and an implicit call for action" (p. 17). They defined *distress* as a subjective complaint or a complaint that could be inferred from manifest behavior (e.g., the anxiety experienced during panic attacks); they defined *disability* as functional impairment across a wide range of activities (e.g., inability to concentrate when depressed); and they defined *disadvantage* as the negative sequelae occurring when the individual interacts with aspects of the physical or social environment (e.g., anorgasmia).

Recently, Wakefield (1992a, 1992b) has offered some penetrating critiques of the DSM conceptualization of disorder. Some DSM disorders (e.g., premature ejaculation) do not necessarily result in impairment in a *wide* range of activities, but may be limited to single areas of functioning. Wakefield has argued that the concept of disorder needs to incorporate better the notion of *harmful dysfunction,* defined as the "failure of a mechanism in the person to perform a natural function for which the mechanism was designed by natural selection" (1992a, p. 236). Wakefield's postulate is reminiscent of King's (1945) simple definition of *normal*—"that which functions in accordance with its design" (p. 494). In the discussion that follows, we consider the original DSM criteria, particularly the requirements of distress and disability, and Wakefield's more recent notion of harmful dysfunction.

Do Children with Gender Identity Disorder Manifest Distress?

Spitzer and Endicott (1978) spent little time elaborating on the concept of distress, perhaps because the subjective complaints of adults are what usually bring them to the attention of clinicians. Moreover, most psychiatric disorders in adults consist of complaints that are, in Wakefield's (1992a) terms, "in the person."

Yet the concept of distress is surely more complicated than this. Several psychiatric disorders common in adults may cause subjective distress only in reaction to specific conflict with the external world (e.g., antisocial personality disorder). In these cases, it is questionable whether distress is simply "in the person." The concept of distress is also intertwined with theoretical agendas. Biological psychiatrists might argue that distress is the result of faulty "hard-wiring" of the organism. Psychoanalytic psychiatrists might argue that distress is the result of a complex interplay of intrapsychic conflicts, with developmental roots. Social constructionists, the contemporary gadflies of psychiatry, are disdainful of the notion of intrapersonal distress except as a response to social oppression. In their view, one can never be the architect of one's own misery.

Regarding children in general, the concept of distress is even more complicated. Is the concept of distress "adultocentric"? Wakefield (1992a), for example, argued that some child psychiatric diagnoses, such as conduct disorder, may be a "rational" response to environmental parameters (e.g., uncaring parents).

Regarding children with gender identity disorder, we need to ask two interrelated questions: Are they distressed by their condition, and, if so, what is the source of the distress? On the first question, there are two broad views. The first view is that the children become distressed about their cross-gender behavior only after it has been interfered with (Stoller, 1975). For example, a little girl becomes angry and cries when told that she cannot become a boy, or a little boy becomes upset when told that he cannot wear his pink dress to school. Stoller (1966, 1975) generally took the position that marked cross-gender identification (in boys) is ego-syntonic because the alleged familial psychodynamics that produce it are systemically syntonic. Green (1974), Rekers (1977b), and others have emphasized that the distress results largely from social ostracism, particularly by peers.

The second view is that the distress is caused by other psychopathology in the child and in the family. Coates and Person (1985), for example, claimed that gender identity disorder is a "solution" to specific forms of psychopathology in the child (particularly separation anxiety and "annihilation" anxiety) that are induced by familial psychopathology. For those who uphold this view, the driven, repetitive, compulsive, and rigid patterns of cross-gender behavior are related to such psychopathological processes.

It is conceivable that both views are correct or that one or the other better fits individual cases. (We discuss both views in greater detail in Chapter 5.) The latter view, however, is more compatible with the notion of inherent distress, whereas the former fits better with the notion that social pathology creates individual pathology. From a clinical standpoint, it has been our experience that from a very early age many youngsters with gender identity disorder feel a sense of discomfort regarding their status as boys or girls, which matches nicely with the DSM notion of distress. Using a semistructured gender identity interview schedule (Zucker, Bradley, Lowry Sullivan, et al., 1993), a clinician obtained the following responses from a 4-year-old boy (IQ = 104) who, prior to the assessment, had informed his parents that he was "dead" and was now a particular girl in a currently popular film for children:

INTERVIEWER (I): Are you a boy or a girl?
CHILD (C): Boy.
I: Are you a girl?
C: Yes.
I: When you grow up, will you be a Mommy or a Daddy?
C: Mommy.
I: Could you ever grow up to be a Daddy?
C: No.
I: Are there any good things about being a boy?
C: No.
I: Are there any things that you don't like about being a boy?
C: Yes.
I: Tell me some of the things that you don't like about being a boy.
C: Because I hate it. 'Cause we get to do stupid, sitting down.
I: Do you think it is better to be a boy or a girl?
C: Girl.
I: Why?
C: Because it's fun—they sit around and talk.

I: In your mind, do you ever think that you would like to be a girl?

C: Yes.

I: Can you tell me why?

C: I don't know. . . . Because we get to sit around and talk and do everything that girls need to do.

I: In your mind, do you ever get mixed up and you're not really sure if you are a boy or a girl?

C: I am a girl.

I: Tell me more about that.

C: (*No response.*)

I: Do you ever feel more like a girl than like a boy?

C: It's too late. Because I'm already a girl. Because I hate being a boy.

I: You know what dreams are, right? Well, when you dream at night, are you ever in the dream?

C: I don't have dreams.

I: Do you ever think that you really are a girl?

C: Yes.

I: Tell me more about that.

C: (*Runs out of test room to return to his mother in the reception area.*)

The distress experienced by this youngster appears quite palpable.[2]

Do Children with Gender Identity Disorder Manifest Disability?

Spitzer and Endicott (1978, p. 23) stated that disability must be shown in "more than one area of functioning," in order to avoid *a priori* decisions as to what areas of human activity are basic or essential. There is little need to quibble about this concept of disability when we consider DSM diagnoses such as major depressive disorder, in which social and occupational functioning are grossly impaired. But surely the concept of disability becomes fuzzier when we consider other kinds of DSM diagnoses. For example, as noted earlier, several sexological DSM diagnoses do not necessarily result in generalized impairment (Wakefield, 1992a).

For children in general, the definition of disability may be too stringent, perhaps because on the whole their conditions are less disabling than adult conditions (although a childhood condition such as autistic disorder is as disabling as any adult condition). If we skirt around the issue of extensiveness of disability, we can ask in a narrower way whether children with gender identity disorder show "disability." In several domains, it might be argued that they do. For example, children with gender identity disorder seem to have more trouble with basic cognitive concepts concerning their gender. We (Zucker, Bradley, Lowry Sullivan, et al., 1993) found that children with gender identity disorder were more likely than controls to misclassify their own gender, which, given the ubiquity of gender as a social category, surely must lead to confusion in their social interactions (cf. Maccoby, 1988). Several empirical studies have shown that children with gender identity disorder have as much general behavioral psychopathology as do other children with clinical problems (for a fuller review of this literature, see Chapter 5). And lastly, the peer relations of children with gender identity disorder (particularly boys) appear impaired, as we have noted in Chapter 2.

Conclusion

A conceptual analysis of gender identity disorder as disorder leads, of course, to other questions. For example, sociobiologists routinely ask, with respect to both proximate and ultimate causes, why there is such a "thing" as gender identity. Bowlby's (1969) exegesis of infantile attachment is the best-known example of this line of inquiry in developmental psychiatry and psychology. Phylogenetically, the function of attachment in the human's "environment of evolutionary adaptedness" was protection; ontogenetically, that function has been claimed to provide the infant with a sense of felt security that encourages exploration of the social and physical environment and promotes autonomous functioning (for discussions of this, see Hay, 1980; Sroufe & Waters, 1977).

Can similar analyses prove profitable in understanding gender identity? Unfortunately, little attention has been given to this question. The ubiquity of gender as a social category suggests its importance for the organization of social life. Given the relation that gender has with later eroticism, a degree of parsimony is obtained by relating the phylogenetic function to reproduction. The connection between gender socialization and eroticism in nonindustrialized societies, where socialization is more formally ritualized, has been lucidly described (e.g., Herdt, 1990a; Herdt & Stoller, 1990). This, of course, leads full circle to the question of the deviance of homosexuality (and, indirectly, gender identity) in evolutionary terms. Bowlby (1969, pp. 130–131), for example, argued that in homosexuality there is an "error" in the stimulus that activates a sexual behavior sequence (i.e., the "object" is a same-sex person instead of an opposite-sex person). But contemporary sociobiologists have not reached agreement on an evolutionary explanation of homosexuality, and the explanations of its potentially adaptive functions that have been proposed seem difficult to verify empirically (e.g.,

Kirsch & Weinrich, 1991; Ruse, 1981; Weinrich, 1987). However, whether or not consensus regarding the phylogenetic function of sexual orientation is reached, one could still argue that the capacity to form pair bonds (either heterosexual or homosexual) enhances the potential for intimacy, which in a gregarious species such as ours is sure to promote better adaptive functioning for the individual.

ASSESSMENT

Psychological Testing

Since the early 1970s, a number of assessment techniques have been developed for use with children with gender identity disorder. These techniques include structured parent interviews regarding specific sex-typed behaviors (Green, 1987; Roberts, Green, Williams, & Goodman, 1987; Zuger & Taylor, 1969); parent-report questionnaires that cover a range of sex-typed behaviors (Bates & Bentler, 1973; Bates, Bentler, & Thompson, 1973; Green, 1976, 1987; Meyer-Bahlburg, Sandberg, Yager, Dolezal, & Ehrhardt, 1994; Zucker, Bradley, Doering, & Lozinski, 1985); measurement of overt (Doering, Zucker, Bradley, & MacIntyre, 1989; Green, Fuller, Rutley, & Hendler, 1972; Rekers & Yates, 1976; Zucker, Doering, Bradley, & Finegan, 1982) and covert (Green & Fuller, 1973a; Zucker, Doering, Bradley, Alon, & Lozinski, 1984) sex-typed play in standardized situations; observation of sex-typed motoric behavior (Bates, Bentler, & Thompson, 1979; Green, Neuberg, & Finch, 1983); assessment of gender constancy development (Zucker, Kuksis, & Bradley, 1988); sex-typed indices on the Draw-a-Person (DAP) (Green, Fuller, & Rutley, 1972; Skilbeck, Bates, & Bentler, 1975; Zucker, Finegan, Doering, & Bradley, 1983) and Rorschach (Zucker, Lozinski, Bradley, & Doering, 1992; Tuber & Coates, 1985) tests; and a structured interview schedule pertaining to cognitive and affective gender identity confusion (Zucker, Bradley, Lowry Sullivan, et al., 1993).

The techniques are summarized in Table 4.6. Generally, these measures have shown significant differences between the index group of gender-referred children and the controls, which have included siblings, children with other psychiatric problems, and normal children. Using parent interview data, for example, Green (1987) found that a discriminant-function analysis required 6 of 16 sex-typed behaviors to classify correctly all boys as members of either the feminine group or the male control group. Such evidence of discriminant validity was an important

TABLE 4.6. Description of Assessment Techniques

Reference	Measure/technique	Content	Original/additional references
Green (1976, 1987)	Parent report	Gender identity, gender role behaviors	Roberts et al. (1987)
Green et al. (1982)	Parent report	Gender identity, gender role behaviors	
Bates & Bentler (1973)	Parent report	Sex-typed games and activities	Doering (1981); Klein & Bates (1980); Meyer-Bahlburg, Feldman, & Ehrhardt (1985); Pleak et al. (1989); Rekers & Morey (1990); Sandberg & Meyer-Bahlburg (1994); Zucker et al. (1985); modified by Meyer-Bahlburg, Sandberg, Dolezal, & Yager (1994)
Bates et al. (1973)	Parent report	Gender role behaviors	Bates et al. (1979); Meyer-Bahlburg, Feldman, & Ehrhardt (1985); Pleak et al. (1989); modified version reported by Zucker et al. (1980)
Zucker & Bradley (this volume)	Parent report	Gender identity, gender role behaviors	Modified from Elizabeth & Green (1984)
Bates et al. (1973)	Parent report	Activity level/extraversion	Modified version, Zucker & Bradley (this volume)
Green, Fuller, Rutley, & Hendler (1972)	Free play	Masculine and feminine sex-typed play	
Rekers & Yates (1976)	Free play	Masculine and feminine sex-typed play	Doering et al. (1989); Rekers & Morey (1990); Zucker et al. (1982, 1985)

60

Green, Fuller, & Rutley (1972)	IT Scale for Children	Projective measure of sex-typed preferences	Rekers, Rosen, & Morey (1990)
Green & Fuller (1973)	Fantasy play	Masculine and feminine fantasy play (stories)	
Zucker, Doering, et al. (1984)	Fantasy play	Masculine and feminine fantasy play (stories)	Cramer & Hogan (1975); Erikson (1951)
Green, Fuller, & Rutley (1972)	Draw-a-Person	Sex of first figure drawn; heights of same-sex and opposite-sex persons; content analysis	Rekers, Rosen, & Morey (1990); Skilbeck et al. (1975); Zucker et al. (1983)
Zucker et al. (1988)	Gender constancy	"Stages" of gender constancy development	Slaby & Frey (1975); Emmerich et al. (1977)
Zucker, Lozinski, et al. (1992)	Rorschach	Sex-typed responses; gender confusion	Tuber & Coates (1985)
Zucker, Bradley, Lowry Sullivan, et al. (1993)	Gender identity interview	Cognitive and affective gender identity confusion	

Note. These assessment measures are the most readily accessible for clinical assessment. All have shown at least some discriminant validity; that is, they have distinguished gender-referred children from normal, sibling, and/or clinical controls. Some of the measures are appropriate for both boys and girls, whereas others (e.g., Bates et al., 1973) have been validated only for boys.

TABLE 4.7. Sex-Typed Behavior Assessment Protocol in the Child and Adolescent Gender Identity Clinic, Clarke Institute of Psychiatry

Measures	Reference	Controls[a]	Published/unpublished results
	Parent measures		
Revised Gender Behavior Inventory for Boys	Zucker et al. (1980)	S,C,N	Zucker et al. (1980, 1985)
Play and Games Questionnaire	Bates & Bentler (1973)	S,C,N	Zucker et al. (1985)
Activity Level/ Extraversion	Zucker et al. (1980)	S,C,N	This volume
Gender Identity Questionnaire (modified)	Elizabeth & Green (1984)	S,C,N	This volume
	Child measures		
Draw-a-Person test	Jolles (1952)	S,C,N	Zucker et al. (1983)
Rorschach test	Zucker, Lozinski, et al. (1992)	S,C,N	Zucker, Lozinski, et al. (1992)
Free-play test (modified)	Rekers & Yates (1976)	S,C,N	Zucker et al. (1982, 1985)
Gender constancy tests	Slaby & Frey (1975); Emmerich et al. (1977)	S,C	Zucker et al. (1988)
Dramatic Productions Test	Cramer & Hogan (1975)	S,C	Zucker et al. (1984)
Gender Identity Interview	Zucker, Bradley, Lowry Sullivan, et al. (1993)	C,N	Zucker, Bradley, Lowry Sullivan, et al. (1993)

[a]Control groups administered these measures: S, siblings; C, clinical controls; N, normal controls.

step in establishing gender identity disorder as a distinct child psychiatric condition (cf. Rutter, 1978).

In our research, psychological testing using some of these assessment measures has proved useful in distinguishing gender-referred children from controls. Table 4.7 shows the assessment protocol that we employ in our clinic. At the time of the assessment, the parents are given these questionnaires (and others) to complete, and the children are administered these tasks during a day of psychological testing. Table

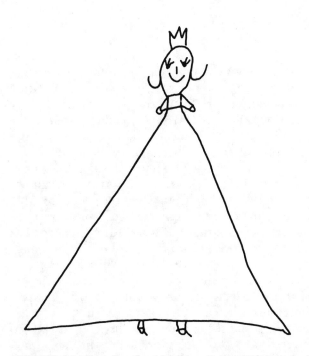

FIGURE 4.1. Drawing of a girl (left) and a boy (right) on the DAP test by an 8-year-old boy with gender identity disorder. Note the marked difference in height. The youngster remarked that the boy was drawn with a "dress on" because he "didn't know how" to draw pants.

4.7 also provides the references for the published or unpublished results for these measures.

For the practitioner, it is important to recognize that the discriminating power of individual tests is not perfect. For example, consider the DAP test, a relatively simple and probably crude marker of gender identification. On this test, children are asked to draw a person and then to identify the person's sex. Normative research has long shown that a large proportion of both boys and girls draw a person of their own sex first in response to this request (Brown, 1979; Heinrich & Triebe, 1972; Jolles, 1952; Tolor & Tolor, 1974). In contrast, three studies showed that children with gender identity disorder were more likely than controls to draw an opposite-sex person first (Green, Fuller, & Rutley, 1972; Skilbeck et al., 1975; Zucker et al., 1983). The percentages of gender problem versus control subjects in the three studies who drew an opposite-sex person first were 57% versus 24%, 32% versus 6%, and 61% versus 20%, respectively.

Although significant in each study, the false-negative rate was considerably higher than the false-positive rate. The high rate of false negatives may be interpreted in several ways. First, given the nominal nature of the measure, the probability of an "incorrect" response is 50% by chance alone. It is also likely that gender-referred children vary in the degree to which they are cross-gender-identified, and this may contribute to more variance on psychological testing. On the DAP test, for example, we found that 72.5% of the gender-referred children who met the complete DSM-III criteria for gender identity disorder drew an opposite-sex person first, in contrast to only 30.4% of the gender-referred children who did not meet the complete criteria (see Table 4.4); thus, the false-negative rate was lower within the more extreme group. The nominal nature of the DAP test precludes any type of continuous measurement; however, other potential indices of sex-typed reactions on the DAP are amenable to more refined analyses. We (Zucker et al., 1983) found that gender-referred children drew taller opposite-sex persons than same-sex persons, whereas controls tended to draw taller same-sex persons than opposite-sex persons. Skilbeck et al. (1975) found that gender-referred boys provided more details in their drawings of females than in their drawings of males, which is a common observation noted in therapy with these boys (Coates, 1985). In general, drawings of males and females are of qualitative, clinical use in understanding the gender representations of children with gender identity disorder (see Figures 4.1–4.3).

Because many clinicians may not be in a position to carry out a complete psychological test battery using available measures, Table 4.8 summarizes the age-related correlations that we have found for several of the measures listed in Table 4.7. It can be seen that the largest age effect, accounting for 18% of the variance, was on the free-play test. In this test, the child is presented with stereotypical masculine and feminine toys and dress-up apparel, and an observer records the duration of play from behind a one-way mirror.

What is the explanation for the age effects? Do they reflect a bona fide reduction in cross-gender identification? Do they mean that the child's cross-gender behavior is going "underground" as he or she becomes more aware of negative social responses by significant others? Is the problem a measurement issue, in that the techniques used to assess gender identity and gender role in older children are either inappropriate or too transparent to elicit valid responses? It may well be that to some extent all of these explanations are correct, and the clinician will have to decide which explanations are most accurate in individual cases.

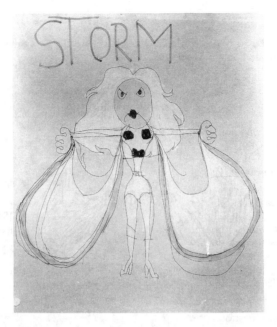

FIGURE 4.2. Spontaneous drawing of a popular female wrestler by an 11-year-old boy with gender identity disorder. The boy's mother, who had died when he was 5 years old, was described by the father as an alcoholic with a violent temper, and who was fond of professional wrestling.

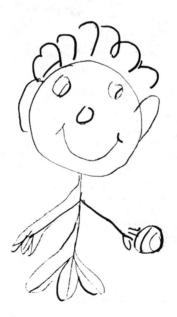

FIGURE 4.3. Drawing of a boy on the DAP test by a girl with gender identity disorder. Note the presence of the third leg.

TABLE 4.8. Measures of Gender Identity and Gender Role: Correlations with Age in Children with Gender Identity Disorder

Measures	r	p[a]	n
Parent measures			
Revised Gender Behavior Inventory for Boys[b]			
Factor 1 (Masculinity)	−.07	n.s.	156
Factor 2 (Femininity I)	−.12	n.s.	156
Factor 3 (Femininity II)	−.33	.001	156
Factor 4 (Mother's Boy)	.25	.002	156
Play and Games Questionnaire[c]			
Scale 1 (Feminine/Preschool)	−.27	.001	156
Scale 2 (Masculine, Nonathletic)	.11	n.s.	156
Scale 3 (Masculine, Athletic)	.28	.001	156
Enjoyment (Scale 1)	−.18	.020	156
Enjoyment (Scale 2)	−.02	n.s.	156
Enjoyment (Scale 3)	−.16	.044	156
Activity Level/Extraversion	−.25	.002	156
Gender Identity Questionnaire[d]	−.21	.019	123
Child measures			
Draw-a-Person test			
Percentage opposite-sex persons drawn first	−.29	.001	188
Height of same-sex person – height of opposite-sex person (in centimeters)	.12	n.s.	186
Rorschach test			
Number of same-sex responses – number of cross-sex responses	.11	n.s.	178
Free-play task			
Percentage of cross-sex play	−.41	.001	166
Gender Identity Interview			
Factor 1 (Affective Gender Confusion)	−.33	.000	107
Factor 2 (Cognitive Gender Confusion)	−.36	.000	107

[a]Two-tailed.
[b]This questionnaire can be used only with boys.
[c]This questionnaire was used with both the boys and the girls, but the data pertain only to the correlations for boys.
[d]On this questionnaire, the total score reflects more sex-atypical behavior.

Sex Differences

We have noted in Chapter 3 that boys are much more likely than girls to be referred for concerns regarding gender identity development. The CBCL data (see Figure 3.6) suggested that girls may be required to display more extreme cross-gender behavior than are boys before an assessment is sought. To test this hypothesis in more detail, we compared the sexes on several measures of sex-typed behavior. For each measure, we first tested for corresponding sex differences on four demographic variables: age, IQ, parents' social class, and parents' marital status. There were no sex differences in IQ and parents' marital status; however, there were some significant sex differences in age and/or social class, so these were covaried as appropriate.

The results are shown in Table 4.9. Of seven sex-typed measures,

TABLE 4.9. Sex Differences on Measures of Gender Identity and Gender Role Behavior

Measures	Boys			Girls			
	M	*SD*	*n*	*M*	*SD*	*n*	*p*
Parent measure							
Gender Identity Questionnaire[a]	2.9	0.5	108	2.7	0.5	15	.041[b]
Child measures							
Draw-a-Person test							
Percentage opposite-sex persons drawn first	51.5	—	163	76.0	—	25	.038
Height of same-sex person – height of opposite-sex person (in centimeters)	–0.4	3.4	161	–0.3	3.1	25	n.s.
Rorschach test							
Number of same-sex responses – number of cross-sex responses	–0.8	3.9	155	–0.9	6.9	23	n.s.[c]
Free-play task							
Percentage of same-sex play – cross-sex play	–0.1	0.7	145	–0.5	0.4	21	.007
Gender Identity Interview							
Factor 1 (Affective Gender Confusion)[d]	0.7	0.6	93	0.9	0.5	14	.049[b]
Factor 2 (Cognitive Gender Confusion)[d]	0.2	0.5	93	0.3	0.5	14	n.s.[d]

Note. The numbers of boys and girls who were administered each sex-typed measure varied somewhat, so these comparisons were based on different numbers of youngsters. *p* values are based on *t* tests.
[a]Absolute range = 1.0–5.0 (lower score more sex-atypical).
[b]Age and social class covaried.
[c]Age covaried.
[d]Absolute range = 0–2 (higher score more deviant).

four showed significant sex differences. In all cases, the girls showed more extreme cross-gender behavior than did the boys. It should be recalled, however, that the proportion of boys and girls who met the complete DSM criteria for gender identity disorder did not differ significantly (see Table 4.3).

Taken together, these findings suggest that the sex differences in sex-typed behavior are primarily attributable not to false-positive referrals of boys, but to the fact that referred girls on average are somewhat more extreme than referred boys in their cross-gender identification. In our view, the most parsimonious explanation of this pattern is that a sex-related threshold effect influences parental motivation to seek out a clinical assessment.

Parent Interview

The clinical interview with the child's parents should establish whether or not the DSM-IV criteria for gender identity disorder have been met. Table 4.10 summarizes some key areas in which clinical judgments are

TABLE 4.10. Clinical Rating Form for the Core Behavioral Features of Gender Identity Disorder of Childhood

---

1. *Identity Statements*
___ Child frequently states the wish to be of the opposite sex or that he or she is a member of the opposite sex (e.g., "I want to be a girl, I am a girl," or "I want to grow up to be a Mommy, not a Daddy").
___ Child occasionally states the wish to be of the opposite sex.
___ Child rarely states the wish to be of the opposite sex.
___ Child does not state the wish to be of the opposite sex.

2. *Anatomic Dysphoria*
___ Child frequently states a dislike of his or her sexual anatomy (e.g., "I don't like my penis"; "I want a penis, not a vagina") or demonstrates this behaviorally (e.g., in a boy, sitting to urinate to simulate having female genitalia; in a girl, standing to urinate to simulate having male genitalia).
___ Child occasionally states a dislike of his or her sexual anatomy or demonstrates this behaviorally.
___ Child rarely states a dislike of his or her sexual anatomy or demonstrates this behaviorally.
___ Child never states a dislike of his or her sexual anatomy or demonstrates this behaviorally.

3. *Cross-Dressing*
___ Child frequently cross-dresses (e.g., in boys, use of mother's clothes, such as dresses, high-heeled shoes, jewelry, and makeup; simulation of long hair with towels. In girls, refusal to wear culturally typical feminine clothing and use of clothing, such as boys' pants and shirts, to simulate a masculine appearance;

TABLE 4.10 (*Continued*)

often desire hair to be very short, in accordance with masculine convention).
___ Child occasionally cross-dresses.
___ Child rarely cross-dresses.
___ Child never cross-dresses.

4. *Toy and Role Play*
___ Child prefers to play with toys and to engage in roles stereotypically associated with the opposite sex (e.g., in boys, a preference for female dolls, such as Barbie or Gem, role play as a female, emulation of female superheroes; drawings invariably are of women. In girls, a preference for male dolls, such as GI Joe or male Transformers, role play as a male, emulation of male superheroes; drawings invariably are of men).
___ Child plays with toys and engages in roles that are both stereotypically masculine and feminine.
___ Child avoids toys and roles that are stereotypically associated with his or her sex but does not engage in toy or role play associated with the opposite sex.
___ Child prefers neutral activities (e.g., drawing, making music) and does not engage in either same-sex or cross-sex toy or role play.
___ Child prefers to play with toys and to engage in roles stereotypically associated with own sex.

5. *Peer Relations*
___ Child prefers to play with opposite-sex peers.
___ Child is a loner or is rejected.
___ Child plays with both same-sex and opposite-sex peers.
___ Child prefers to play with same-sex peers.

6. *Mannerisms*
___ Child frequently displays motoric movements and speech characteristics that are associated with the opposite sex, either in "natural" or "exaggerated" form (e.g., in boys, this includes hand movements, hip control, elevated pitch and lisp; in girls, this includes low voice projection).
___ Child occasionally displays motoric movements and speech characteristics that are associated with the opposite sex.
___ Child rarely displays motoric movements and speech characteristics that are associated with the opposite sex.
___ Child never displays motoric movements and speech characteristics that are associated with the opposite sex.

7. *Rough-and-Tumble Play*
___ In boys, there is an aversion to rough-and-tumble play or participation in group sports, such as hockey, football, and soccer. There is often a concern regarding physical injury. In girls, there is a strong attraction to rough-and-tumble play and group sports, particularly with boys.
___ In boys, there is no interest in rough-and-tumble play or participation in group sports, but the accompanying fear is not present.
___ In boys, there is an interest in rough-and-tumble play or participation in group sports. In girls, such interests are not dependent on a male peer group, but, rather, are expressed in more typical ways (e.g., mixed-sex teams, all-girl teams).

Note. From Zucker (1992b, pp. 327–328). Copyright 1992 by Lawrence Erlbaum Associates, Inc. Reprinted by permission. These behavioral features have been drawn from a variety of sources, including Green (1974, 1987), Rekers (1977a), Stoller (1968b), Zucker (1985), and Zuger (1966).

required. This information should be sufficient for a diagnostic decision. For the purpose of diagnosis, the interviewer should consider only the child's current behaviors, such as those displayed during the past 6 months. From a developmental perspective, however, it is also important to understand the course of these behaviors, including their onset and any changes that have occurred over time. It is not unusual, for example, to find that an older child may have had a history of expressing cross-sex wishes but that these are no longer expressed, despite the presence of other cross-gender behaviors.

Child Interview

A clinical interview with the child is also useful in establishing the presence of gender-dysphoric feelings and confusion about his or her status as a boy or a girl. Although such an interview is not required for diagnosis, it provides a qualitative impression of the child's conflictual issues, and thus may be helpful in planning a treatment program. We have developed a semistructured gender identity interview schedule that can be of use in organizing the child interview (Table 4.11). (For an example of such an interview, see pp. 56–57.)

Influence of Informant

In making a diagnostic decision, we have relied primarily on parents to act as informants during the clinical assessment. We have not formally relied on what the child has to say. The degree of informant concordance in reporting psychiatric symptomatology in children has become a topic of increasing interest over the past few years (e.g., Edelbrock & Costello, 1988; Gutterman, O'Brien, & Young, 1987). There is some evidence that better concordance (e.g., between mother and child) is found for symptoms that are concrete, observable, and unambiguous (e.g., Herjanic & Reich, 1982). For example, the Diagnostic Interview for Children and Adolescents contains two items related to gender identity: cross-dressing and wishing to be of the opposite sex. Herjanic and Reich (1982) reported a kappa of .33 for cross-dressing, but a kappa of only .10 for wishing to change sex. The low kappa values for both items can be partially explained by their relatively low frequency of occurrence, but the difference between the two values seems consistent with Herjanic and Reich's general finding regarding such item characteristics as relative observability.

TABLE 4.11. Gender Identity Interview for Children (Boy Version)

1. Are you a boy or a girl? BOY___ GIRL___
2. Are you a (opposite of first response)?___
3. When you grow up, will you be a Mommy or a Daddy?
   MOMMY___ DADDY___
4. Could you ever grow up to be a (opposite of first response)? YES___ NO___
5. Are there any good things about being a boy? YES___ NO___
   If YES, say: Tell me some of the good things about being a boy.
   (Probe for a maximum of three responses.)
   If YES or NO, ask: Are there any things that you don't like about being a
   boy? YES___ NO___
   If child answers YES, say: Tell me some of the things that you don't like about
   being a boy. (Probe for a maximum of three responses.)
6. Do you think it is better to be a boy or a girl? YES___ NO___ Why?
   (Probe for a maximum of three responses.)
7. In your mind, do you ever think that you would like to be a girl?
   YES___ NO___
   If YES, ask: Can you tell me why? (Probe for a maximum of three responses.)
8. In your mind, do you ever get mixed up and you're not really sure if you are a
   boy or a girl? YES___ NO___
   If YES, say: Tell me more about that. (Probe until satisfied.)
9. Do you ever feel more like a girl than like a boy? YES___ NO___
   If YES, say: Tell me more about that. (Probe until satisfied.)
10. You know what dreams are, right? Well, when you dream at night, are you
    ever in the dream? YES___ NO___
    If YES, ask: In your dreams, are you a boy, a girl, or sometimes a boy and
    sometimes a girl? BOY___ GIRL___ BOTH___ NOT IN DREAMS___
    (Probe regarding content of dreams.)
11. Do you ever think that you really are a girl? YES___ NO___
    If YES, say: Tell me more about that. (Probe until satisfied.)

Note. From Zucker, Bradley, Lowry Sullivan, et al. (1993, p. 448). Copyright 1993 by Lawrence Erlbaum Associates. Reprinted by permission.

On occasion, we have found that parents were surprised to learn that their child wished to be of the opposite sex. In some of these cases, the child had been referred at the suggestion of a professional (e.g., a teacher) who was concerned about the child's gender identity development. In others, there appeared to be an element of parental denial, since other members of the family (e.g., siblings) were aware of the child's cross-sex desires. In all of these cases, the diagnosis was informant-dependent. In general, however, it has been our experience that parents are usually very good informants regarding their child's gender identity development.

Clinical Issues

In this section, we describe the format of our clinical assessment procedure and discuss technical issues that we have encountered over the years. (For very similar views on these matters, see Coates & Wolfe, in press.)

Preparation for Evaluation

An assessment process can be said to begin when the parents, perhaps at the suggestion of a professional (e.g., a teacher, a family physician), make the decision to seek a psychiatric/psychological evaluation. Achenbach (1979) noted that it is invariably parents, not children, who make this decision—a situation that differs dramatically from the referral process as it is normally initiated with adult patients (except when an adult is so impaired that he or she is unable to activate a referral, when the referral is court-ordered, etc.). In our experience, Achenbach's (1979) observation is almost always valid. Over the years we have encountered only one youngster, a 6-year-old girl, who formally activated the referral. She asked her mother whether she could see "a doctor" because she felt so unhappy about being a girl.

When one works in a hospital setting (as we do), a parent or a referring professional typically contacts an intake worker, who does the initial paperwork. In the majority of cases, this procedure is straightforward and the family is informed about the availability of services, the waiting list, and so on. Because of the high visibility of the Clarke Institute within the mental health field in Toronto, referring professionals often refer complex or specialized cases to our child service; over the years, awareness of our gender identity clinic has become reasonably widespread. In addition, many professionals feel that they lack the specialized training needed to conduct a gender identity assessment and are often grateful that we are available to do so. This is not surprising, in light of the low prevalence of gender identity disorder and the inherent anxieties elicited by issues of sex and gender.

Over the past several years, we have observed an interesting change in some of our referrals—namely, that some of the parents who contact us about an assessment profess a rather marked ambivalence about it. (We presume that parents who are even more ambivalent or are not concerned never call.) The ambivalence seems to revolve around four manifest issues: (1) Is their child's behavior really a problem? (2) How do they broach the topic with their child? (3) Does their child need to participate in the assessment? and (4) Will the assessment damage their child? In such situations, we have found that it is better for one of us (rather than the intake worker) to initiate the assessment process by exploring these questions over the telephone (cf. Hazell, 1992). A working assumption that led us to this position is that the parental ambivalence is, in most cases, "part of the problem"; that is, it is correlated with family variables that, at the least, have perpetuated the child's gender identity confusion (detailed consideration of family factors is given in Chapters 5 and 7). We have found that for most of such ambivalent cases, the initial telephone contact (usually several calls) has proved extremely helpful in reducing parental anxiety and establishing what might be called an "assessment alliance" with the family. Nevertheless, the clinician should recognize that initial ambivalence may well signal a poor prognosis for a family's capacity eventually to enter treatment.

CASE EXAMPLE 4.2

Ben was a 5-year-old boy whose mother contacted us after speaking with the family physician. Ben lived with his upper-middle-class parents, an older brother, and an infant sister. During an intake telephone interview, Ben's mother began by stating that both she and her husband were "concerned" about him, but quickly added, "It's more our problem than his." She went on to make some rather disjointed remarks: that Ben had always been a "difficult child . . . we're intelligent . . . my husband's convinced he's homosexual." She then described various aspects of Ben's gender identity development, indicating marked cross-gender identification. Ben preferred girls as playmates; his favorite toy was a dollhouse; he role-played only as a female (e.g., a queen, a princess) and wanted to be a ballet dancer; his drawings were always of beautiful females; he enjoyed cross-dressing and rejected stereotypical masculine clothing (e.g., sweatshirts with sports logos); he avoided rough-and-tumble play; and he wanted to be a girl. When Ben's mother was asked how she thought Ben felt about being a boy, she said, "God, I have no idea." Regarding his clothing, she said that because of the colors there "wasn't a [boy's] snowsuit in the city" that he would wear. In general, she felt that Ben's cross-gender identification "permeate[d] his whole attitude."

Ben's mother then talked about her husband's refusal to let Ben take ballet lessons. When asked her view on this, she commented, "I prefer ballet to hockey . . . it's more beautiful, profound. . . . He is what he is, I want him to be happy. . . . We've worked hard to make him happy, it's been hell." She said that Ben's "pretty face" and curly hair had often resulted in his being mistaken for a girl. She then reiterated that Ben had always been a difficult child, and that he had been a "miserable baby." In fact, she recalled that she had taken him for a psychiatric assessment at the age of 2 because of this. The report from that assessment indicated that she found him to be "precocious" but "unhappy, constantly crying, and fussing." She reported that he had "sudden mood swings and when he did not get his own way crie[d] continuously." The report noted that "All methods of coping have failed. Mother is quite depressed and is seeking relief and help." It indicated that Ben's mother felt guilty because she found more pleasure in her older son, and that she complained about not being able to spend time with the older son because of Ben's "difficult and demanding behaviors." The report also noted that Ben's father, an executive at a successful business, would spend some evenings during the week at a hotel because Ben's crying kept him from sleeping through the night at home and "he need[ed] to be rested for his work." The report ended with a recommendation of treatment to focus on "the pathology of [the] mother–child relationship." The parents chose not to follow this recommendation.

On the basis of the information provided during the intake interview, an assessment was recommended. Ben's mother agreed to this, but she then indicated that she did not want to "get him involved." She expressed a lot of anxiety about this, commenting, "If we start poisoning his dollhouse. . . . I don't want to hurt him. . . . The whole thing fills me with anxiety."

Given Ben's mother's profound unease about bringing him for an assessment, we initially met with the parents alone. After meeting with us, the parents chose to allow Ben to participate in the assessment process. The assessment left little doubt in our minds that he was a profoundly unhappy youngster whose marked cross-gender identification was accompanied by a variety of socioemotional and relationship difficulties. Although Ben's parents seemed to find the assessment process useful and accepted (in principle) some of our recommendations, they did not pursue the recommendations that Ben be seen in individual therapy and that they should participate in parental counseling. From our standpoint, the parents' decision not to pursue therapy was troubling, since we felt that we had established a good working relationship with them and because they had indicated a willingness to pursue therapy at a second feedback/interpretive session.

Although it is important to be aware of parental ambivalence about the assessment process, such ambivalence is not necessarily an indication that parents will reject a recommendation for treatment when it is warranted. We have had experience with a number of other parents who chose to pursue therapy, despite the intense anxiety activated by the assessment process.

Assessment Sequence

In our clinic, we typically ask all members of a family to attend the initial assessment interview. On occasion, we see families without older siblings if the parents feel that these siblings would unnecessarily stigmatize the identified patient (e.g., by teasing). This occurs rarely, but when it does, the older siblings (usually male) often have their own difficulties, and the family in general has not functioned particularly well. It has rarely been a problem for us to involve fathers; this was apparently a difficulty commonly encountered by clinicians seeing families a generation ago (e.g., Stoller, 1979). Perhaps this reflects some kind of cohort effect in either clinician or family expectations. For the very ambivalent families of the kind described above, we meet with parents alone to establish whether they wish to pursue the assessment, and if they do, we arrange for subsequent visits with the child.

Over the past few years, we have become more aware of the importance of clarifying with the parents what information about the reason for the assessment they will provide to their child. In the majority of cases, the parents are able to tell their child directly about the reason for the assessment (e.g., that they wish to understand why their child wants to be of the opposite sex). Again, this issue is more complex with the ambivalent cases. Typically, the parents are at a loss about how to introduce the assessment process. For example, one mother wanted to tell her 4-year-old son that they were going to see a "friend" of a relative who happened to work at the Clarke Institute. Usually, the parents are quite vague with their child, stating that they are going to see someone to talk about how family members get along with one another. Our approach is to encourage the parents to provide their child with more explicit information about the reason for the assessment. Usually, they are able to tell their child that they are going to see a "talking doctor who knows a lot about children" and is going to help him or her understand why "you might not be so happy about being a boy (girl)." Some parents, particularly mothers, find it helpful when they are told to emphasize to their child that "no one is angry with you—we just want to understand how you are feeling."

During our initial assessment interview, we review the child's gender identity development and other aspects of the child's development, and we inquire about aspects of the family matrix in general. After this interview, the parents are seen separately and the child is interviewed individually. The parents are then seen individually on subsequent visits to take their own life history and to inquire about family issues that were not covered in the family assessment. The child is also seen for psychological testing (as described above). Then, at an interpretive/feedback session, we provide our opinion and treatment recommendations.

In our experience, several questions usually need to be addressed during the assessment process. It is not uncommon for parents to inquire about the availability of biological tests. Such an inquiry may reflect either a vague belief that some kind of physical anomaly explains their child's problem, or an explicit conviction about etiology (such connections are usually professed by more educated parents). Our response to the inquiry is always contextual, based on our hunches about the parents' belief systems. For example, if parents ask about "chromosome testing," we will explain that in the absence of an intersex condition the karyotyping of the sex chromosomes is unlikely to be informative (see also Chapter 6). At the same time, we can begin to discuss the complexity of biological influences on psychosexual differentiation, while pointing out that current technology does not permit tests of certain biologically based hypotheses. From a more dynamic perspective, a clinician should recognize that questions about biological factors may well be part of a parental belief system. For example, one mother of an 11-year-old boy with a long history of gender identity disorder had taken him to an endocrinologist because she believed he had a small penis. When told that the length of the boy's penis was within normal limits, she remained unconvinced and wondered about the competence of the physician. Further exploration revealed that the mother hoped that her son was "really a girl" and could have his penis removed. The mother commented that *it would be easier for her* if he was a girl, since she had no idea how to help him with his feelings.

Another question that usually needs to be addressed concerns our opinion about the accuracy of the referral. Some parents acknowledge the hope that we will say that nothing is "wrong," that they were "overreacting," or the like. For some families, then, we provide a provisional opinion at the end of the initial interview. Perhaps because of the nature of our clinic and its setting, it is rare for us to assess a false-positive case. Thus, our initial feedback is really part of alliance building with the family. Typically, we will indicate to the parents that we think that they made the correct decision in coming to talk to us; that we think their child is struggling with gender identity issues; and that we believe it would be helpful to continue the assessment process. We attempt in most cases to defer our full opinion until the end of the assessment process.

A number of parents ask whether their child will ultimately want to change his or her sex, and a greater number ask whether their child will ultimately become gay, lesbian, or homosexual. These questions can be answered in a factual manner based on the formal clinical and research literature to date (see Chapters 9 and 10), but they also need to be understood contextually. For example, some parents are extremely upset (for various reasons) about the prospect that their child will develop a homosexual orientation. On the other hand, some parents indicate that they have no concern about this and just want their child to be happy. For parents who are anxious about the likelihood of their child's becoming homosexual, it is often necessary to do extended clinical work to uncover and work through the sources of their anxiety. But we also attempt to shift the focus of their concern to the child's current discomfort about his or her status as a boy or a girl, and to indicate that this is the area in which they can be directly helpful. This recommendation usually deflects the parents' longer-term concern. An absence of longer-term parental concerns can be understood in various ways. For some parents, such an absence may reflect complex dynamic issues pertaining to sex and gender in general, including an insensitivity about their child's current gender identity conflict, in which case extended clinical work centering on these issues is often necessary. For other parents, however, acceptance of their child's eventual sexual orientation reflects a genuine empathy. In these instances, the parents recognize the distinction between gender identity and sexual orientation, and indicate that helping their child feel better as a boy or a girl is their primary goal. We will consider these issues in more detail in Chapter 9.

NOTES

1. The members of the DSM-III Advisory Committee on Psychosexual Disorders were Anke A. Ehrhardt, Diane S. Fordney-Settlage, Richard C. Friedman, Paul H. Gebhard, Richard Green, Helen S. Kaplan, Judith B. Kuriansky, Harold I. Lief, Jon K. Meyer, John Money, Ethel S. Person, Lawrence Sharpe, Robert L. Spitzer, Robert J. Stoller, and Arthur Zitrin. The members of the DSM-III-R Subcommittee on Gender Identity Disorders were Anke A. Ehrhardt, David McWhirter, Heino F. L. Meyer-Bahlburg, John Money, Ethel S. Person, Robert L. Spitzer, Janet B. W. Williams, and Kenneth J. Zucker. The members of the DSM-IV Subcommittee on Gender Identity Disorders were Susan J. Bradley (Chair), Ray Blanchard, Susan Coates, Richard Green, Stephen B. Levine, Heino F. L. Meyer-Bahlburg, Ira B. Pauly, and Kenneth J. Zucker.

2. As an aside, it might be noted that many sexological diagnoses in the DSM-III- R do not include felt distress as a criterion (see, e.g., Gert, 1992). Pedophilia is probably a good example. Wakefield (1992a) has suggested that women with inhibited female orgasm probably constitute a heterogeneous group, of which only a proportion experience felt distress regarding the lack of orgasmic experience in their life histories.

CHAPTER 5

Associated Psychopathology

Comorbidity—that is, the presence of two or more psychiatric disorders—occurs frequently among children referred for psychiatric evaluation. Assuming that the putative comorbid conditions actually represent distinct disorders, it is important to know for various reasons (e.g., prevention and treatment planning) whether one condition increases the risk for the other condition or whether the conditions are caused by distinct or overlapping factors (Caron & Rutter, 1991; Verhulst & Koot, 1992). In this chapter, we review the literature on associated psychopathology or behavioral difficulties among children with gender identity disorder.

Several measurement approaches have been employed to address this matter, including standardized behavior problem questionnaires (e.g., Bates et al., 1973, 1979; Rekers & Morey, 1989b, 1989c), ratings of social behavior in structured situations (Bates et al., 1979) and on questionnaires (Zucker, 1985), assessment of personality functioning and structure on projective tests (Coates & Tuber, 1988; Goddard, 1986; Goddard & Tuber, 1989; Ipp, 1986; Kolers, 1986; Tuber & Coates, 1985, 1989), and ascertainment of other psychiatric disorders (Coates & Person, 1985). Almost all of this work has focused on boys.

The greatest amount of information on general behavior problems comes from parent-report data obtained via the Child Behavior Checklist (CBCL). On the CBCL, each of 118 items is rated on a 3-point scale ranging from 0 to 2 for frequency of occurrence. In the standardization of the CBCL, factor analysis was performed on six sex × age groupings (4–5 years, 6–11 years, and 12–16 years). Two broad-band factors were identified, termed Internalizing and Externalizing. Across the six groups, there were also common and unique narrow-band factors (see, e.g., Achenbach, 1978; Achenbach & Edelbrock, 1979). Internalizing disorders have been characterized as disturbances of emotion or behavioral deficits (e.g., depression, social withdrawal, anxiety), whereas Externalizing disorders have been characterized as disturbances of conduct or behavioral excesses (e.g., aggression, hyperactivity). Several attempts have been made to map the similarity of these dimensional categories of disorder onto more formal DSM diagnoses (e.g., Achenbach, 1980; Cicchetti & Toth, 1991; Edelbrock & Costello, 1988).

CBCL DATA ON BOYS WITH GENDER
IDENTITY DISORDER

Parent-Report Data

In our own research, we have made extensive use of data from the CBCL (e.g., Zucker, 1985, 1990b). Table 5.1 presents maternal-report data for 161 gender-referred boys and 90 male siblings (of both our male and female probands) for five CBCL indices of disturbance: the number of elevated narrow-band scales ($T > 70$), the number and sum of items rated 1 or 2, and T scores for the Internalizing and Externalizing broad-band scales.[1] On all five indices, the gender-referred boys had significantly higher levels of behavioral disturbance (all p's < .001). Table 5.1 also shows that the boys with gender identity disorder had significantly higher Internalizing T scores than Externalizing T scores, t (160) = 3.01, p = .003, whereas the male siblings did not, $t < 1$.

CBCL ratings were also available from 117 fathers of the 161 boys, and the mother–father correlations were significant for all five indices (r's ranged from .41 to .58, all p's < .001). The strength of these correlations was consistent with the findings of many other studies that have assessed the concordance of parent ratings (Achenbach, McConaughy, & Howell, 1987).

Table 5.2 presents the CBCL data as a function of two age groupings (4–5 and 6–11 years). It can be seen in Table 5.2 that the boys aged 4–5 had a higher average IQ, were more likely to be from a higher social class background, and were more likely to be living in two-parent, intact families (all p's < .001). Accordingly, the comparisons between the two age groupings were conducted with these demographic variables covaried. For three of the disturbance ratings (number of elevated narrow-band scales, the sum of items rated 1 or 2, and the Externalizing T), the boys aged 4–5 with gender identity disorder had significantly lower disturbance ratings than did their counterparts aged 6–11 (all p's < .05); for the other two ratings (number of items rated 1 or 2 and

TABLE 5.1. Maternal Ratings of Behavioral Disturbance on the CBCL of Boys with Gender Identity Disorder and Male Siblings

Measures	Gender identity disorder ($n = 161$)		Siblings ($n = 90$)	
	M	*SD*	*M*	*SD*
No. elevated narrow-band scales	1.8	2.3	0.8	1.6
Number of items[a]	34.9	16.6	25.5	15.2
Sum of items[b]	43.2	24.8	30.1	21.0
Internalizing *T*	60.7	10.1	53.9	10.8
Externalizing *T*	59.2	10.7	54.4	9.9
Age (in years)	7.0	2.4	7.5	2.9
IQ	108.5	15.4	107.3[c]	15.4
Social class	42.4	15.2	43.7	14.4
Marital status				
Both parents	110 (*n*)		64 (*n*)	
Mother only/reconstituted	51 (*n*)		26 (*n*)	

[a]Absolute range = 0–118.

[b]Absolute range = 0–236.

[c]$n = 21$. In our research, we assessed systematically the IQ of siblings from the first 36 families evaluated; after that, sibling IQs were obtained only if there was a particular research issue of interest or if it was clinically indicated.

the Internalizing *T*), the differences approached significance (both *p*'s < .10).

In both age groupings, the boys with gender identity disorder differed slightly, albeit significantly, from the male siblings with regard to age and social class (see Table 5.2). Accordingly, the comparisons were conducted with age and social class covaried. In the group aged 4–5, three of the disturbance ratings for the boys with gender identity disorder (the number and sum of items and the Internalizing *T* score) were significantly higher than those of the male siblings (*p*'s ranged from < .003 to .05). In the group aged 6–11, all five indices of disturbance were significantly different (all *p*'s < .01).

The difference in degree of behavioral disturbance between the two age groupings was also reflected in the percentage of boys whose CBCL sum score fell in the clinical range (> 90th percentile). Of the 67 boys aged 4–5 with gender identity disorder, only 14 (20.9%) boys had a total Behavior Problem score in the clinical range, compared to 4 (12.9%) of 31 male siblings—a nonsignificant difference. In contrast, 58 (61.7%) of the 94 boys aged 6–11 with gender identity disorder had scores in the clinical range, compared to only 17 (28.8%) of 59 male siblings, $\chi^2 = 14.41$, $p < .001$. Thus, the older boys with gender identi-

TABLE 5.2. Maternal Ratings of Behavioral Disturbance on the CBCL for Boys with Gender Identity Disorder and Male Siblings as a Function of Age Grouping

| Measures | 4–5 years[a] | | | |
| | Gender identity disorder ($n = 67$) | | Siblings ($n = 31$) | |
	M	SD	M	SD
No. elevated narrow-band scales	0.8	1.4	0.3	0.8
Number of items	29.1	13.2	21.3	12.7
Sum of items	33.7	16.8	24.7	17.2
Internalizing *T*	57.5	9.6	49.9	10.4
Externalizing *T*	55.1	9.4	50.6	10.1
Age (in years)	4.8	0.7	4.4	0.7
IQ	114.9	13.0	112.7[c]	13.5
Social class	49.5	13.0	43.1	15.1
Marital status				
Both parents	58 (*n*)		25 (*n*)	
Mother only/reconstituted	9 (*n*)		6 (*n*)	

| Measures | 6–11 years[b] | | | |
| | Gender identity disorder ($n = 94$) | | Siblings ($n = 59$) | |
	M	SD	M	SD
No. elevated narrow-band scales	2.5	2.5	1.0	1.9
Number of items	38.9	17.7	27.6	16.1
Sum of items	49.7	27.4	32.9	22.4
Internalizing *T*	62.8	10.0	55.9	10.5
Externalizing *T*	62.0	10.7	56.4	9.3
Age (in years)	8.5	1.9	9.2	2.0
IQ	103.5	15.8	102.3[d]	16.0
Social class	37.1	14.8	43.9	14.1
Marital status				
Both parents	52 (*n*)		39 (*n*)	
Mother only/reconstituted	42 (*n*)		20 (*n*)	

[a]Several boys in each group were 3 years old. Their CBCL profiles were computed using the norms for 2- to 3-year-olds (Achenbach, Edelbrock, & Howell, 1987), but were prorated to adjust for the smaller number of items on the questionnaire.

[b]Several boys in each group were 12 years old. Their CBCL profiles were computed using the norms for 12- to 16-year-olds.

[c]$n = 10$.

[d]$n = 11$.

ty disorder were about three times as likely as their 4- to 5-year-old counterparts to have a CBCL sum score in the clinical range.

For the boys aged 4–5 with gender identity disorder, the Internalizing T score was significantly higher than the Externalizing T score, t (66) = 2.68, p = .009; however, the difference between the two broadband scales for the boys aged 6–11 was not significant, t (93) = 1.58, p = .118. For the male siblings in both age groupings, the Internalizing and Externalizing T scores did not differ significantly.

The CBCL narrow-band scales for the two groups of boys by age grouping are displayed in Figure 5.1. We computed t tests for each narrow-band scale, with age and social class covaried (see above). Among the boys aged 4–5, the boys with gender identity disorder had a significantly higher T score than the male siblings on only one of the eight narrow-band scales, Immature (p < .05). In contrast, the boys aged 6–11 with gender identity disorder had significantly higher T scores than the male siblings on seven of the nine narrow-band scales: Schizoid–Anxious, Depressed, Uncommunicative, Obsessive–Compulsive, Social Withdrawal, Hyperactive, and Aggressive (p's ranged from < .01 to .001).

Table 5.3 shows the percentage of boys with gender identity disorder, the male siblings, and the referred and nonreferred groups from the standardization sample who had narrow-band scale scores in the clinical range (> 98th percentile). Among the boys aged 4–5 with gender identity disorder, the percentage with narrow-band elevations was generally more similar to that of the nonreferred sample than to the referred sample. Among the boys aged 6–11 with gender identity disorder, however, the percentage with narrow-band elevations was quite similar to that of the referred sample, particularly with regard to the Internalizing scales, the Social Withdrawal scale, and one of the Externalizing scales, Aggressive. The percentage of gender-referred boys with elevated Hyperactive and Delinquent subscales was substantially lower than the percentage of referred boys from the standardization sample with elevations on these scales.

Comparisons with Pair-Matched Clinical Controls

Table 5.4 presents maternal-report data for 46 gender-referred boys pair-matched to 46 clinical control boys who had participated in several research studies conducted in our clinic (Birkenfeld-Adams, 1995; Doering, 1981; Mitchell, 1991). Pairs were matched as closely as possible with regard to age (±1 year), IQ (±15 points), parents' social class (Hollingshead, 1975), and parents' marital status (two parents vs.

TABLE 5.3. Percentage of Boys with Narrow-Band Scales in the Clinical Range (*T* > 70)

	4–5 years			
Narrow-band scales	Gender identity disorder (*n* = 63)	Siblings (*n* = 27)	Referred (*n* = 100)	Nonreferred (*n* = 100)
Social Withdrawal	12.7	3.7	37.0	3.0
Depressed	20.6	3.7	37.0	4.0
Immature	7.9	3.7	42.0	3.0
Somatic Complaints	9.5	3.7	25.0	3.0
Sex Problems	14.3	7.4	14.0	0.0
Schizoid	1.6	3.7	14.0	2.0
Aggressive	12.7	7.4	61.0	6.0
Delinquent	7.9	3.7	29.0	2.0

	6–11 years			
Narrow-band scales	Gender identity disorder (*n* = 94)	Siblings (*n* = 59)	Referred (*n* = 300)	Nonreferred (*n* = 300)
Schizoid–Anxious	34.0	11.9	31.0	3.0
Depressed	21.3	5.1	31.0	2.0
Uncommunicative	37.2	20.3	44.0	6.0
Obsessive–Compulsive	28.7	11.9	30.0	2.0
Somatic Complaints	19.1	13.6	14.0	2.0
Social Withdrawal	42.6	8.5	28.0	2.0
Hyperactive	17.0	6.8	34.0	3.0
Aggressive	34.0	13.6	43.0	2.0
Delinquent	13.8	11.9	40.0	4.0

Note. Data for the nonreferred and referred samples from Achenbach and Edelbrock (1983, p. 64).

mother only/reconstituted). The two groups did not differ significantly on any of the five CBCL indices of disturbance.

Teacher-Report Data

Since the Teacher's Report Form (TRF) of the CBCL became available (Achenbach & Edelbrock, 1986; Edelbrock & Achenbach, 1984), we have also collected teacher ratings on the gender-referred boys. TRF data were obtained for 67 (75.2%) of 89 boys. Parents of 21 other boys did not give consent to contact the teacher, and the form for 1 boy was not returned by his teacher. An additional 13 boys were not yet in school, and thus TRF ratings on them were not available.

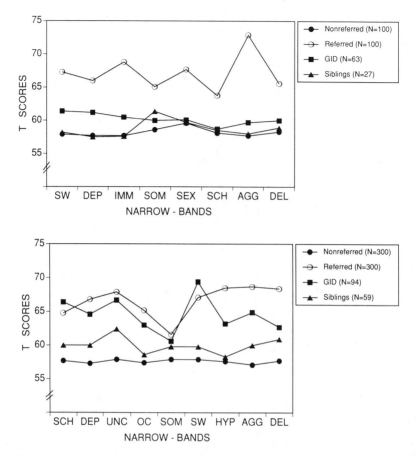

FIGURE 5.1. Top panel: Narrow-band factors on the CBCL, 4- to 5-year-old boys. SW, Social Withdrawal; DEP, Depressed; IMM, Immature; SOM, Somatic Complaints; SEX, Sex Problems; SCH, Schizoid; AGG, Aggressive; DEL, Delinquent. Bottom panel: Narrow-band factors on the CBCL, 6- to 11-year-old boys. SCH, Schizoid–Anxious; DEP, Depressed; UNC, Uncommunicative; OC, Obsessive–Compulsive; SOM, Somatic Complaints; SW, Social Withdrawal; HYP, Hyperactive; AGG, Aggressive; DEL, Delinquent. GID, gender identity disorder. Nonreferred and referred group data are from the standardization study (Achenbach & Edelbrock, 1983, Appendix D).

In the standardization sample (see Achenbach & Edelbrock, 1986), one age grouping included boys aged 6–11 years, so we divided our sample into two age groupings: 6–11 years and 4–5 years. These data are presented in Table 5.5. For the 41 boys aged 6–11 with gender identity disorder, the sum of the items on the TRF was midway between that of the referred boys and that of the nonreferred boys in the standardization sample. The Internalizing T score was nearly identical to

TABLE 5.4. Maternal Ratings of Behavioral Disturbance on the CBCL for Boys with Gender Identity Disorder and Pair-Matched Clinical Controls

Measures	Gender identity disorder ($n = 46$)		Clinical controls ($n = 46$)	
	M	SD	M	SD
No. elevated narrow-band scales	2.5	2.7	2.3	2.3
Number of items	38.8	18.2	42.2	15.5
Sum of items	50.1	27.2	53.5	25.6
Internalizing T	63.6	10.2	63.2	8.5
Externalizing T	62.2	11.1	65.8	9.2
Age (in years)	6.9	2.2	6.9	2.3
IQ[a]	11.3	2.1	12.1	2.1
Social class	38.1	14.7	40.7	12.8
Marital status				
Both parents	24 (n)		27 (n)	
Mother only/reconstituted	22 (n)		19 (n)	

[a]Based on four subtests from the Wechsler Intelligence Scale for Children—Revised (WISC-R), the WISC—Third Edition (WISC-III), the Wechsler Preschool and Primary Scale of Intelligence (WPPSI), or the WPPSI—Revised (WPPSI-R) (average = 10; absolute range = 1–19).

TABLE 5.5. Ratings of Behavioral Disturbance on the TRF for Boys with Gender Identity Disorder

Measures	Gender identity disorder				Nonreferred, 6–11 years ($n = 300$)		Referred, 6–11 years ($n = 300$)	
	4–5 years ($n = 26$)		6–11 years ($n = 41$)					
	M	SD	M	SD	M	SD	M	SD
No. elevated narrow-band scales	0.2	0.7	0.9	1.4	—	—	—	—
Number of items	20.6	15.1	34.6	21.5	—	—	—	—
Sum of items	25.6	23.8	46.8	32.8	22.3	22.9	65.8	31.9
Internalizing T	57.5	7.1	61.2	9.6	52.3	8.3	62.2	8.7
Externalizing T	51.7	9.0	58.4	9.4	52.2	9.2	65.6	8.9

Note. Data for the nonreferred and referred samples from Achenbach and Edelbrock (1986, Appendix C, p. 160).

that of the referred sample, whereas the Externalizing T score was nearly identical to that of the nonreferred sample. Of the 41 boys, 19 (46.3%) had a total Behavior Problem score in the clinical range.

For the 26 boys aged 4–5 with gender identity disorder, there was considerably less behavioral disturbance, although the Internalizing T score fell midway between the T scores of the nonreferred and referred samples. Of the 26 boys, only 3 (11.5%) had a total Behavior Problem score in the clinical range. (These analyses need to be treated with caution, since the gender-referred boys aged 4–5 were below the age range of the standardization sample.)

Table 5.5 also shows that in both age groupings, the Internalizing T score was significantly higher than the Externalizing T score (t's = 4.0 and 2.3, p's < .001 and .03, respectively).

For those youngsters on whom both maternal-report and teacher-report data were available (n = 64), the correlations were significant for all five indices of disturbance (r's ranged from .40 to .63, all p's < .001). In general, these correlations were stronger than those typically found between parent and teacher reports (Achenbach, McConaghy, & Howell, 1987).

Profile Patterns

Achenbach and Edelbrock (1983; see also Edelbrock & Achenbach, 1980) employed cluster analysis to develop a "taxonomy of profile patterns" from CBCL data. Their goal in employing this classification approach was to detect similarities among profiles of individual children. Because they sought to identify variations in the behavior problem patterns of children with significant socioemotional difficulties, they conducted the original CBCL analyses on only the referred sample in the standardization study (see Achenbach & Edelbrock, 1983, Chap. 8). For each sex × age grouping, intraclass correlations were calculated and then subjected to centroid cluster analysis, from which profile types were identified and labeled. Intraclass correlations can range from –1.00 to 1.00. A score of .00 represents the mean of the referred sample in the standardization study, and the end points represent ±1 *SD*.

Table 5.6 shows the mean intraclass correlations for the profile types of our boys aged 4–5 and 6–11 with gender identity disorder, respectively. For the boys aged 4–5, the profile type most similar to the referred sample was Depressed–Social Withdrawal. The profile types least similar to the referred sample were Aggressive–Delinquent, Aggressive, and Sex Problems (for the last profile, this is artifactual, since

TABLE 5.6. Mean Intraclass Correlations of Profile Types on the CBCL for Boys with Gender Identity Disorder

Profile types	M	SD
4- to 5-year-olds (*n* = 41)		
Depressed–Social Withdrawal	.04	.38
Somatic Complaints	−.16	.27
Immature	−.13	.35
Sex Problems	−.28	.39
Schizoid	−.16	.35
Aggressive	−.28	.29
Aggressive–Delinquent	−.42	.26
6- to 11-year-olds (*n* = 77)		
Schizoid–Social Withdrawal	.04	.37
Depressed–Social Withdrawal–Aggressive	−.20	.33
Schizoid	.16	.38
Somatic Complaints	.02	.40
Hyperactive	−.33	.34
Delinquent	−.29	.32

Note. Profile types are listed in the order presented by Achenbach and Edelbrock (1983). Intraclass correlations were calculated only if the sum of items rated as a 1 or a 2 exceeded 25 (see Edelbrock & Achenbach, 1980).

we intentionally scored as "0" the two gender identity items that loaded on the Sex Problems factor). For our boys aged 6–11, the profile types most similar to the referred sample were Schizoid, Schizoid–Social Withdrawal, and Somatic Complaints; the profile types least similar to the referred sample were Hyperactive, Delinquent, and Depressed–Social Withdrawal–Aggressive. For both age groupings, the lack of similarity to the Externalizing profile types was stronger than the similarity to the Internalizing profile types.

Summary

Overall, the CBCL data showed that the boys with gender identity disorder were comparable to pair-matched clinical controls with regard to degree of behavioral disturbance, but were in general more disturbed than the male siblings. In the group aged 6–11, the boys with gender identity disorder were more disturbed than were the nonreferred boys in the CBCL and TRF standardization samples, but this difference was not apparent in the group aged 4–5. The patterning of behavioral disturbance indicated a predominance of internalizing symptomatology; this is consistent with the findings of investigators who have used a different behavior problem questionnaire (Rekers & Morey, 1989c; Sreenivasan, 1985), observational ratings of "body constriction" (Bates et al., 1979), clinical diagnoses of separation anxiety and dysthymia (Coates & Person, 1985), and maternal report of behavioral inhibition or shyness (Coates, Wolfe, & Hahn-Burke, 1994). Nevertheless, inspection of the CBCL and TRF distributions shows that there was tremendous range in the extent of CBCL psychopathology. We provide information later on some correlates of this diversity, but first we attempt to provide a richer account of the CBCL data by discussing representative profiles along with clinical data taken from the psychiatric assessment. The selected profiles consist of randomly selected youngsters with a CBCL sum score that was ≥ 1 *SD* below the clinical cutoff, at the clinical cutoff, or ≥ 1 *SD* above the clinical cutoff for the respective age groupings.

Case Vignettes of 4- to 5-Year-Old Boys

CASE EXAMPLE 5.1

Marcus was 5 years old with an IQ of 125. He was referred by the family physician because of maternal concern about his gender identity development; his father professed no concern about this, but chose to participate in the assessment to please his wife. Marcus lived with his parents, two older siblings, and one younger sibling. On the Hollingshead index, the family's social class ranking was a II.

On the CBCL, Marcus's mother identified 13 items as characteristic of his behavior, which summed to 13, well below the clinical cutoff. Both the Internalizing *T* score (45) and the Externalizing *T* score (38) were also well below the clinical cutoff. The ratings by the father closely matched those of the mother.

The absence of CBCL psychopathology was generally consistent with our clinical impression of Marcus's functioning. He did well in kindergarten, and neither of his parents felt that he showed major difficulties at home. Like many other boys with gender identity disorder, he was described by his mother as very sensitive. His mother regarded him as compliant, perhaps too compliant. In an individual interview, Marcus described a poor relationship with his father, which both parents acknowledged. Marcus's father spent long hours away from home involved in the service of a social cause. He was often sarcastic in his interactions with his son, and Marcus complained to us that his father was "always mad" because, in his view, his father didn't "like . . . Mom any more." Marcus's father acknowledged that his interactional style with his children made them feel that he was ready to "draw blood," although he was not physically punitive. Marcus felt that his mother rarely got mad at him, but said that he could generally tell if she was angry by her "mad face," which made him feel "ugly and scared." At one point he asked rhetorically, "Why does everyone have to be mad?" On the Rorschach test, Marcus's sensitivity to affect was also apparent in his numerous references to fire, smoke, and volcanoes. The protocol also contained responses that shifted unpredictably between benevolent and malevolent interactions (e.g., "People playing . . . they were going to throw water on him," "Spiders . . . spitting at each other . . . they were fighting . . . no . . . they were kissing . . . that's how they kiss, if they can't kiss like us, they spit").

Marcus had a very close relationship with his mother. Since his older siblings were several years his senior, his mother had been able to spend a lot of time with him, which she greatly enjoyed. Her unplanned pregnancy with his younger sister, however, left her feeling extremely depressed, and Marcus was quite jealous of the sister's arrival in the family. Interestingly, Marcus's mother noted that he was extremely sensitive to any perceived discrimination against or criticism of boys. For example, he was very distressed by a nursery rhyme that favored girls. Lastly, Marcus had required corrective surgery at the age of 2 years for a circumcision that was done poorly at the time of his birth. The restraints and postoperative pain had been very upsetting for him. During our assessment, Marcus could not say much about his memory of this procedure, but when asked how he could tell the difference between boys and girls, he became anxious and spent a considerable amount of time looking under the couch "for something."

It was our impression that Marcus was a sensitive and anxious youngster, but that this did not interfere with his general functioning. He was clearly free of gross psychopathology. Although his mother had suffered from significant depression upon becoming pregnant when he was 2, she had functioned much better before that, which contributed to a good beginning for him. There was, however, a clear need to help Marcus with his jealous feelings, his fragility over perceived criticism, and his poor relationship with his father. Apart from the gender identity disorder, there were no DSM-III-R diagnoses.

CASE EXAMPLE 5.2

Jeremiah, a 4-year-old with an IQ of 135, was referred at the suggestion of a professional at his school. He lived with his parents, who were in a common-law relationship. His father was divorced and had three children from this earlier union, with whom he was in periodic contact. On the Hollingshead index, the family's social class ranking was a III.

On the CBCL, Jeremiah's mother identified 34 items as characteristic of his behavior; this summed to 37, which fell 6 points below the clinical cutoff. His Internalizing T score (58) was somewhat lower than his Externalizing T score (63), which was just below the clinical cutoff of 64. Jeremiah's father, however, reported very few behavioral difficulties in him—identifying only 9 items, which summed to 9.

Apart from Jeremiah's cross-gender identification, which was profound, his parents reported no other behavioral or psychological concerns. Jeremiah was described by his kindergarten teacher as having a "bubbly personality . . . obedient, mature, kind, and considerate of others." Jeremiah's mother described him as "bright, delightful." There was no evidence for any DSM-III-R diagnosis other than the gender identity disorder.

As noted above, Jeremiah's Externalizing T score on the mother's form was just below the clinical cutoff. This was of interest, since there was no clinical evidence that he was an undercontrolled youngster in the sense found in the disruptive behavior disorders. In this case, maternal characteristics seemed to loom large in accounting for this. During the assessment, it was observed how "controlling" Jeremiah's mother was. She looked at him constantly; he would "check" with her before responding to questions or offering his own spontaneous comments; and she was considerably more forceful than her common-law husband. Although the parents seemed to care about each other, they talked casually about separating because of constant quarreling. Jeremiah's mother had profound ambivalence about his cross-gender identification in the sense that she was quite unsure whether it was a problem, and she strongly reinforced his feminine behaviors (by buying him female dolls, allowing him to cross-dress, etc.). In contrast, Jeremiah's father was very worried about his gender identity development, commenting, for example, that it was inappropriate to allow him to wear dresses on the street. During an intake telephone interview, Jeremiah's mother had said that she would leave her partner if he continued questioning her about Jeremiah's cross-gender behavior. She indicated forcefully that it would not bother her in the least if Jeremiah developed a homosexual orientation. Asked how she would feel if he were to seek sex reassignment, she answered that this was fine with her as long as he was happy.

It was our clinical opinion that Jeremiah's mother had a great deal of ambivalence regarding men and masculinity, and that it was probably very difficult for her to tolerate any signs of masculinity in Jeremiah. It is therefore conceivable that his relatively high Externalizing T score reflected her low tolerance for behaviors that she may have interpreted as aggressive, with their concomitant masculine association. There was some evidence for this in Jeremiah's Rorschach protocol, which vacillated between idealized representations of females and highly aggressive, destructive ones (e.g., "wicked witches" who killed). It was also of note that on each of the three days that Jeremiah was seen, he did not want to go home with his mother, wishing to remain with the female examiners who were involved in his evaluation.

CASE EXAMPLE 5.3

Trevor, an only child who lived with his mother, was 5 years old and had an IQ of 129. He was referred because of his mother's concern about his gender identity development. His parents had separated when he was 2.5 years old. On the Hollingshead index, the family's social class ranking was a II.

On the CBCL, Trevor's mother identified 47 items as characteristic of his behavior. These items summed to 62, which was in the clinical range. Trevor's Internalizing T score (76) was substantially higher than his Externalizing T score (64), but both were in the clinical range.

Trevor was an extremely attractive, fine-featured youngster. One of the subjects in our study of physical attractiveness (described in Chapter 6), he had higher attractiveness ratings than any other subject. He was described by his mother as extremely precocious, particularly with regard to verbal skills.

In addition to possessing a marked cross-gender identification, Trevor was an anxious youngster, and was prone to become quite absorbed in fantasy that was not always easy to understand. He occasionally used a security blanket to which he had become attached as an infant. During the initial assessment, his mother had a great deal of difficulty in separating from him; in contrast, he seemed to ignore his mother. During his individual interview, Trevor was very anxious and nervous and engaged in arm flapping. He completed a very complicated puzzle, but showed no pleasure in his success.

The family history indicated that Trevor's father had never been invested in his care. Trevor's parents had long been estranged; according to his mother, his father used alcohol excessively and was erratic in his occupational functioning. Trevor's mother had been quite depressed for much of his infancy and early childhood, although she was able to function successfully in her work. In addition to dysthymia, Trevor's mother had borderline personality traits, particularly with regard to affects and interpersonal relations. She did not, however, have a history of impulsive behavior.

Trevor was assessed prior to the publication of the DSM-III. Apart from the gender identity disorder diagnosis, he was given the DSM-II diagnosis of overanxious reaction of childhood.

Case Vignettes of 6- to 11-Year-Old Boys

CASE EXAMPLE 5.4

Carl was 6 years old with an IQ of 114. He was referred by the family physician because of parental concern about his gender identity development. He lived with both of his parents and a younger brother. On the Hollingshead index, the family's social class ranking was a III.

On the CBCL, Carl's mother identified 20 items as characteristic of his behavior, which summed to 23, well below the clinical cutoff. The Internalizing T score (59) was substantially higher than the Externalizing T score (46). The number and sum of items reported by the father were quite similar to the maternal ratings. Despite the low total sum score, the Schizoid–Anxious narrow-band score on the mother's form fell just below the clinical cutoff, and the Uncommunicative narrow-band score was in the clinical range. The narrow-band scales on the paternal form were, however, all within the normal range.

Apart from his marked cross-gender identification, Carl's parents reported only one other behavioral concern—enuresis, which occurred both during the day and at night. He did well at school and showed no overt signs of separation anxiety; however, he had a transitional object, a teddy bear, with which he still slept at night. His parents felt that he was quite shy, very different from his brother, whom they described as aggressive and difficult to manage. His brother also suffered from a major articulation disorder, although his IQ was in the high-average range.

Carl's parents reported several marital problems. His father felt that his wife was "domineering," which he resented and dealt with by avoidance (e.g., walking out of the house during conflicts). In turn, Carl's mother reported that she held things in and was angry at her husband when he walked out. She complained that men had it easier than women. Despite acknowledging these difficulties in their marriage, Carl's parents denied chronic, overt marital discord.

The CBCL profile of an internalizing youngster was consistent with observations we made during the clinical interview. Carl was quite inhibited and had trouble answering questions and remaining focused. He interpreted as real fighting what his parents had described as "play fighting." He indicated that in his view his mother was "always" the boss. He also indicated being worried when his father spanked his brother. When asked to make up a story, it was about "people looking for their mothers."

It was our impression that Carl was a temperamentally inhibited youngster, upset by his perception of parental quarreling. We speculated that he was sensitive to his mother's professed resentment toward men, and worried by his father's anger and disciplinary style with his brother. His enuresis seemed in part related to his anxious state. A DSM-III diagnosis of enuresis was given, and we queried whether he also met the criteria for overanxious disorder.

CASE EXAMPLE 5.5

Charles was 8 years old with an IQ of 106. He was referred at the suggestion of a friend of his mother, who had been an employee at the Clarke Institute and knew about our clinic. He lived with both of his parents and a younger sibling. On the Hollingshead index, the family's social class ranking was a III.

On the CBCL, Charles's mother identified 40 items as characteristic of his behavior, which summed to 51 and fell in the clinical range. The Internalizing T score (71) was in the clinical range and was substantially higher than the Externalizing T score (58). The ratings provided by the father, however, contrasted sharply with those provided by the mother: He identified only 23 items as characteristic of Charles's behavior; these summed to 23, which was well below the clinical cutoff. Both the Internalizing T score (57) and the Externalizing T score (53) were below the clinical cutoff.

The maternal CBCL profile of a markedly internalizing youngster was very consistent with clinical observation. In our view, the paternal profile seemed to underestimate the difficulties that Charles was experiencing. This seemed related to the father's general style during the assessment, which was to minimize any concerns about Charles in particular or the family in general.

During the initial assessment with the family, Charles spent the first 45 minutes of the interview sitting on the arm of his mother's chair, on her lap, or behind her. He seemed to have a strong need to be in close proximity to his mother, and several members of our team commented that his behavior was reminiscent of Harlow's classic photographs of frightened rhesus macaques.

Apart from his cross-gender identification, Charles's mother commented during an initial intake telephone interview that he was "very insecure." There was a 2-year history of encopresis, and Charles talked about "hating school" because of peer teasing. He also worried that if he attended school, he might "miss something" at home and someone might come there and hurt his mother. He did not like to be separated from her and worried that she might die if she went away on a trip. On the way home after the initial interview, Charles said to his mother that he was "holding a lot of things in" that he had never told anyone, including fear of his stuffed animals and of his closet door when it was ajar. He also said to his mother that he thought the assessment had to do with his parents' wanting him to be "sent away." This seemed related to his literal interpretation of comments his mother would make to him when she became frustrated with his behavior: "Maybe go live with someone else. . . . We'll let someone who doesn't have anything come and live in your room."

Charles was felt to be anxious and withdrawn during psychological testing. His fingernails were noted to be extensively bitten. His eye contact with the female examiner was poor. On the Rorschach, he provided only 11 responses, which was consistent with his constricted psychological state.

The DSM-III-R diagnoses were functional encopresis (secondary type) and separation anxiety disorder.

CASE EXAMPLE 5.6

John was 11 years old with an IQ of 107. He was referred at the suggestion of a maternal aunt, whom school authorities concerned about him had apparently contacted. John lived with his mother and her parents. His father (a distant maternal cousin) and mother had separated before he was 2, and he had not seen his father since then. His mother believed that his father lived on the street and suffered from a chronic psychiatric disorder, possibly schizophrenia. On the Hollingshead index, the family's social class ranking was a IV.

On the CBCL, John's mother identified 74 items as characteristic of his behavior; these summed to 126, well within the clinical range. The Internalizing T score (81) and Externalizing T score (84) were both in the clinical range.

Apart from his cross-gender identification, John had shown long-standing difficulties in his social and emotional development. About a year prior to the assessment, the family decided to have him live with his maternal aunt, who felt that she might be able to handle his difficulties better than the mother did. He had never been able to establish friendships with children his age. He often played with his cousins, who were substantially younger, and he delighted in being extremely bossy and dictatorial with them. His aunt stated that he "lived in a world of his own" and that on occasion he would laugh for no apparent reason, which scared her. His school functioning was poor, possibly complicated by the fact that English was his second language. He was socially withdrawn and immature, often spending hours watching cartoons on television. He was preoccupied with religion, which provided him with some comfort. He had engaged in compulsive handwashing for several years and was very concerned about dirt. When his mother talked about this during the assessment, he became very anxious and politely asked for permission to leave the room so that he could wash his hands, stating that he was feeling "uncomfortable." His mother also appeared to have obsessional concerns about cleanliness, although at the time of the assessment it was unclear whether she met formal diagnostic criteria. John's DSM-III diagnoses were schizoid disorder of childhood and obsessive–compulsive disorder.

CBCL DATA ON GIRLS WITH GENDER IDENTITY DISORDER

Parent-Report Data

To date, the empirical literature has provided virtually no systematic data on possible associated psychopathology in girls with gender identity disorder. Table 5.7 presents maternal-report data for 24 gender-referred girls and 76 female siblings (of both our female and male probands) for the same five CBCL indices of disturbance described earlier for boys. On all five indices, the gender-referred girls had significantly higher levels of behavioral disturbance (p's ranged from $< .006$ to .025). For the two groups of girls, the Internalizing T and Externalizing T scores did not differ significantly from each other.

Table 5.8 presents the CBCL data as a function of two age groupings, 4–5 and 6–11 years. The girls aged 4–5 with gender identity disorder had substantially lower disturbance ratings than did their counterparts aged 6–11, whereas the female siblings in the two age groupings did not. In the group aged 4–5, the girls with gender identity disorder did not differ significantly from the female siblings on any of the disturbance indices. By contrast, in the group aged 6–11, the girls with gender identity disorder had significantly higher levels of disturbance than the female siblings on four of the five indices with social class covaried (all p's $< .05$).

Of the 8 girls aged 4–5 with gender identity disorder, only 1 (12.5%) had a total Behavior Problem score in the clinical range, compared to 4 (17.4%) of 23 female siblings—a nonsignificant difference. In contrast, 11 (68.8%) of the 16 girls aged 6–11 with gender identity disorder had scores in the clinical range, compared to 17 (32.1%) of 53 female siblings, $\chi^2 = 5.43$, $p < .02$. Thus, the older girls with gender

TABLE 5.7. Maternal Ratings of Behavioral Disturbance on the CBCL for Girls with Gender Identity Disorder and Female Siblings

Measures	Gender identity disorder (*n* = 24)		Siblings (*n* = 76)	
	M	*SD*	*M*	*SD*
No. elevated narrow-band scales	2.2	2.7	0.9	1.7
Number of items	35.3	19.1	25.2	16.1
Sum of items	46.0	30.1	30.8	22.5
Internalizing *T*	61.3	11.2	55.1	11.5
Externalizing *T*	60.2	13.7	53.6	11.5
Age (in years)	7.6	2.7	7.8	2.8
IQ	109.4[a]	22.4	99.6[b]	19.7
Social class	38.1	17.4	42.9	16.0
Marital status				
Both parents	16 (*n*)		53 (*n*)	
Mother only/reconstituted	8 (*n*)		23 (*n*)	

Note. For one proband and her two sisters, the mother did not read English, so she could not complete the CBCL. The father could read English, so his data were used. CBCL data for two other probands were not available.

[a]*n* = 23.

[b]*n* = 17. In our research, we assessed systematically the IQ of siblings from the first 36 families evaluated; after that, sibling IQs were obtained only if there was a particular research issue of interest or if it was clinically indicated.

identity disorder were more than five times as likely as their 4- to 5-year-old counterparts to have a CBCL sum score in the clinical range.

For the girls aged 4–5 with gender identity disorder, the Internalizing *T* score tended to be significantly higher than the Externalizing *T* score, $t(7) = 2.24$, $p = .06$, but the two broad-band factors did not differ significantly among the girls aged 6–11. For the female siblings in both age groupings, the Internalizing and Externalizing *T* scores did not differ significantly.

On the CBCL narrow-band scales (Figure 5.2), there were no significant differences between the girls aged 4–5 with gender identity disorder and the female siblings. The girls aged 6–11 with gender identity disorder had significantly higher *T* scores than the female siblings on four of the nine narrow-band scales: Schizoid–Obsessive, Hyperactive, Delinquent, and Cruel (*p*'s ranged from < .003 to .05).

Table 5.8 also shows the CBCL data for girls from the standardization sample. In the group aged 4–5, the girls with gender identity disorder had scores closely comparable to those of the nonreferred sample.

TABLE 5.8. Maternal Ratings of Behavioral Disturbance on the CBCL for Girls with Gender Identity Disorder, Female Siblings, and the Standardization Sample

	4–5 years							
	Gender identity disorder ($n = 8$)		Siblings ($n = 23$)		Nonreferred ($n = 100$)		Referred ($n = 100$)	
Measures	M	SD	M	SD	M	SD	M	SD
No. elevated narrow-band scales	0.1	0.4	0.4	0.9	—	—	—	—
Number of items	24.6	13.4	23.9	14.8	—	—	—	—
Sum of items	27.9	14.9	30.1	21.9	25.2	17.1	58.8	29.1
Internalizing T	54.6	10.7	50.4	11.3	50.8	10.5	66.5	11.3
Externalizing T	48.5	7.5	47.5	9.7	49.8	8.7	61.5	12.8
Age (in years)	4.8	1.0	4.3	1.1	—	—	—	—
IQ	116.8	19.8	97.4[a]	15.6	—	—	—	—
Social class	46.3	12.8	38.5	17.5	—	—	—	—
Marital status								
Both parents	7 (n)		15 (n)		—		—	
Mother only/ reconstituted	1 (n)		8 (n)		—		—	

	6–11 years							
	Gender identity disorder ($n = 16$)		Siblings ($n = 53$)		Nonreferred ($n = 300$)		Referred ($n = 300$)	
Measures	M	SD	M	SD	M	SD	M	SD
No. elevated narrow-band scales	3.3	2.8	1.1	1.9	—	—	—	—
Number of items	40.6	19.6	25.8	16.8	—	—	—	—
Sum of items	55.1	33.1	31.1	23.0	19.9	14.2	58.4	26.2
Internalizing T	64.7	10.2	57.1	11.0	51.3	9.1	67.0	9.1
Externalizing T	66.1	12.3	56.3	11.3	51.0	9.4	68.1	9.5
Age (in years)	9.0	2.2	9.3	1.8	—	—	—	—
IQ	105.5[b]	23.4	100.6[c]	21.7	—	—	—	—
Social class	34.0	18.3	44.8	15.1	—	—	—	—
Marital status								
Both parents	9 (n)		38 (n)		—		—	
Mother only/ reconstituted	7 (n)		15 (n)		—		—	

Note. Data for the nonreferred and referred samples from Achenbach and Edelbrock (1983, Appendix D, pp. 213–214).
[a]$n = 5$. [b]$n = 15$. [c]$n = 12$.

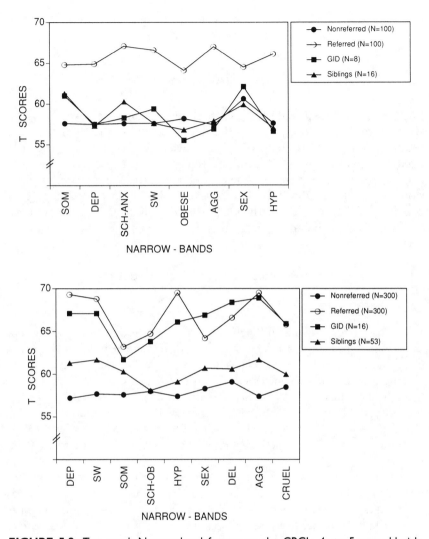

FIGURE 5.2. Top panel: Narrow-band factors on the CBCL, 4- to 5-year-old girls. SOM, Somatic Complaints; DEP, Depressed; SCH-ANX, Schizoid or Anxious; SW, Social Withdrawal; OBESE, Obese; AGG, Aggressive; SEX, Sex Problems; HYP, Hyperactive. Bottom panel: Narrow-band factors on the CBCL, 6- to 11-year-old girls. DEP, Depressed; SW, Social Withdrawal; SOM, Somatic Complaints; SCH-OB, Schizoid–Obsessive; HYP, Hyperactive; SEX, Sex Problems; DEL, Delinquent; AGG, Aggressive; CRUEL, Cruel. GID, gender identity disorder. Nonreferred and referred group data are from the standardization study (Achenbach & Edelbrock, 1983, Appendix D).

In contrast, the girls aged 6–11 with gender identity disorder had scores closely comparable to those of the referred sample.

Summary

In general, the CBCL data for girls parallel the data for boys. The girls were more disturbed than were the female siblings, although this was found only for the group aged 6–11. As was true for the boys, the girls aged 6–11 were comparable to the referred group, whereas the girls aged 4–5 were comparable to the nonreferred group in the standardization sample (Achenbach & Edelbrock, 1983). Below we attempt to provide a richer account of the CBCL data by discussing representative profiles along with clinical data taken from the psychiatric assessment.

Case Vignettes of 4- to 5-Year-Old Girls

CASE EXAMPLE 5.7

Erika was 5 years old with an IQ of 109. Her parents sought an assessment because of their concern about her gender identity development. She was an only child who lived with her parents and her paternal grandparents. On the Hollingshead index, the family's social class ranking was a I.

On the CBCL, Erika's mother identified 9 items as characteristic of her behavior, which summed to 10, well below the clinical cutoff. Both the Internalizing T score (39) and the Externalizing T score (41) were also well below the clinical range. The father's report on the CBCL was consistent with the mother's.

Apart from Erika's marked cross-gender identification, her parents reported no behavioral or emotional concerns. Regarding her gender identity development, they were particularly concerned about her preoccupation with aggressive fantasy. In her overt behavior, however, she was not at all aggressive, unlike youngsters with the disruptive behavior disorders.

The absence of parent-reported psychopathology on the CBCL contrasted strikingly with aspects of Erika's behavior during an individual clinical interview and with her responses on the Rorschach test. In the clinical interview, Erika was clearly preoccupied with aggressive fantasy. She was also very controlling in her interactions with the female interviewer. She talked at great length and often seemed to diverge considerably from the questions posed to her. It appeared to us that her need to control the interviewer reflected her underlying anxiety. Her Rorschach protocol was extremely disorganized and poorly modulated. It was one of the more disturbed protocols that we have encountered. On Card II, for example, Erika's free associations were as follows:

"Eeeps. How did she . . . Oh, this is a church . . . and this is a fire explod-ing and this is a man, he used to be alive, he exploded. And the church ex-ploded. [The examiner then noted that he could not follow Erika's next verbalizations because of the rapidity of her speech. Erika then inverted the card.] I think *you* had it the wrong way. Oh, it's half a bat and half a man. Oh, how long have we been in here? Are we going to have lunch soon? If you show me the next blot . . . Okay, let's get on with the show [said impatiently]."

The inquiry for Card II yielded further evidence of Erika's disorganization and internal agitation.

"[*What made it look like a church?*] Oh, let me show you the card again. Maybe *you* don't understand. Oh, maybe I don't want the church. This is not really the church, I don't want it to be a church. It's E Jickle. You can explode electricity. Oh, man and woman. [The examiner noted that Erika was 'rambling' at this point and that he could not keep up with her ver-balizations.] Oh, we're just making this up, just pretend. This is a big hole. You know when you make a big hole [points to DS5]. I can't keep it in my mind. I can't focus it. Sometimes E Jickle . . . sometimes E Power electric spreads all over the place and you can't see it. Sometimes . . . when you have a blackout. It won't hurt anybody. That's all I know. Next. [*Erika, I'd like you to go back to the church that you said you saw. What made it look like a church to you?*] I can't focus it in my mind with-out the card. Oh, here's the steeple. . . . Do you see all this . . . the black? Well, it can be exploding. And this man, he was near it. And here are his eyes, his nose, and his mouth. [*They were all blown up?*] Yep. The man's eyes . . . somebody found his eyeballs. And this is not true. This is pre-tend. Somebody found his eyes and took them to the doctor and the doc-tor ran away. . . . He was so scared. That's all I can tell you about that picture, okay? Okay? Okay? [*What made it seem like a church explod-ed?*] That's one thing I really don't know 'cause I forgot what I said. [*You said before that the black made it look like it exploded.*] Here are the two men running away from . . . can't you see that they are running? [Erika began to swing a small brass bell on a string that she was wearing around her neck. She said, 'I can tell you whether I'm going to have a baby boy or a baby girl. See? If the bell swings like this (laterally), it's going to be a baby girl. If it swings like this (in a circle), that means a boy.' Erika then pretended to hypnotize the examiner with the bell.]"

From an interpretive point of view, Erika's need to emphasize that her Rorschach responses were "just pretend" can be understood as an attempt to gain some control over what seemed to be a frightening experience for her. Prognostically, one could argue that this was also a favorable sign, in that there was some capacity to distance herself from very primitive feelings.

The family history provided some clues to understanding Erika's internal anxiety and need to control. Several months after Erika's birth, her mother had awakened on her own birthday physically paralyzed. She was taken to the hospital and diagnosed as suffering from postpartum depression. In the hospital, she was treated pharmacologically and with electroconvulsive therapy. Since that time, she had been in treatment with a psychiatrist whose approach was almost exclusively pharmacological. At the time of our assessment, Erika's mother informed us that she was feeling better. Over time, we learned much more about her psychological state and history. Her mother had died when she was 12, and she subsequently became the victim of an incestuous relationship with her father, which continued through his second marriage up until the time she left home in her late adolescence. She seemed to suffer from an empty depression and marked dependency, and she had the features of borderline personality disorder with the exception of overt anger and rage. Erika's father was a very quiet man with an obsessional character structure. He was chronically dissatisfied with his life. Erika's mother felt that he viewed fatherhood as an interference with his life goals and that he took this "resentment" out on his daughter. The course of our clinical involvement in this case never confirmed this perception, although it is likely that Erika experienced his "broodiness" as a source of threat.

The extended paternal family also revealed clues about Erika's development. A paternal sister was markedly gender-dysphoric, to the point that she had once sought sex reassignment. She was refused on the grounds that she was "really" a lesbian. The sister's gender dysphoria and sexual orientation were a source of great embarrassment and shame to her family and were never discussed. (Although we never met Erika's aunt, she was apparently very supportive of the therapeutic process, and on one occasion she referred a friend to us for an assessment.) Erika's paternal grandparents played a strong role in her early development. As noted earlier, Erika's family lived with these grandparents, and they had done a lot of the caregiving during the mother's depression. Erika's parents felt that the grandmother was chronically depressed and disliked women. She had made a suicide attempt at the time of Erika's birth, which was never discussed. Erika's parents also felt that the grandparents were extremely competitive and aggressive with Erika, and they believed that this contributed to her cross-gender identification.

CASE EXAMPLE 5.8

Nancy was 4 years old with an IQ of 143. She was referred by the family physician because of parental concern about her gender identity development. She lived with her parents and a younger brother. On the Hollingshead index, the family's social class ranking was a III.

On the CBCL, Nancy's mother identified 36 items as characteristic of her behavior. These summed to 39, which was 4 points below the clinical cutoff. The Internalizing T score (62) fell just below the clinical cutoff and was higher than the Externalizing T score (58). The number and sum of items identified by the father were quite similar to the mother's ratings.

Apart from Nancy's marked cross-gender identification, her parents did not report major concerns about her current behavioral or emotional development.

Despite the relatively stable nature of the family at the time of assessment, the clinical history revealed that the first 2 years of Nancy's life had in fact been difficult. The parents described their situation then as having been very unhappy and stressful. At that time they lived in the country, and Nancy's mother felt very isolated. She described Nancy as having been a colicky baby who did not like to be held. She said that Nancy had been a "very serious" infant "who never smiled until age 2." She recalled feeling very "disappointed" and "rejected" because Nancy was not a cuddly baby and seemed unresponsive to her efforts at soothing. Despite Nancy's lack of positive response to her mother, she showed marked stranger anxiety and separation anxiety, crying without a pause during brief separations. This created tension with the extended family, which included many paternal aunts who blamed the parents because they were living "way out in the middle of nowhere." Nancy's mother described herself as "having been terrible, very depressed" during this 2-year period. She experienced her husband as uncommunicative; she felt that her problems with Nancy were resulting in part from her own deficiencies; and living in the country made her feel trapped. She decided to return to work part-time when Nancy was 6 months old because of the difficulties she was experiencing, particularly in her parenting role.

During our assessment, Nancy spent almost all of her time with her mother and had little contact with or regard for her father. The parents recalled that between the ages of 12 and 18 months Nancy had been very "antagonistic" to her father, which he found frustrating. They described the situation as having been intolerable, to the point that Nancy and her father "couldn't look at each other." Nancy's father said, "I have a personality in which I need to be liked," and he commented with some regret that he had probably exacerbated the situation by becoming "childish" and retaliatory with Nancy. Interestingly, when Nancy was about 2, she was cared for on a part-time basis by a relative who had two older sons. Her parents felt that she liked to be with these boys, who, however, would "antagonize and razz" her. Nancy seemed to have experienced this as a rejection. In general, Nancy's mother described her as extremely "sensitive" and as "crumbling" to peer pressure.

At 2.5 years of age, Nancy was enrolled in nursery school, but she was so separation-anxious that her mother withdrew her. Her parents felt that even up to the present, she had great difficulty separating from her mother. This was observed when we attempted to interview her individually. She was quite upset, crying and clinging to her mother's leg. She agreed to being seen only if her brother could remain with her in the room. Once separated, however, she was able to relax and talk openly about her feelings with the female examiner. By the end of the interview, she said that she liked the female interviewer "better" than her mother and that she did not wish to leave the room to be reunited with her parents.

In our conceptualization of Nancy's early history, it seemed to us that although her parents were free of gross psychiatric disorder, the first 2 years of her life had in fact been compromised by several factors. First, Nancy's connectedness to her mother was adversely affected by her difficult temperament (fussy, hard to soothe, etc.), and this problem was exacerbated by the mother's view that her difficulties in interchanges with her daughter stemmed from her own failings. Second, Nancy's relationship with her father also seemed to become quite conflictual when he began to perceive her as rejecting him. It was our impression that Nancy's self-confidence was shaky by the time she was 2 years of age, and that this may have contributed to her great difficulty in adapting to nursery school and to her strong reaction to exclusion by the two sons at the home where she was being cared for. It was at about this time that Nancy began to manifest signs of cross-gender identification. In our clinical interview with her, one aspect of her fantasy play concerned a boy who protected the "scared king and queen" from a dragon by fighting him off with his sword. In that fantasy, the boy felt no fear.

Apart from the gender identity disorder, there were no DSM-III-R diagnoses, although it was noted that Nancy was subthreshold for separation anxiety disorder.

Case Vignettes of 6- to 11-Year-Old Girls

CASE EXAMPLE 5.9

Eva was 6 years old and lived with a younger sibling and her parents. The referral was initiated by her mother, who had been episodically concerned about her gender identity development. On the Hollingshead index, the family's social class ranking was a I.

On the CBCL, Eva's mother identified 38 items as characteristic of her behavior, which summed to 38. This fell somewhat below the clinical range; however, the Internalizing T score (67) was in the clinical range and was somewhat higher than the Externalizing T score (60).

The CBCL profile of an internalizing youngster was consistent with clinical observation. Eva was described by her mother as "sensitive" and "quick to tears." Eva's mother also felt that she had low self-esteem and was very sensitive to comments made by other children. On school days, she tended to be clingy and tearful, and was avoidant in new situations where she might be singled out. There had been a 3-month wait before Eva could be seen. During this time, there had been several extensive telephone discussions with her mother. In these conversations, her mother made no mention of what proved to be a severe marital crisis: Eva's parents had separated briefly because of an event involving her father. In the course of the assessment, Eva's father blocked every effort to explore the marital relationship and commented bluntly that it had no bearing on his daughter's development. He seemed to minimize the extent of Eva's gender dysphoria and refused to return after the initial visit. However, Eva's mother continued to attend the assessment sessions, although she would not permit Eva to be seen for psychological testing. During the initial interview, Eva fought back tears when the interviewer gently commented on the parents' "separation."

Because the parents were reluctant to let us assess Eva comprehensively, only a provisional DSM-III-R diagnosis of adjustment disorder with depressed mood was given.

CASE EXAMPLE 5.10

Sammy was 8 years old with an IQ of 94. At the time of the assessment, she lived in a residential treatment setting. On the Hollingshead index, her social class background was a V.

On the CBCL, Sammy's child care worker identified 84 items as characteristic of her behavior, which summed to 141, well within the clinical range. Both the Internalizing *T* score (79) and the Externalizing *T* score (89) were also well within the clinical range.

Apart from her marked cross-gender identification, Sammy manifested pervasive socioemotional disturbance. Her life had been characterized by extreme instability. Her mother had come from a very disturbed family and had spent many years under the care of child welfare authorities. At the time of Sammy's birth, she had been an amphetamine addict, a heavy user of barbiturates, and a prostitute. Sammy's father was her mother's pimp; her parents never lived together. When Sammy was 2, the mother felt unable to cope with parenting and turned her child's care over to the father. After this, the father would demand sex from the mother before allowing her to see Sammy. When living with her father, Sammy was surrounded by older half-brothers from his previous liaisons and, according to reports from other agencies, was subjected to severe physical abuse. On numerous occasions, she also saw her father physically abuse her mother. When she was 5, she was in her father's apartment when his current partner shot him in the face with a revolver. She was then taken into care. At the time of our assessment, Sammy was in terror that her father might find her and take her away again, and she ruminated about finding a gun and a penis so that she could protect herself and her mother.

The DSM-III-R diagnoses were functional enuresis (nocturnal), oppositional defiant disorder, and overanxious disorder. A reactive attachment disorder was also queried. Sammy showed profound impairment in her personality functioning, which suggested a serious risk for later character pathology.

OTHER MEASURES OF ASSOCIATED PSYCHOPATHOLOGY

Social Competence

The CBCL also contains a section on social competence, which assesses functioning in three areas: Activities (amount and quality of the child's participation in sports, hobbies, and games, and jobs and chores), Social (membership and participation in organizations, number of friends and contacts with them, and behavior with others and alone), and

School (performance in academic subjects, placement in a special class, grade failure, and problems in the school setting). There is also a total Social Competence score. Achenbach and Edelbrock (1981, p. 60) reported that the four social competence T scores correlated only modestly with CBCL behavioral psychopathology, so that to some extent they constituted independent measures of child functioning.

The top portion of Table 5.9 presents our social competence data for gender-referred boys, male siblings, clinical control boys, and normal control boys. The clinical and normal control boys were participants in several research studies conducted in our clinic, as noted earlier. On all four scales, the normal controls were significantly younger than the other three groups, who did not differ from one another (the age difference existed mainly because some of the normal boys were part of a study that called for children to be 3–6 years of age). For the School T score, there were also group differences in parents' social class and marital status; accordingly, these variables were covaried as appropriate.

One-way analyses of variance showed that the normal controls had higher social competence ratings on all four scales than the other three groups, with $p < .05$ for two scales and $p < .10$ for the other two (Table 5.9).

Social competence data were also available for the girls with gender identity disorder and the female siblings. Regarding demographic variables, the two groups differed in social class only with regard to the School scale, so it was covaried (fewer girls had School T scores, since it is not computed for children under the age of 6 years). The girls with gender identity disorder had significantly lower social competence scores than the female siblings on two of the scales: Social ($p < .02$) and the total score ($p < .03$) (see the bottom portion of Table 5.9).

Projective Testing

Several researchers have utilized the Rorschach test to assess aspects of ego functioning, including object relations and thought disturbance, in boys with gender identity disorder (e.g., Goddard, 1986; Goddard & Tuber, 1989; Ipp, 1986; Kolers, 1986; Tuber & Coates, 1985, 1989). As might be apparent, these studies have been guided by ideas derived from psychoanalytic theory about personality development. On different scales for measuring Rorschach responses, boys with gender identity disorder have, on average, shown more impairment than normal controls (Goddard & Tuber, 1989; Ipp, 1986; Kolers, 1986; Tuber & Coates, 1989). However, both Ipp (1986) and Kolers (1986) found that

TABLE 5.9. Maternal Ratings of Social Competence on the CBCL

	Boys					
Measures	Gender identity disorder	Siblings	Clinical controls	Normal controls	F	p^a
Activities T						
M	48.3	48.5	48.1	51.5	2.6	.055
SD	8.5	7.2	8.9	5.5		
n	156	85	45	56		
Social T						
M	42.0	45.5	43.8	44.0	2.2	.085
SD	10.8	9.9	10.1	11.2		
n	156	85	45	56		
School T						
M	44.0	45.1	41.1	52.1	4.6	.004
SD	10.0	10.1	10.5	5.9		
n	93	59	27	31		
Total T						
M	44.8	46.7	45.9	51.3	3.7	.012
SD	11.2	11.4	13.7	11.4		
n	155	85	45	56		

	Girls			
Measures	Gender identity disorder	Siblings	t	p
Activities T				
M	48.0	49.2	<1	n.s.
SD	7.0	7.1		
n	24	67		
Social T				
M	39.6	45.0	2.4	.017
SD	9.7	9.2		
n	24	67		
School T				
M	41.5	47.4	1.5	.130[b]
SD	13.6	8.6		
n	16	52		
Total T				
M	42.1	47.4	2.3	.022
SD	8.6	9.8		
n	24	67		

[a]For the Activities T score, Duncan's multiple-comparison procedure showed that the normal controls (NC) had a significantly higher score than the boys with gender identity disorder (GID), the siblings, and the clinical controls (CC); all p's < .05. For the Social T score, there were no significant differences at $p < .05$. For the School T score, NC > GID = siblings = CC at $p < .05$. For the Total T score, NC > GID = siblings = CC at $p < .05$.
[b]With social class covaried.

the siblings of the gender-referred boys were equally impaired, and Goddard and Tuber (1989) found that gender-referred boys with a diagnosis of separation anxiety disorder were, by and large, no more disturbed than clinic-referred boys with that diagnosis.

As with the CBCL data on general behavior problems, boys with gender identity disorder appear as disturbed as clinical controls but more disturbed than normal controls. In contrast to the CBCL data, proband–sibling differences were not found by Ipp (1986) and Kolers (1986)—a discrepancy that can be resolved only by further empirical work. Unfortunately, the studies conducted to date have not examined correlations between the Rorschach test and other measures of impairment, such as data available from the CBCL and TRF. But, like the CBCL data, the projective findings suggest that with regard to general psychopathology, boys with gender identity disorder are more similar to than different from clinical control boys.

ON THE RELATION BETWEEN ASSOCIATED PSYCHOPATHOLOGY AND GENDER IDENTITY DISORDER

Although some might construe our focus on parent-report data on behavior problems as a relatively narrow, even superficial, approach to assessment of psychopathology, it is our view that the CBCL data give preliminary support to previous clinical observations that gender identity disorder in both boys and girls is, on average, associated with other behavioral difficulties. It must be asked, then, what connection (if any) these difficulties have with the gender identity disorder itself. As proposed elsewhere (Zucker & Green, 1992), three models have been considered to account for the association. Because these models were developed primarily with boys in mind, we restrict the discussion accordingly.

The first model holds that the child's marked cross-gender behavior is the target of social ostracism (particularly by peers), and that this is the mechanism leading to the display of general psychopathology (Rekers, 1977b; cf. Green, 1974; Green et al., 1980).

The second model implicates the role of parental influences, such as psychiatric disorder, erratic child-rearing practices, and marital discord, in the child's gender development. In general, this view considers the genesis of the gender identity disorder in the context of more global problems in the child's development and familial psychopathology (e.g., Bates et al., 1974; Chiland, 1988). Coates (1985, 1990, 1992) and her colleagues (e.g., Coates et al., 1991; Coates & Person, 1985; Coates & Wolfe, 1995; Marantz & Coates, 1991; Rainbow, 1986; Sherman, 1985), who have discussed this view in some detail, have advanced a specific hypothesis—namely, that separation anxiety (which is activated by uneven maternal availability) plays a pivotal role in the development of gender identity disorder in boys. According to Coates and Person (1985), severe separation anxiety precedes the feminine behavior of the boys, which emerges in order "to restore a fantasy tie to the physically or emotionally absent mother. In imitating 'Mommy' [the boy] confuse[s] 'being Mommy' with 'having Mommy.' [Cross-gender behavior] appears to allay, in part, the anxiety generated by the loss of the mother" (p. 708).

The last model suggests that parental influences play a role in both the general psychopathology and the gender identity disorder, but that different aspects of parental behavior are involved. In this view, the relation between parental influences and general psychopathology in boys with gender identity disorder could be explained, for example, by aspects of parental functioning that are diagnostically nonspecific, such as marital discord and psychiatric disorder. Other parental variables, such as reinforcement or tolerance of feminine behavior and atypical psychosexual parental traits, which may be diagnostically specific (cf. Green, 1987), lead directly to the gender identity disorder; the disorder, in turn, is associated with general psychopathology through the mechanism of social ostracism.

Although this last model suggests that gender identity disorder and general psychopathology may be influenced by distinct parental influences, it could also be argued that these two facets of parental influence may be related. For example, parents with extensive marital discord or personality disorder may be less mobilized psychologically to intervene in their child's cross-gender behavior, which increases the likelihood of subsequent exposure to social ostracism.

These three models may be summarized as follows:

1. Gender identity disorder→general psychopathology.
2. Parental influences→general psychopathology→gender identity disorder.
3. Parental influences→general psychopathology.
   Parental influences→gender identity disorder→general psychopathology.

Below, we review the limited empirical data thus far available as a basis for evaluating these models.

Model I

We have provided some evidence that supports the first model (Zucker, 1990b). It was hypothesized that extent of general psychopathology would be correlated with age, since social ostracism would be expected to exert a stronger effect over time. Using the five CBCL indices of behavioral disturbance (see above), we found that age was in fact significantly correlated with degree of CBCL psychopathology in our sample of 161 gender-referred boys (r's ranged from .28 to .42, all p's < .001).

The age of the boys was also significantly correlated with three other demographic variables (IQ and parents' social class and marital status), in that younger boys were brighter, more likely to be from a higher social class background, and more likely to be living with both of their parents. In turn, these three demographic variables were also significantly correlated with CBCL psychopathology (absolute r's ranged from .21 to .43) and with one another. The simple correlations indicated that children with lower IQ, whose parents were of lower socioeconomic status, and who came from "nonintact" or reconstituted families (i.e., their parents were separated, divorced, or remarried, or the boys had been adopted in childhood) had more CBCL psychopathology.

To test whether age contributed unique variance to CBCL psychopathology, we performed multiple-regression analyses with the four demographics as predictor variables and with the CBCL indices as criterion variables. For all five CBCL indices, age and parents' social class and/or marital status contributed unique variance (Table 5.10).

The age effect was examined further by dividing the gender-referred boys as a function of two CBCL age groupings, 4–5 years and 6–11 years. Table 5.3 shows the CBCL disturbance indices, and Figure 5.1 shows the CBCL narrow-band subscales as a function of age grouping. It can be seen that the boys aged 4–5 with gender identity disorder were closely comparable to the nonreferred boys from the standardization sample, but not to the referred boys. In contrast, the boys aged 6–11 with gender identity disorder were closely comparable to the referred boys but not to the nonreferred boys, particularly for the Internalizing narrow-band scales. A very similar pattern was observed when we analyzed our TRF data (Figure 5.3).

In another set of analyses (following Zucker, 1990b), the relation between age and CBCL psychopathology was examined as a function of whether or not the boys met the complete DSM-III criteria for gender identity disorder. Age was more strongly correlated with CBCL psychopathology in the subgroup of boys (n = 90) who met the complete criteria (mean age = 5.9 years; r's ranged from .40 to .50) than in the

TABLE 5.10. Demographic Predictors of CBCL Psychopathology in Boys with Gender Identity Disorder (*n* = 161)

Criterion measures	Significant predictor variables[a]
No. elevated narrow-band scales	Step 1: Marital status (R^2 = .19) Step 2: Age ($R^2\Delta$ = .09)
Number of items	Step 1: Social class (R^2 = .14) Step 2: Marital status ($R^2\Delta$ = .03) Step 3: Age ($R^2\Delta$ = .02)
Sum of items	Step 1: Social class (R^2 = .15) Step 2: Age ($R^2\Delta$ = .05) Step 3: Marital status ($R^2\Delta$ = .03)
Internalizing *T*	Step 1: Social class (R^2 = .09) Step 2: Age ($R^2\Delta$ = .03)
Externalizing *T*	Step 1: Social class (R^2 = .13) Step 2: Age ($R^2\Delta$ = .03) Step 3: Marital status ($R^2\Delta$ = .02)

Note. The four demographic variables entered were age, IQ, parents' social class, and parents' marital status.
[a]*p*'s ranged from < .05 to < .001.

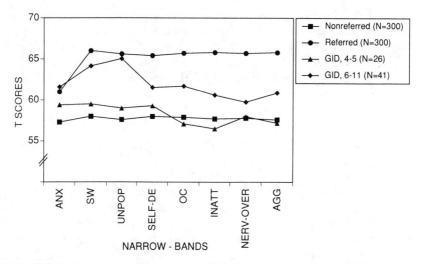

FIGURE 5.3. Narrow-band factors on the TRF, 6- to 11-year-old boys. ANX, Anxious; SW, Social Withdrawal; UNPOP, Unpopular; SELF-DE, Self-Destructive; OC, Obsessive–Compulsive; INATT, Inattentive; NERV-OVER, Nervous–Overactive; AGG, Aggressive. GID, gender identity disorder. Nonreferred and referred group data are from the standardization study (Achenbach & Edelbrock, 1986).

subgroup of boys (n = 65) who did not meet them (mean age = 8.2 years; r's ranged from .16 to .27).

A more direct measure of social ostracism—the extent to which the boy was called a "sissy" (as gauged by maternal report)—was equally correlated with CBCL psychopathology in the two diagnostic subgroups (r's ranged from .34 to .53). Multiple-regression analysis showed that age was the best predictor of psychopathology in the subgroup that met the complete DSM-III criteria (β's ranged from .40 to .50), whereas being called a "sissy" was the best predictor of psychopathology in the non-DSM-III group (β's ranged from .39 to .53). Although the two subgroups were equally likely to be called a "sissy," Zucker (1990b) suggested that younger children probably had less familiarity with the abstract label "sissy" than the older children; this may have accounted in part for the label's stronger impact on the non-DSM-III group, which was, as noted above, over 2 years older than the DSM-III group. It is also possible that the impact of being called a "sissy" was less in the DSM-III group, since, because of their younger age, they probably had experienced such putative teasing for a shorter period of time.[2]

Model 2

At least two lines of evidence are required to support the second model. First, it must be shown that there is a greater degree of parental psychopathology and dysfunction in families of boys with gender identity disorder than in control families. Then the specific influence of that psychopathology and dysfunction on the genesis of the gender identity disorder must be shown.

The Occurrence of Parental Psychopathology/Dysfunction

On the first point, several empirical studies have provided relevant information. On standardized interview and self-report measures, Marantz and Coates (1991) found that the mothers of boys with gender identity disorder showed more signs of psychopathology than did the mothers of demographically matched normal boys, including more pathological ratings on the Diagnostic Interview for Borderline Patients (Gunderson, Kolb, & Austin, 1981) and the Beck Depression Inventory (Beck, Ward, Mendelson, Mock, & Erbaugh, 1961). On the Structured Clinical Interview for DSM-III (Spitzer, Williams, Gibbon, & First, 1992; Williams et al., 1992), Wolfe (1990) reported a high rate of psychiatric disorder in both the mothers and fathers of boys with gender identity disorder, although the strength of this study was limited by the absence of a concurrent control group. Other studies of boys with gender identity disorder also implicate family dysfunction, as judged by rates of parental separation and divorce (Coates, 1985; Rekers & Swihart, 1989), prior parental contact with the mental health profession (Rekers, Mead, Rosen, & Brigham, 1983), and parental overprotectiveness (Bates et al., 1974).

Over the past several years, our group has collected systematic data on maternal psychopathology, marital discord, and child-rearing practices, some of which were reported by Mitchell (1991). The assessment protocol is shown in Table 5.11. As of this writing, data have been analyzed for 63 mothers of gender-referred boys, 13 clinical control boys, and 24 normal boys. The clinical and normal control boys, all of whom were participants in Mitchell's (1991) study, were pair-matched to the gender-referred boys for age and for parents' social class and marital status. For IQ, it was also possible to pair-match in advance a majority of the clinical controls.

Table 5.12 shows that the three groups were well matched on the demographic variables. On the CBCL, the probands and the clinical controls were significantly more disturbed than the normal control boys. On the Gender Identity Questionnaire (see Table 4.8), the probands were more deviant than the two control groups, which did not differ from each other.

Table 5.13 and Figure 5.4 summarize the results for the maternal measures. On several of the measures of psychopathology, the mothers of the boys with gender identity disorder differed significantly from the mothers of the normal control boys; the clinical control mothers had scores that fell midway between those of the other two groups. There were no between-group differences on the measure of marital discord.

TABLE 5.11. Maternal Assessment Protocol

Measures	Reference
Symptom Checklist 90—Revised	Derogatis (1983)
Inventory to Diagnose Depression	Zimmerman & Coryell (1987)
Diagnostic Interview for Borderline Patients	Gunderson & Kolb (1978)
Diagnostic Interview Schedule	Robins et al. (1981)
Dyadic Adjustment Scale	Spanier (1976)
Child-Rearing Practices Report	Block (1981); Trickett & Susman (1988)
Recalled Childhood Gender Identity Scale	Mitchell & Zucker (1991)

TABLE 5.12. Demographic Characteristics and Ratings of Behavioral Disturbance on the CBCL

Measures	Gender identity disorder ($n = 63$)		Clinical controls ($n = 13$)		Normal controls ($n = 24$)		p
	M	SD	M	SD	M	SD	
Child's age (in years)	6.4	2.0	6.3	1.9	5.9	1.8	n.s.
Child's IQ[a]	11.4	2.1	11.6	2.6	12.1	1.8	n.s.
Social class[b]	43.9	13.6	40.5	13.2	43.1	11.8	n.s.
Marital status							
Both parents	45 (n)		6 (n)		17 (n)		n.s.
Mother only/ reconstituted	18 (n)		7 (n)		7 (n)		
No. elevated narrow-band scales	1.7	2.4	1.9	2.1	0.3	1.0	.0165
Number of items	35.4	15.6	39.9	16.0	20.5	13.8	.0001
Sum of items	43.7	22.7	50.6	24.6	23.2	16.9	.0001
Internalizing T	61.5	9.6	62.4	8.1	49.0	8.9	.0001
Externalizing T	60.1	10.0	65.4	11.8	49.3	9.8	.0001

[a]Based on four subtests from the WISC-III, WISC-R, or WPPSI-R (average = 10).
[b]Hollingshead's (1975) four-factor index of social status (absolute range = 8–66).

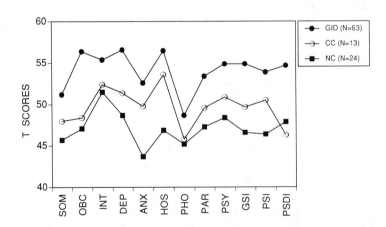

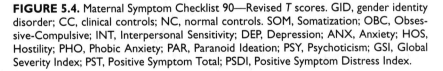

FIGURE 5.4. Maternal Symptom Checklist 90—Revised T scores. GID, gender identity disorder; CC, clinical controls; NC, normal controls. SOM, Somatization; OBC, Obsessive-Compulsive; INT, Interpersonal Sensitivity; DEP, Depression; ANX, Anxiety; HOS, Hostility; PHO, Phobic Anxiety; PAR, Paranoid Ideation; PSY, Psychoticism; GSI, Global Severity Index; PST, Positive Symptom Total; PSDI, Positive Symptom Distress Index.

TABLE 5.13. Measures of Maternal Psychopathology, Marital Discord, and Child-Rearing Practices

Measures	Gender identity disorder (*n* = 63)		Clinical controls (*n* = 13)		Normal controls (*n* = 24)		*F* or χ^2	*p*
	M	*SD*	*M*	*SD*	*M*	*SD*		
Inventory to Diagnose Depression[a]	13.2	9.6	11.6	8.5	9.3	8.5	1.6	n.s.
Diagnostic Interview for Borderline Patients[b]								
Social Adaptation	1.6	0.5	1.7	0.5	1.9	0.2	6.4	.002
Impulse Action Patterns	0.1	0.3	0.0	0.0	0.0	0.0	1.2	n.s.
Affects	0.8	0.8	0.3	0.8	0.4	0.7	4.0	.022
Psychosis	0.03	0.2	0.0	0.0	0.0	0.0	<1	n.s.
Interpersonal Relations	0.5	0.7	0.2	0.4	0.5	0.5	<1	n.s.
Total scale score	3.0	1.6	2.2	1.3	2.8	1.0	1.8	n.s.
Diagnostic Interview Schedule (number of diagnoses)[c]	1.7	1.7	0.6	1.0	0.8	0.7	5.5	.005
Dyadic Adjustment Scale (total score)[d]	98.0	22.4	93.0	21.5	102.0	27.1	<1	n.s.
Child-Rearing Practices Report[e]								
Authoritarian Control	2.6	0.5	2.7	0.5	2.4	0.4	2.2	.113
Enjoyment of Child and Parenting Role	5.4	0.8	5.2	0.5	5.8	0.5	4.0	.022
Autonomy	5.0	0.5	4.9	0.7	5.1	0.4	1.4	n.s.

[a]Absolute range = 0–88.
[b]Absolute range for five subscales = 0–2; for total score = 0–7.
[c]Absolute range = 0–26.
[d]Absolute range = 0–151.
[e]Absolute range for each scale = 1–7.

On the Child-Rearing Practices Report (CRPR), there was a between-group difference on the Enjoyment of Child and Parenting Role factor, as well as a trend on the Authoritarian Control factor. On the Enjoyment of Child factor, the mothers of the clinical controls were significantly less likely than the mothers of the normal controls to indicate that they enjoyed their children and the parenting role; the mothers of the probands had a score between that of the other two groups. On the Authoritarian Control factor, the clinical control mothers were most authoritarian and the normal control mothers were least authoritarian. Again, the mothers of the probands had a score between that of the other two groups.

Overall, these data lend some support to the hypothesis that clinic-referred boys with gender identity disorder come from families in which there are, on average, greater levels of parental and familial dysfunction than in the families of normal controls. However, these results must be viewed with caution, since only two studies have used a concurrent, demographically matched normal control group (Marantz & Coates, 1991; Mitchell, 1991; Mitchell, Zucker, Bradley, & Lowry Sullivan, 1995) and only one study (our own) has included a clinical control group.[3] Our preliminary data suggest that the mothers of boys with gender identity disorder are probably more similar to than different from the clinical control mothers, thus leaving open the question of specificity of maternal dysfunction vis-à-vis gender identity disorder. It would appear, however, that we may be in a position to conclude that general parental psychopathology is a nonspecific risk factor in the development of gender identity disorder (cf. Marantz, 1984).

The Hypothesized Role of Separation Anxiety

As noted earlier, the specific role of separation anxiety disorder vis-à-vis gender identity disorder has been one of the psychological pathways invoked to explain the influence of parental dysfunction. Coates and Person (1985) based this argument, in part, on their finding that of 25 boys with a DSM-III diagnosis of gender identity disorder, 15 (60%) boys also met the DSM-III criteria for separation anxiety disorder. Thacher (1985), for example, described a 3-year-old boy seen in Coates's clinic who was, according to his mother, "depressed and listless and unable to separate from her without becoming exceedingly upset" (p. 4). The clinical history revealed a great deal of parental psychopathology and marked marital discord, characterized by periodic separations, chronic quarreling, and physical violence. In this context, the boy's mother noted the emergence of various cross-gender behaviors, including his insistence that he "was a girl with a vagina" (p. 4, italics omitted). It is possible, then, that boys with marked separation anxiety use representational markers of a maternal object (e.g., cross-dressing) to deal with their anxiety. The following vignette offers a clinical illustration of the possible relation between separation anxiety and the emergence of symptoms of gender identity disorder.

CASE EXAMPLE 5.11

Darnell was a 5-year-old boy with an IQ of 128. He was referred by a child psychiatrist who had previously assessed and treated an older brother for symptoms suggestive of oppositional defiant disorder and a "difficult temperament." Darnell was born at a time when his parents were experiencing increased marital discord, which was characterized primarily by increasing withdrawal on his father's part. There was little overt marital discord. His father spent long periods of social time away from the family and experienced a strong absence of sexual desire (including impotence) toward his wife, who reported that her previous sexual relationships had always been fulfilling. Darnell's parents separated a couple of times before his second birthday and separated for the last time when he was 2 years old. Darnell's mother was a sensitive parent, accomplished in her profession, and free of gross psychopathology; by her late childhood, however, the quality of her family's life had been adversely affected by her father's emergent alcoholism.

For most of Darnell's life, the routine of his family was extremely stressful. He experienced several changes in babysitters, his father's prolonged absences, and frequent brief separations from his mother, whose profession required her to be away from the family for several days at a time. Darnell's mother described him as sensitive and having considerable difficulty separating from her (e.g., at nursery school). She felt that he had low self-esteem, manifested, for example, by frequent self-deprecatory remarks (e.g., "I hate myself").

Darnell's cross-gender behavior began in the context of the chronically stressful family situation. When Darnell was 4, his mother became involved with another man (whom she eventually married), who reported that when she was out of town, he would come home from work and often find Darnell cross-dressed. That Darnell's cross-dressing and other feminine behaviors increased during his mother's absence was therefore fairly compelling, at least as judged by the observations of his stepfather-to-be. By age 4, Darnell had also developed an intellectual interest in geography, often looking at globes or maps of the world. During the assessment, the interviewer commented to him that by learning about the world, he was able to "keep track of . . . Mom." Darnell smiled and nodded affirmatively.

Elsewhere, Zucker and Green (1991) noted several methodological and interpretive caveats regarding the Coates and Person (1985) data on separation anxiety. The interview procedure used to assess separation anxiety was not described, and information on interrater reliability was not given. Moreover, the diagnoses of separation anxiety and gender identity disorder were made concurrently at the time of assessment, so it is unclear whether separation anxiety actually preceded the emergence of gender identity disorder, as called for by the model. On this point, there is only clinical impression, not empirical verification. As noted by Marantz and Coates (1991), it remains unclear why cross-gender behavior should follow the emergence of separation anxiety, since not all boys with separation anxiety disorder develop gender identity disorder and not all boys with gender identity disorder develop separation anxiety disorder. In other words, the "choice of symptoms" to cope with separation anxiety is not readily apparent.

Despite these methodological and interpretive problems, Coates and Person's (1985) diagnostic impression regarding the high rate of separation anxiety disorder among boys with gender identity disorder is consistent with the more general finding noted earlier that boys with gender identity disorder show a predominance of internalizing psychopathology. For example, even among our boys aged 4–5 with gender identity disorder, who were clearly less disturbed than their counterparts aged 6–11, there was a predominance of internalizing behavior on both the CBCL and TRF (see Tables 5.2 and 5.5).

Lowry and Zucker (1991; Lowry Sullivan, Zucker, & Bradley, 1995) attempted to assess the presence of separation anxiety among a consecutive series of gender-referred boys. When this study was begun, we were not satisfied with the extant measures of separation anxiety; for example, although some semistructured interviews, such as the Diagnostic Interview for Children and Adolescents (Herjanic & Reich, 1982) and the Interview Schedule for Children (Kovacs, 1983), contained questions on separation anxiety, they did not cover all of the items described in DSM-III. Thus, we simply transformed the DSM-III criteria for separation anxiety disorder into structured interview questions that could be answered by mothers as "yes," "sometimes," or "no" (Table 5.14). This interview schedule was administered to the mothers of 85 gender-referred boys (mean age = 6.3 years). A "conservative" diagnosis of separation anxiety disorder was given if the mother answered "yes" to questions in three of the nine content domains, as required in the DSM-III. A "liberal" diagnosis of separation anxiety disorder was given if the mother answered "sometimes" or "yes" to questions in three of the nine content domains. For the majority of the protocols, interscorer reliability was available from audiotape. Without resolution, interscorer agreement exceeded 95% for specific questions and was 100% for final diagnostic decisions. Internal consistency of the interview schedule yielded an acceptable Cronbach's alpha of .78. Across the 21 items, the mean sum was 5.3 (SD = 5.0, range = 0–22).

Of the 85 boys, 54 (63.5%) were judged to meet the complete DSM-III diagnostic criteria for gender identity disorder; the remaining 31 (36.5%) all showed signs of gender identity disorder but did not meet the complete criteria. Of the 54 boys who met the complete criteria for gender identity disorder, 11 (20.4%) boys met the conservative standard for separation anxiety disorder, compared to 3 (9.7%) of the

TABLE 5.14. Separation Anxiety Disorder Interview Schedule

Instruction to mother: "Please answer each question with a 'Yes,' 'Sometimes,' or 'No.'"

Time frame to interviewer: Behavior should pertain to the past 6–12 months.

1a. Does [name of child] worry in an unrealistic way about something harmful happening to you?

1b. Does _____ worry in an unrealistic way that you will leave and not return?

2a. Does _____ worry in an unrealistic way that he will get lost from you?

2b. Does _____ worry in an unrealistic way that he will get kidnapped?

2c. Does _____ worry in an unrealistic way that he will get killed?

2d. Does _____ worry in an unrealistic way that he will be the victim of an accident?

3a. Is _____ reluctant to go to school so he can stay with you at home?

3b. Does _____ refuse to go to school so he can stay with you at home?

4a. Is _____ reluctant to go to sleep unless you are next to him?

4b. Does _____ refuse to go to sleep unless you are next to him?

4c. Is _____ reluctant to sleep away from home (friend or relative) because he wants to remain with you at home?

4d. Does _____ refuse to sleep away from home (friend or relative) because he wants to remain with you at home?

5a. Does _____ avoid being alone (e.g., playing) at home because he wants to be with you?

5b. Does _____ get upset if he cannot follow you around the house?

6. Does _____ have repeated nightmares involving the theme of separation from you?

7. On school days, does _____ complain of physical problems like stomachaches, headaches, nausea, or vomiting?

8a. When _____ knows that the two of you are going to be separated (e.g., when you leave for work, or go out for the evening, etc.), does he get very upset?

8b. When the two of you are separated (e.g., when you leave for work, or go out for the evening, etc.), does _____ get very upset?

9a. When _____ is not with you, does he seem to be withdrawn?

9b. When _____ is not with you, does he seem to be sad?

9c. When _____ is not with you, does he seem to be having a hard time concentrating on his school work or in his play?

Note. The nine content domains reflect the DSM-III criteria for separation anxiety disorder (American Psychiatric Association, 1980, p. 53).

31 boys who did not meet the complete criteria for gender identity disorder—a nonsignificant association ($\chi^2 < 1$). When the liberal standard was used, however, there was a relation between the presence of gender identity disorder and separation anxiety disorder. Of the 54 boys who met the complete criteria for gender identity disorder, 33 (61.1%) boys met the liberal criteria for separation anxiety disorder, compared to only 9 (29.0%) of the 31 boys who did not meet the complete criteria for gender identity disorder ($\chi^2 = 6.9$, $p < .01$, two-tailed).

Other analyses showed that the boys who met the criteria for separation anxiety disorder were comparable to the boys who did not with regard to age, IQ, and parents' social class, but were more likely to come from mother-only or "reconstituted" families (Table 5.15). For the entire group, the number of separation anxiety traits scored as "sometimes" or "yes" correlated significantly, albeit modestly, with the CBCL Internalizing T score ($r = .30$, $p < .01$), but not with the CBCL Externalizing T score ($r = .18$, n.s.).

Because the boys who met the complete DSM criteria for gender identity disorder were significantly younger than the boys who did not meet the complete criteria and came from a higher social class background, and because marital status was associated with the liberal standard for separation anxiety disorder, we correlated the DSM diagnosis for gender identity disorder with our interview diagnosis of separation anxiety disorder after partialing out age, social class, and marital status. The correlation was significant, $r(80) = .33$, $p = .002$ (two-tailed), suggesting that the relation between the diagnoses was not substantially confounded by the differences in demographic characteristics.

Although these results do not clarify the causal relation between separation anxiety and gender identity disorder, they provide some support for the notion that boys with gender identity problems may well manifest difficulties in the area of separation anxiety. It should be recognized, however, that our assessment of separation anxiety requires further validation in its own right. The more conservative standard for separation anxiety revealed no significant association with gender identity disorder. The more liberal standard revealed a significant associa-

TABLE 5.15. Relation between "Liberal" Diagnosis of Separation Anxiety Disorder and Demographic Characteristics

	Separation anxiety disorder				
	Yes ($n = 42$)		No ($n = 43$)		
Demographics	M	SD	M	SD	p
Age (in years)	6.0	1.8	6.5	2.0	n.s.
IQ	108.3	13.9	112.2	13.5	n.s.
Social class	43.5	13.8	46.7	12.9	n.s.
Marital status					
Both parents	27 (n)		38 (n)		.018
Mother only/					
reconstituted	15 (n)		5 (n)		

tion with gender identity disorder; it is likely that this cutoff was over-inclusive, however, since the "prevalence" rate was substantially higher than the rate usually reported in the epidemiological literature, even if one assumes that separation anxiety may be overrepresented among boys with gender identity disorder (see Bernstein & Borchardt, 1991). We are inclined, therefore, to view our liberal definition of separation anxiety as a dimensional trait measure rather than a true measure of this disorder. We hope that further work in this area can take advantage of the more recent developments in the use of structured interview techniques to assess anxiety disorders in children (see, e.g., Bell-Dolan & Brazeal, 1993; Klein & Last, 1989; Silverman, 1991).

The possibility that boys with gender identity disorder are prone to anxiety, and more specifically to separation anxiety, raises the question of a linkage between attachment relations with the mother and psychosexuality. Normative separation anxiety peaks at about 18 months (Kotelchuck, Zelazo, Kagan, & Spelke, 1975)—a time not too distant from the developmental period in which the signs of both typical and atypical gender development first appear (e.g., Fagot, 1985a). It is also known that anxious or insecure attachments, as conceptualized and measured by proponents of ethological attachment theory (e.g., Ainsworth, Blehar, Waters, & Wall, 1978), can be assessed by 12 months of age. Thus, it is conceivable that a temporal model connecting insecure attachment and gender identity disorder could be studied longitudinally. The rarity of frank gender identity disorder would make this task expensive and almost impossible to carry out; however, recent advances in the assessment of attachment relations during the preschool years (Bretherton & Waters, 1985; Greenberg, Cicchetti, & Cummings, 1990) suggest a more feasible preliminary strategy—formal assessment of the quality of mother–child attachment relationships in boys with gender identity disorder who are referred during the preschool years.

Birkenfeld-Adams (1995) has now completed such a study in our clinic. Preliminary analyses were consistent with the hypothesis that insecure attachments would be overrepresented in boys with gender identity disorder. But boys referred for other clinical problems also showed high rates of insecure attachments, which was consistent with previous research showing that preschool boys with disruptive behavior disorders are insecurely attached (DeKlyen, 1992; Greenberg, Speltz, & DeKlyen, 1993; Greenberg, Speltz, DeKlyen, & Endriga, 1991; Speltz, Greenberg, & DeKlyen, 1990). At best, then, it would seem that an insecure attachment might be conceptualized as a nonspecific risk factor in the development of gender identity disorder. Other factors are clearly required, and this matter is considered more fully in Chapters 6–8.

Model 3

As discussed above, the third model suggests that distinct parental influences may be related to the associated psychopathology and gender identity disorder, respectively. In this section, we examine data for the part of the model that attempts to identify correlates of general psychopathology in the child. Several aspects of maternal behavior were studied: composite measures of both psychopathology and child-rearing practices, marital discord, and recalled maternal childhood gender identity, respectively. The simple correlations between the maternal and demographic variables and three CBCL indices of psychopathology are shown in Table 5.16.

Three regression analyses were then performed with the maternal and demographic variables as predictors and the CBCL indices as criterion variables. Table 5.17 shows the results. The strongest and most consistent predictor of CBCL psychopathology was the composite measure of maternal psychopathology. The child's age also contributed unique variance to all three indices, and maternal child-rearing style contributed unique variance on one index. Marital discord, recalled maternal gender identity, and the three other demographic variables were unrelated to degree of child psychopathology.

When these analyses were repeated with the mothers of the clinical and normal controls, similar results were obtained. For the simple correlations (Table 5.18), the only major difference was that the relation

TABLE 5.16. Simple Correlations between Maternal Behaviors/Demographic Variables and CBCL Psychopathology in Boys with Gender Identity Disorder ($n = 63$)

Maternal measures/ demographics	CBCL variables		
	Sum of items	Internalizing T	Externalizing T
Psychopathology (composite)	.59*	.52*	.40*
Marital discord	.13	.18	.15
Child-rearing style			
Authoritarian	.21	.10	.16
Enjoyment	−.59*	−.41*	−.40*
Autonomy	−.39*	−.26*	−.30*
Recalled gender identity			
Factor 1	.03	−.04	.08
Factor 2	−.04	−.13	.01
Age of child	.35*	.35*	.29*
IQ	−.26*	−.24	−.20
Social class	−.32*	−.27*	−.28*
Marital status	−.26*	−.19	−.25*

*$p < .001$–$.05$ (two-tailed).

TABLE 5.17. Predictors of CBCL Psychopathology in Boys with Gender Identity Disorder (*n* = 63)

Criterion measures	Significant predictor variables[a]
Sum of items	Step 1: Maternal psychopathology (R^2 = .35) Step 2: Age ($R^2\Delta$ = .11) Step 3: Child-rearing practices ($R^2\Delta$ = .06)
Internalizing *T*	Step 1: Maternal psychopathology (R^2 = .27) Step 2: Age ($R^2\Delta$ =.11)
Externalizing *T*	Step 1: Maternal psychopathology (R^2 = .24) Step 2: Age ($R^2\Delta$ = .07)

Note. Eight predictor variables were entered: age, IQ, social class, marital status, maternal psychopathology (composite), marital discord, child-rearing practices (composite), and recalled maternal childhood gender identity (composite).
[a]*p*'s ranged from < .05 to < .001.

TABLE 5.18. Simple Correlations between Maternal Behaviors/Demographic Variables and CBCL Psychopathology (Full Sample, *n* = 100)

Maternal measures/ demographics	CBCL variables		
	Sum of items	Internalizing *T*	Externalizing *T*
Psychopathology (composite)	.56*	.53*	.48*
Marital discord	.24*	.33*	.27*
Child-rearing style			
Authoritarian	.23*	.17	.24*
Enjoyment	−.59*	−.46*	−.48*
Autonomy	−.35*	−.26*	−.32*
Recalled gender identity			
Factor 1	−.00	−.02	.03
Factor 2	−.06	−.05	−.04
Age of child	.34*	.32*	.34*
IQ	−.36*	−.29*	−.32*
Social class	−.27*	−.18	−.29*
Marital status	−.20*	−.18	−.22*

*p < .001–.05 (two-tailed).

between marital discord and CBCL psychopathology was also significant. For the regression analyses (Table 5.19), the strongest and most consistent predictor of CBCL psychopathology was the composite measure of maternal psychopathology. The child's age also contributed unique variance to all three indices; maternal child-rearing style and

TABLE 5.19. Predictors of CBCL Psychopathology in Boys (Full Sample, $n = 100$)

Criterion measures	Significant predictor variables[a]
Sum of items	Step 1: Maternal psychopathology ($R^2 = .32$)
	Step 2: Child-rearing practices ($R^2\Delta = .09$)
	Step 3: Age ($R^2\Delta = .05$)
	Step 4: IQ ($R^2\Delta = .02$)
Internalizing T	Step 1: Maternal psychopathology ($R^2 = .28$)
	Step 2: Age ($R^2\Delta = .07$)
	Step 3: Marital discord ($R^2\Delta = .03$)
	Step 4: IQ ($R^2\Delta = .03$)
Externalizing T	Step 1: Maternal psychopathology ($R^2\Delta = .23$)
	Step 2: Age ($R^2\Delta = .08$)
	Step 3: Child-rearing practices ($R^2\Delta = .05$)

Note. Eight predictor variables were entered: age, IQ, social class, marital status, maternal psychopathology (composite), marital discord, child-rearing practices (composite), and recalled maternal childhood gender identity (composite).
[a]p's ranged from $< .05$ to $< .001$.

child's IQ contributed unique variance on two indices; and marital discord contributed unique variance on one index. Recalled maternal gender identity and the three other demographic variables were unrelated to degree of child psychopathology.

These data suggest that some of the variance in CBCL psychopathology among boys with gender identity disorder is accounted for by risk factors commonly found in child psychiatric disorders in general. Thus, whatever role (if any) these risk factors play in the genesis of the gender identity disorder, they are clearly of some direct relevance to an understanding of the associated psychopathology observed in boys with this disorder, and thus have obvious implications for treatment (see Chapter 9).

Our data are, of course, subject to important caveats. Given that the maternal and child psychopathology measures were both provided by the mothers, we are concerned about the possibility of informant bias. However, a recent literature suggests that mothers with emotional or psychiatric problems do not necessarily overreport psychopathology in their children (for a review, see Richters, 1992). Nevertheless, it is important to have independent assessments of the child's psychopathology (e.g., by fathers or teachers) as a check on the validity of the maternal data. The father- and teacher-report CBCL data described earlier provide some relevant confirmatory information.

Another issue is the confidence we can place in our data regarding direction of effects. Some of the maternal measures (e.g., the Symptom

Checklist 90—Revised, the Dyadic Adjustment Scale, and the CRPR) may reflect concurrent maternal behaviors and attitudes, rather than maternal characteristics that precede the emergence of child psychopathology as measured by the CBCL. On the other hand, some of the measures reflect patterns of maternal functioning that cover longer periods of time (e.g., the Diagnostic Interview Schedule). Our clinical impression has been that the maternal measures probably reflect enduring patterns of functioning rather than simply state characteristics. In addition, there is certainly a literature that documents in a more prospective fashion the important role played by parental behaviors in the development of child psychopathology. Nevertheless, one could make the case that the maternal impairment is more a reaction to than a cause of the child's psychopathology. Although these need not be mutually exclusive (i.e., both could be contributory), there is one indirect test of the "child effects" hypothesis. If maternal impairment is simply a reaction to the child's psychopathology, one might predict a correlation of maternal impairment with the child's age, since the chronicity of the child's psychopathology should have a stronger impact on the mother's functioning over time. As it turns out, the child's age was unrelated to all our measures of maternal impairment.

GENERAL SUMMARY

In summary, this chapter has considered the evidence for the presence of associated psychopathology in children with gender identity disorder. On average, children with gender identity disorder appear to show as much general psychopathology as is shown by other children referred for clinical problems. There appears to be support for clinical observations that internalizing psychopathology is overrepresented among boys with this disorder. Multiple factors, including social ostracism and familial risk variables, appear to account for the associated psychopathology. At present, the evidence regarding the causal role played by this general psychopathology in the development of the gender identity disorder is inconclusive, but this is an issue that we explore further in the next three chapters.

NOTES

1. It will be recalled from Chapter 3 that two items on the CBCL specifically pertain to cross-gender behavior (item 5, "Behaves like opposite sex," and item 110, "Wishes to be of opposite sex"). It has also been our experience that certain other items on the CBCL are endorsed in a manner that reflect the child's

cross-gender identification. For example, a parent might endorse item 84 ("Strange behavior") and then provide an example such as "Thinks he's a girl." For all of the analyses reported here, these items were scored as 0's to avoid any artificial inflation of the disturbance indices.

2. Among the girls with gender identity disorder, we calculated correlations between the CBCL indices of disturbance and the demographic variables of age, IQ, and parents' social class and marital status. Social class was the only demographic variable that correlated with the disturbance indices (r's ranged from $-.40$ to $-.63$), indicating that girls from lower social class backgrounds had higher disturbance ratings. Because the demographic variables were correlated, we conducted multiple-regression analyses, as was done with the boys. Social class was the only significant predictor of disturbance. Although the sample size was small, it is of interest that age was not related to degree of disturbance. To the extent that age reflects increasing social ostracism, this mechanism did not appear to predict degree of disturbance, as was the case for boys. This finding is consistent with our previous discussion of the differential degree of social ostracism experienced by boys and girls with gender identity disorder (see Chapters 2–4). Unfortunately, for girls, unlike boys, we do not have a more direct measure of putative social ostracism (see above).

3. Rainbow (1986) compared a small number of mothers of boys who had both gender identity disorder and separation anxiety disorder ($n = 5$) with mothers of boys who had only separation anxiety disorder ($n = 5$). However, the gender identity disorder sample appears to be unrepresentative of the larger sample from which it was drawn (cf. Marantz, 1984; Marantz & Coates, 1991), so these data were not considered here.

CHAPTER 6

Etiology: Biological Research on Gender Identity Disorder and Related Psychosexual Conditions

Sexologists in the biological and social sciences have devoted considerable attention to identifying the determinants of psychosexual differentiation. There are those who argue that these determinants are predominantly biological, psychological, or sociological. There are others who advocate integrative or interactionist analyses, such as the currently popular "biopsychosocial" perspective. Most researchers, however, tend to test rather specific hypotheses—pieces, so to speak, of the etiological puzzle. In this chapter, we evaluate critically the etiological (or quasi-etiological) research concerning possible biological influences on gender identity disorder in children and allied psychosexual conditions, including gender identity disorder (transsexualism) in adults, homosexuality, and certain intersex conditions.

At the outset, it should be explained why etiological studies of allied psychosexual conditions might inform us about the etiology of gender identity disorder in children. This is particularly important with regard to biological research, since so little work of this type has been conducted on children with gender identity disorder. In our view, the reason is relatively straightforward: Gender identity disorder in children is associated both with gender identity disorder (transsexualism) and with homosexuality in adults (see Chapter 3). Although these associations are not perfect, the relations are strong enough that information about the origins of one of these conditions might provide clues about the origins of the others.

EARLY BIOLOGICAL RESEARCH

The search for biological correlates and determinants of psychosexual differentiation in humans has been a slow, complex process. Several hypotheses have led to dead ends. In the 1930s, for example, it was suggested that homosexual men were genetically female (Lang, 1940).[1] Techniques for karyotyping the sex chromosomes, which were developed in the mid-1950s (Moore & Barr, 1955), quickly laid this idea to rest (Pare, 1956, 1965; Pritchard, 1962). Although the occasional case report has documented an anomalous sex chromosome pattern in an adult with gender identity disorder (e.g., James, Orwin, & Davies, 1972; Taneja, Ammini, Mohapatra, Saxena, & Kucheria, 1992), the vast majority have the normal XX or XY complement (Barr & Hobbs, 1954; Hoenig & Torr, 1964). Two samples of boys with gender identity disorder all had normal sex chromosomes (Green, 1976; Rekers, Crandall, Rosen, & Bentler, 1979).

More recently, the H-Y sex-determining antigen (Polani & Adinolfi, 1983) was claimed to be reversed in transsexual adults (Eicher et al., 1981). There was an apparent partial replication by Engel, Pfäfflin, and Wiedeking (1980), but subsequent attempts were nonconfirmatory (Ciccarese, Massari, & Guanti, 1982; Wachtel et al., 1986). As noted by Hoenig (1981; 1985a, pp. 53–61), more stringent testing conditions by the original research team resulted in a failure to replicate, and there were high rates of false positives. Research in this area has since ceased.

A final example of a false lead concerns the relation between systemic (peripheral) sex hormone levels and sexual orientation. Several decades ago, it was assumed that some homosexual men had levels of male-typical sex hormones that were depressed; accordingly, many such men were injected with androgens, in the expectation that this would shift their sexual arousal pattern from men to women. The injections only increased their sex drive for men (Barahal, 1940). As more sensitive assays became available, there were reports on hormonal patterns consistent with the hypothesis, but when research designs became more rigorous and potential confounds (e.g., recreational drug use) were eliminated, the bulk of the evidence was nonconfirmatory. Similar results have been obtained in homosexual women, and this line of research has also petered out (for reviews, see Meyer-Bahlburg, 1977, 1979, 1982, 1984, 1993b).

Despite such false starts, the study of biological variables remains a central endeavor in contemporary sexological research, guided by different and perhaps more sophisticated models of psychosexual differentiation.

BEHAVIOR GENETICS

Several well-known research designs are available to assess the potential influence of genes on behavioral traits (Kendler, 1993; Plomin, 1994). These include the *family history* method, in which the trait of interest is assessed within families (e.g., among siblings), and the *twin study* method, in which concordance rates for a trait are compared between monozygotic (MZ) and dizygotic (DZ) twins. If a trait is familial and/or more prevalent in MZ than in DZ twins, then it is possible that genetic influences are involved. But since in most family and twin studies individuals are reared together, psychosocial factors may be equally plausible with regard to transmission (the more powerful design, in which twins are reared apart, is much more difficult to execute for obvious reasons). But as a first step in establishing consistency with a genetic hypothesis, familiality or MZ > DZ must be demonstrated.

Familiality and Gender Identity Disorder in Children

Among children with gender identity disorder, there has been little evidence for familiality. Clinical data from several centers have yielded very low concordance rates among nontwin siblings (S. Coates, personal communication, July 23, 1993; Green, 1974, 1987). In our clinic, we have assessed only one family in which three male siblings were concordant for gender identity disorder. Case reports of both MZ twins (Chazan, 1995, Chap. 4; Green & Stoller, 1971) and DZ twins (Esman, 1970) have all been discordant for gender identity disorder. Green (1987, Chap. 8) later described his pair as substantially discordant for sexual orientation. In our clinic, we have assessed five pairs of DZ twins (age range = 3–8 years). Three of these were male–male pairs; one was a male–female pair; and the remaining pair, described in detail elsewhere (Zucker et al., 1987), consisted of a true hermaphrodite (with a karyotype of 45 X, 47 XYY; assigned at age 5 weeks to the female sex) and a normal genetic female. All five of the pairs were discordant for gender identity disorder. One pair of MZ twin males has also been evaluated, and they too were discordant for gender identity disorder. A second pair of MZ twin males was described by their mother during an intake telephone interview as concordant for gender identity disorder, but the parents chose not to pursue a comprehensive assessment. Lastly, Zuger (1989) reported an unremarkable prevalence of homosexuality in the first- and second-degree male (4%) and female (1%) relatives of 55 child and adolescent males with gender identity disorder.

Familiality and Gender Identity Disorder in Adults

Familiality for gender identity disorder (transsexualism) in adults has not been well studied. Although case reports have documented the occurrence of both concordance and discordance among twin and non-twin siblings (reviewed in Hoenig, 1985a; see also Garden & Rothery, 1992; Gooren, Frants, Ericksson, & Rao, 1989; Joyce & Ding, 1985), the number of cases is small and clinical experience suggests that familiality is rare (R. Blanchard, personal communication, August 1, 1993).

Familiality and Sexual Orientation

Over four decades ago, Kallmann (1952a, 1952b) reported a 100% concordance rate for homosexuality among MZ twin males and a 15.4% concordance rate among DZ twin males. Ten years later, Schlegel (1962) reported similar concordance rates in a German sample. After Kallmann's study, a sprinkling of case reports on MZ twins reared together were published in the English-language literature, in which there was no strong pattern favoring concordance over discordance for homosexuality. Interestingly, some of the reports on the discordant male pairs noted that the homosexual twin had shown behavioral signs of femininity during childhood, whereas the heterosexual twin had not (e.g., Friedman, Wollesen, & Tendler, 1976; McConaghy & Blaszczynski, 1980; Zuger, 1976). The sporadic nature of the case report literature, the presence of discordant cases, methodological criticisms of Kallmann's data (Rosenthal, 1970, pp. 250–255), and a general antipathy toward genetic research in the decades after World War II (Rosenthal, 1970) lessened interest in the potential contribution of genetics to the development of sexual orientation and, indirectly, gender identity. Recent studies, however, have sparked renewed attention to genetic influences, and much of this work has been guided conceptually by advances in the field of behavior genetics (e.g., Plomin & Daniels, 1987; Plomin & Rende, 1991).[2]

Eckert, Bouchard, Bohlen, and Heston (1986) described two pairs of MZ twin males who had been reared *apart*: One pair was primarily discordant for homosexuality, but the other pair was concordant, and when these twins were reunited in adulthood, they became sexual partners! Four female MZ twin pairs, also reared apart, were all discordant for homosexuality. Whitam, Diamond, and Martin (1993) also described two pairs of MZ male twins who had been reared apart; one pair was concordant for homosexuality and the other pair was discordant, although the discordant pair also had sexual relations for a time.

Using larger samples of male and female twins reared together, sev-

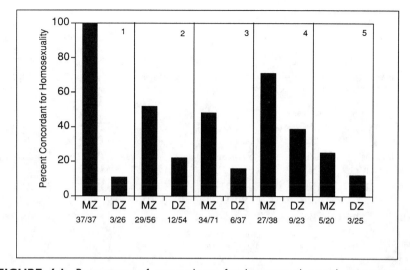

FIGURE 6.1. Percentages of concordance for homosexual sexual orientation in monozygotic (MZ) and dizygotic (DZ) twin pairs in which the index twin was homosexual and then the unknown sexual orientation of the cotwin was assessed. 1, Kallmann (1952a, 1952b); 2, Bailey and Pillard (1991); 3, Bailey et al. (1993); 4, Whitam et al. (1993); 5, King and McDonald (1992).

eral studies (summarized in Figure 6.1) have shown significantly greater concordance rates for homosexuality in MZ twins than in DZ twins. In addition, several studies (summarized in Table 6.1) have assessed the concordance for sexual orientation among nontwin siblings reared together, and the results of these studies also implicate a familial factor (see also Pattatucci & Hamer, in press). Because the concordance rates for sexual orientation were greater among MZ twins than among DZ twins, these studies were consistent with (though not proof of) a genetic influence. That sexual orientation is not "purely" genetic, however, might be inferred from the simple observation of the far from perfect concordance among the MZ twins.

In addition to reporting simple concordance rates, Bailey and Pillard (1991) and Bailey, Pillard, Neale, and Agyei (1993) calculated the magnitude of heritability using a standard model-fitting procedure. The model provided estimates for heritability, shared-environment influence, and nonshared-environment influence.[3] In both studies, heritability estimates were generally high under a range of assumptions. In contrast, shared-environment estimates were low, generally close to zero; however, nonshared-environment estimates usually fell in between the heritability and shared-environment estimates and, in some cases, were as strong as the heritability estimates.

Chapter 6

TABLE 6.1. Sibling Concordance for Sexual Orientation

		Heterosexual probands		Homosexual probands	
Study		HT siblings	BS/HS siblings	HT siblings	BS/HS siblings
			Male probands		
Pillard et al.	Brothers	49 (92.5%)	4 (7.5%)	46 (71.9%)	18 (28.1%)
(1982)	Sisters	60 (95.2%)	3 (4.8%)	43 (93.5%)	3 (6.5%)
Pillard &	Brothers	53 (96.4%)	2 (4.6%)	53 (77.9%)	15 (22.1%)
Weinrich (1986)	Sisters	61 (91.0%)	6 (9.0%)	44 (91.7%)	4 (8.3%)
Bailey (1989)	Brothers	84 (100%)	0 (0.0%)	113 (79.0%)	30 (21.0%)
	Sisters	69 (100%)	0 (0.0%)	119 (90.2%)	13 (9.8%)
Bailey & Pillard	Brothers	—	—	—	—	129 (90.1%)	13 (9.2%)
(1991)					
Bailey & Bell	Brothers	226 (95.8%)	10 (4.2%)	455 (91.0%)	45 (9.0%)
(1993)	Sisters	229 (99.1%)	2 (0.9%)	462 (97.1%)	14 (2.9%)
Hamer et al.	Brothers	—	—	—	—	90 (86.5%)	14 (13.5%)
(1993a)					
Total	Brothers	412 (96.3%)	16 (3.7%)	886 (86.8%)	135 (13.2%)
	Sisters	419 (97.4%)	11 (2.6%)	668 (95.2%)	34 (4.8%)
			Female probands		
Bailey (1989)	Brothers	57 (95.0%)	3 (5.0%)	26 (86.7%)	4 (13.3%)
	Sisters	53 (89.8%)	6 (10.2%)	19 (79.2%)	5 (21.8%)
Pillard (1990)	Brothers	44 (100%)	0 (0.0%)	30 (83.3%)	6 (16.7%)
	Sisters	47 (88.7%)	6 (11.3%)	45 (75.0%)	15 (25.0%)
Bailey & Bell	Brothers	108 (100%)	0 (0.0%)	185 (88.1%)	25 (11.9%)
(1993)	Sisters	91 (100%)	0 (0.0%)	176 (93.6%)	12 (6.4%)
Bailey &	Brothers	80 (98.8%)	1 (2.2%)	102 (92.7%)	8 (7.3%)
Benishay (1993)	Sisters	81 (97.6%)	2 (2.4%)	87 (87.9%)	12 (12.1%)
Bailey et al.	Brothers	—	—	—	—	99 (95.2%)	5 (4.8%)
(1993)	Sisters	—	—	—	—	63 (86.3%)	10 (13.7%)
Total	Brothers	289 (98.6%)	4 (1.4%)	442 (90.2%)	48 (9.8%)
	Sisters	272 (95.1%)	14 (4.9%)	390 (87.8%)	54 (12.2%)

Note. HT, exclusively or predominantly heterosexual; BS/HS, bisexual or exclusively homosexual. All siblings were nontwins. In this table, we calculated values based on the largest number of siblings available in each study; this included subjects whose sexual orientation was classified solely on the basis of the proband's knowledge. In some of these studies, siblings were interviewed when possible, but interviews were not attempted in some of the other studies. Each study should be examined directly for details regarding the manner in which sexual orientation was assessed and subsequently classified.

Before we comment further on these estimates and their possible interpretations, several general remarks about the twin studies are in order. It can be seen in Figure 6.1 that the concordance rates varied considerably. King and McDonald (1992) found the lowest concordance rate among MZ twins (25%), but their study was methodologically weak, in that the assessment of sexual orientation was poorly described and none of the subjects were interviewed directly. Whitam et al. (1993) reported the highest concordance rate for MZ twins (71%), but a troubling aspect of their data was that the concordance rate for DZ twins (39%) was not significantly lower than the concordance rate for MZ twins in the Bailey and Pillard (1991) and Bailey et al. (1993) studies (our analyses).

These variations in concordance rates may be partly explained by what behavior geneticists refer to as *ascertainment bias* or *recruitment bias* (Lykken, McGue, & Tellegen, 1987). In all of these studies, subjects were recruited primarily through advertisement in publications directed toward a homosexual readership. Although Bailey and Pillard (1991) and Bailey et al. (1993) discussed in detail the possible sources of bias entailed by this method, it is really impossible to know who does and does not respond to such advertisements. In some respects, this situation is very different from twin research (e.g., on schizophrenia) in which a researcher may have access to all, or almost all, potential subjects (e.g., hospitalized patients). Thus, testing for possible bias really yields only a rough approximation of what that bias might be (Torgersen, 1987).

When twins are reared together, concordance differences between MZ and DZ twins could be accounted for by a greater similarity in life experiences (e.g., parental child-rearing practices) among the MZ pairs. Behavior geneticists have addressed this possibility by assessing environmental variables of potential relevance to the trait under study—the so-called *equal-environment assumption* (see, e.g., Loehlin & Nichols, 1976; Plomin & Daniels, 1987; Plomin & Rende, 1991, pp. 179–182; Reiss, Plomin, & Hetherington, 1991). In general, behavior geneticists have not found strong support for the hypothesis that MZ twins are treated more similarly than DZ twins (Kendler, 1993). Rather, as in the study of ordinary siblings, nonshared-environment influences have been deemed of greater importance; however, it could be argued that tests of the equal-environment assumption have not been particularly strong. For example, being dressed alike or sharing the same room (apparently more common among MZ than DZ twins; see Kendler, 1993) may not be the most potent influences on behavioral development in general and on psychosexual differentiation in particular.

With regard to sexual orientation, no one has actually tried to test the equal-environment assumption directly. More important, one needs to decide in advance what the "trait-relevant" environmental experiences might be (Byne & Parsons, 1993). On this point, one would want to examine any of the putative psychosocial influences on sexual orientation that have been studied in other research contexts. As a simple hypothesis, one might predict that if such influences were important, then in concordant MZ twins both twins would have been exposed to them, but in discordant MZ twins only the homosexual twin would have had such exposure (cf. Dank, 1971). Along these lines, Green and Stoller (1971) tentatively concluded that their pair of MZ twin boys discordant for gender identity disorder had in fact differed with regard to several childhood traits and experiences (e.g., physical appearance at birth, cuddliness, activity level, and illness). The last variable apparently resulted in differences in contact with the parents, and all of these variables were deemed relevant for psychosexual differentiation. It is obvious, however, that rigorous twin studies concerning the possible effects of nonshared-environment influences on psychosexual differentiation remain to be done.

Of course, an ideal twin study design would use a representative sample of twins (e.g., from registries), who would then be assessed regarding their psychosexual development. Buhrich, Bailey, and Martin (1991) employed this strategy in a study of 161 male twin pairs from Australia. The response rate was about 53%. Among the 95 MZ twin pairs, 13 individuals were primarily homosexual. These individuals consisted of 4 twin pairs who were primarily concordant for homosexuality and 5 primarily homosexual twins whose cotwins were not primarily homosexual. Among the 63 DZ twin pairs, 2 individuals were primarily homosexual and neither of their cotwins was also primarily homosexual. Thus, in 4 of 9 MZ twin pairs in which at least one twin was primarily homosexual, this twin had a cotwin who was also primarily homosexual, compared to 0 of 2 DZ twin pairs. Although these percentages are consistent with those obtained in the previously discussed twin studies (in which one starts with a homosexual proband who is also a twin), the results are obviously nonsignificant because of poor statistical power. This points to the technical problem of starting with a twin registry, as considerably larger numbers of pairs are required to test accurately for differences between MZ and DZ twins.

Bailey (1995) has now reported the preliminary results of such a large-scale study, again using twins from Australia. For male twins, the concordance rate for homosexuality was significantly higher in MZ than DZ pairs, thus providing consistency with the results obtained by Bailey and Pillard (1991); however, for female twins, there was no evidence for a greater concordance rate for homosexuality in MZ than

DZ pairs, which thus conflicts with the results obtained by Bailey et al. (1993).

Bell et al. (1981) conjectured that homosexuality in men or women with a childhood cross-gender history might represent a more "constitutional" (i.e., heritable) form of sexual orientation than homosexuality in individuals without such a history. If this conjecture is correct, then a homosexual twin proband with a history of cross-gender behavior should be more likely to have a homosexual cotwin. Bailey and Pillard (1991) and Bailey et al. (1993) tested this hypothesis in their samples of male and female homosexual twins, but found no support for it.

MOLECULAR GENETICS

If one admits the existence of a genetic influence on sexual orientation, its location requires the contribution of molecular genetics. Hamer, Hu, Magnuson, Hu, and Pattatucci (1993a) recently reported the results of such a study. Hamer et al. studied 114 families of homosexual men. In an initial pedigree analysis of 76 homosexual men, they noted increased rates of homosexuality in maternal male relatives. They also observed this pattern of familiality in a selected sample of 38 families that contained two homosexual brothers.

Because a male inherits his X chromosome from his mother, Hamer et al. focused a DNA linkage analysis on that chromosome. Forty families, each of which contained two homosexual brothers, were studied. DNA was typed for 22 markers that spanned the X chromosome. Markers judged specific to sexual orientation were found on the distal portion of Xq28, the subtelomeric region of the long arm of the X chromosome. Of the 40 pairs of brothers, 33 were concordant for all markers and 7 were discordant at one or more loci.

Hamer et al.'s (1993a) study was the first investigation that applied the methodology of molecular genetics to an aspect of psychosexual differentiation. Because other molecular genetic studies pertaining to behavioral traits, such as schizophrenia and bipolar disorder, either had not been replicated or had been invalidated by reanalyses (Mowry & Levinson, 1993), Hamer et al. have emphasized the importance of replication attempts. If their results are found to be valid, the next steps would be to identify the chromosomal mapping of the loci and to isolate the relevant DNA sequences.

Several rapid commentaries on Hamer et al.'s study have been made, including discussion about assumptions of the base rate of homosexuality in the general population and among siblings of homosexual probands and their relevance to the statistical aspects of linkage analysis (Baron, 1993; Fausto-Sterling & Balaban, 1993; King, 1993; Risch, Squires-Wheeler, & Keats, 1993). Uncertainty about the parameters required for linkage analysis could therefore affect the risk of a Type I error (for a rebuttal, see Hamer, Hu, Magnuson, Hu, & Pattatucci, 1993b, 1993c).

Hamer et al.'s study raises fascinating questions. How does one account for the discordant pairs? Will heterosexual brothers of homosexual men prove to be concordant or discordant for the marker? Similarly, what percentage (if any) of heterosexual men will have the same markers? If there is some concordance among heterosexuals, what factors prevent the gene from being expressed? Once it is possible to identify markers in individuals, what percentage of homosexual men (i.e., those without homosexual brothers) will have them? Similarly, will subgroups of homosexual men (e.g., those with a history of childhood cross-gender identification) be more likely to have the markers, as Bell et al. (1981) wondered? Will the markers be detected in transsexuals with a homosexual orientation, but not among transsexuals with a nonhomosexual orientation? Can they be detected in boys with gender identity disorder? What mechanisms are involved that ultimately affect actual behavior? Can markers for sexual orientation in females also be identified? Regarding the last question, Hamer, Hu, Magnuson, Hu, and Pattatucci (1993d) reported that such a study was in progress. A relatively nontechnical account of the Hamer et al. (1993a) study can be found in Hamer and Copeland (1994).

As noted earlier, Hamer et al. (1993a) emphasized the importance of replication efforts. As this volume went to press, Hamer (1995) reported a successful replication with an additional 40 pairs of homosexual brothers, of whom 27 (68%) showed concordance for Xq28 markers. In contrast, Ebers (1995; personal communication, April 10, 1995) reported the preliminary results of another such attempt, in which evidence was not found for the presence of markers specific to sexual orientation on Xq28; however, methodological differences between Ebers's (1995) study and the reports by Hamer (1995) and Hamer et al. (1993a) may account for the discrepancy (see Marshall, 1995).

PRENATAL SEX HORMONES

In animals other than humans, the effects of prenatal and perinatal patterns of sex steroid secretion on the development of sex-dimorphic behavioral development have been extensively studied (Beach, 1981).

Scores of studies—with rodents, ruminants, carnivores, birds, and non-human primates—have shown an important role for hormonal influences on sex-dimorphic behavior (for some reviews, see Arnold & Breedlove, 1985; Baum, 1979; Beach, 1975; Beatty, 1979, 1984, 1992; Breedlove, 1994; Eberhart, 1988; Ellis, 1986; Feder, 1984; Goy & McEwen, 1980; Kelley, 1988; Komisaruk, 1978). Although there is both within- and cross-species variation, the basic principle that the prenatal or perinatal hormonal milieu shapes or induces a predisposition to certain sex-dimorphic behavioral patterns has marshaled a great deal of support.

In many respects, the prenatal hormonal model has been at center stage in elucidating the role of biological factors in psychosexual differentiation (Collaer & Hines, 1995; Meyer-Bahlburg, 1995). This has been so in part because it has been possible to study experimentally the role of sex hormones in many animal species. Such studies have in turn allowed researchers to consider the relevance of animal models for human psychosexual differentiation.

Animal Studies

The Principle of Organizational and Activational Influences

For over 30 years, animal researchers have studied the distinction between organizational and activational influences of the sex steroids. As summarized by Beatty (1992),

> *Activational* effects refer to reversible changes in morphology, physiology, or behavior that depend on the continued presence of the hormone in the body and on the functional integrity of the receptors on which it acts. Within broad limits the age of the organism has only a minor influence on the activational effects of gonadal hormones, which are qualitatively similar from puberty to senescence. In contrast, the *organizational* effects of gonadal hormones produce enduring changes in morphology, physiology, and behavior, which arise from relatively brief exposure to the hormone during a limited period of perinatal development. In all mammals that have been studied, a relatively brief period exists during which the developing organism is responsive to the organizational actions of gonadal hormones. (pp. 85–86, italics added)

What many regard as the watershed study demonstrating this distinction was conducted by Phoenix, Goy, Gerall, and Young (1959; see

TABLE 6.2. Lordosis and Mounting in Hermaphroditic Female Guinea Pigs and Controls

	Control females ($n = 14$)	Hermaphrodites ($n = 9$)	Castrated males ($n = 8$)
Lordosis (maximum median duration, in seconds)	11.3	2.3	2.5
Mounting (mean no.)	0.0	4.4	11.8

Note. Data from Phoenix, Goy, Gerall, and Young (1959).

also Young, Goy, & Phoenix, 1964). Phoenix et al. (1959) injected pregnant guinea pigs with testosterone propionate during most of the gestation. In female offspring, this manipulation created a form of physical pseudohermaphroditism, as judged, for example, by masculinized external genitalia that were virtually indistinguishable from those of normal male offspring. These animals were then gonadectomized after birth. Several comparison groups were also studied, including untreated male and female offspring, which were also gonadectomized. Thus, the postnatal influence of endogenously circulating hormones was eliminated in all three groups.

When the offspring were mature, they were injected with various doses of estradiol benzoate to test for the display of lordosis, a female-typical sexual behavior. Compared to the female controls, the pseudohermaphroditic females showed reduced lordotic responses comparable to the responses of the male controls (Table 6.2). Table 6.2 also shows that the pseudohermaphroditic females were more likely to show mounting, a male-typical sexual behavior, than were the female controls. Phoenix et al. also demonstrated an apparent permanence of these effects, as inferred by their continuation when the animals were older. These results led to the principle that patterns of prenatal hormone exposure "have an organizing action on the tissues mediating mating behavior in the sense of altering permanently the responses females normally give as adults" (Phoenix et al., 1959, p. 379).

The Distinction between Behavioral Masculinization and Defeminization

Over the past few decades, animal researchers have noted that the hormonal mechanisms responsible for the display of male-typical and female-typical behaviors may not be identical across all mammalian species. Thus, two technical terms, *behavioral masculinization* and *behavioral defeminization,* were introduced (Whalen & Edwards, 1967). *Behavioral masculinization* refers to the increased likelihood of male-typical behavior (e.g., intromission); *behavioral defeminization* refers to the decreased likelihood of female-typical behavior (e.g., lordosis).

In a review of these constructs, Baum (1979) concluded that "behavioral masculinization occurs in all mammalian species . . . and that it depends, at least in part, on the action of testicular androgen or its metabolites in the brain during a critical perinatal period. In contrast, the process of behavioral defeminization is not a universal response among all mammals to early androgenic stimulation" (p. 279). The distinction was important because in rats, masculinization and defeminization appear to be highly correlated; however, the two processes in higher mammals, including nonhuman primates, appear to be less so. How these concepts might apply to psychosexual differentiation in humans is discussed below.

Social Influences

Apart from pointing to the predisposing role of prenatal sex hormones, studies with animals have also addressed the importance of the social environment in influencing the display of sex-dimorphic behavior. For example, Harlow and Harlow (1965) noted that biologically normal monkeys reared under conditions of harsh deprivation during infancy "never attain [the heterosexual] stage of beautiful, bounteous bliss" (p. 325). Such monkeys avoided sexual interaction or were grossly inept at it. The therapeutic intervention devised by Harlow and Harlow to ameliorate these sexual deficits was rather gruesome:

> In an effort to overcome this difficulty of our reluctant females, we devised an apparatus called the rape rack. Females artificially postured in this apparatus are acceptable sexual objects to some of our breeding males. . . . The little data we now possess [suggest] that rape-rack experience does not overcome female frigidity—a finding not completely surprising. (p. 329)

The pioneering social deprivation experiments conducted by Harlow and his colleagues played a crucial role in the elaboration of attachment theory (Bowlby, 1969) and in the study of other aspects of psychosocial development. However, in regard to psychosexual development in particular, this work probably shed only a little light on long-term sequelae, since outcome under more normative conditions could hardly be inferred from it.

Over the years, primatologists have gathered a great many behavioral data pertaining to social influences that are relevant to an understanding of sex-dimorphic behavioral development. For example, Lovejoy and Wallen (1988) remarked that "from controlled laboratory studies, it has become apparent that sex differences result from an interaction between a specific rearing environment . . . and an animal's prenatal hormonal milieu" (p. 348). But they also noted that "the relative contributions of the rearing environment and the prenatal hormonal environment appear to vary with the specific behavior under study . . . some sexually dimorphic behaviors, such as mounting and rough play, occur consistently across a wide range of rearing conditions . . . [whereas] other juvenile sex differences, such as aggression and passivity, are only found under specific social conditions" (p. 348). Thus, much recent work has attempted to identify more carefully the environmental conditions that accentuate or attenuate the expression of sex-dimorphic behaviors (e.g., Goy & Wallen, 1979; Meaney, Stewart, & Beatty, 1985; Nieuwenhuijsen, Slob, & van den Werff ten Bosch, 1988; Pomerantz, Roy, & Goy, 1988).

Although considering this literature in detail would be beyond the scope of this book, we should mention a couple of points made in it that may contribute to an understanding of psychosexual differentiation in humans. For example, it is interesting to note that while variations in rearing conditions may attenuate the expression of sex-dimorphic behaviors, we have rarely encountered a report in which there was a reversal or inversion in the expression of a sex difference (e.g., more grooming of infant monkeys by male juveniles than by female juveniles, or more mounting of peers by females than by males).

Along these lines, it is of interest to consider the influence of rearing conditions on the development of "sexual preference" in nonhuman primates. Take, for example, the sex composition of the peer group. Slob and Schenck (1986) studied three feral-born male stump-tailed macaques (*Macaca arctoides*) that were housed together ("isosexual rearing") for 9 years from prepubertal age without any exposure to females. When experimentally tested for their sexual preference as adults, all three preferred novel females, not each other. In animals, then, it seems that whereas a heterosexual orientation can be attenuated or even reversed by hormonal manipulation (e.g., Adkins-Regan, 1988; Bakker, Brand, van Ophemert, & Slob, 1993; Brand, Houtsmuller, & Slob, 1993; Goy & Goldfoot, 1975), similar effects are much more difficult to induce by psychosocial environmental manipulation.

Although it would be intriguing indeed if primatologists could use environmental manipulation to induce cross-gender behavioral preferences (both nonsexual and sexual), such work does not appear to be imminent (cf. Green, 1993). Thus, we are left with the current evidence for interaction effects noted by Lovejoy and Wallen (1988).

Human Studies

Given the important role of prenatal sex hormones in the psychosexual differentiation of animals, it is not surprising that researchers have long sought to determine whether similar effects exist among humans.

Conceptual Issues

At the outset, several conceptual issues should be addressed. Most contemporary researchers recognize that the place of *Homo sapiens* on the phylogenetic scale is such that hormonal influences on some aspects of sex-dimorphic behavior should be less powerful in humans than they are in other animals, particularly as one moves down the evolutionary ladder. As Money (1988, p. 26) has wryly noted, humans are, after all, not "hormonal robots."

Another issue concerns the validity of transposing animal models to human models of sex-dimorphic behavior (e.g., Beach, 1976, 1979a, 1979b; Davidson, 1979). It is unlikely, for example, that there is an appropriate animal model for human gender identity, given its subjective, phenomenological nature. In contrast, there appear to be better animal analogues for gender role behaviors, such as rough-and-tumble play, aggression, and parenting. Regarding sexual behavior, some researchers have been skeptical about the transposition of such behaviors as lordosis and mounting to humans, and there has been considerable debate over semantics. Consider, for example, a man who prefers receptive anal intercourse with another man. Is this a lordotic, female-typical behavior? Is it an example of behavioral demasculinization or feminization? But what about a man who prefers penetrative anal intercourse with another man? Is this an example of masculinization? Or is it feminization because the object of desire is another male? Similarly, is the behavior of a woman who prefers the "superior" position during ventral–ventral sexual interaction with another woman an example of mounting, a male-typical behavior, and therefore masculinization?

A third issue concerns the distinction between sexual behavior per se and sexual orientation. Although homosexual behavior can be observed throughout the animal kingdom (e.g., Gadpaille, 1980; Nadler,

1990; Weinrich, 1980), there is some consensus that under naturalistic conditions a sexual preference for same-sex conspecifics in mature animals—that is, an exclusive homosexual orientation—does not occur (e.g., Adkins-Regan, 1988; Rosenblum, 1990). And, of course, animal models are of minimal utility in understanding the historical and cultural variability in the attributions or meaning-making that humans confer on their sexuality—that is, their sense of self as "heterosexual," "bisexual," or "homosexual."

The Example of Congenital Adrenal Hyperplasia

Congenital adrenal hyperplasia (CAH) nicely illuminates the complexities of hormone–behavior relations in humans. CAH is an inherited, autosomal recessive disorder of adrenal steroidogenesis (White, New, & Dupont, 1987). Among Caucasians, the incidence is about 1 in 5,000–15,000 live births. Because of the excessive production of adrenal androgens, genetic females with this disorder are born with ambiguous or fully masculinized external genitalia. Surgical repair can normalize the appearance of the external genitalia; cortisone replacement therapy, available since 1950, normalizes the malfunctioning endocrine system and, in theory, essentially shuts down the excessive production of adrenal androgen (Money & Ehrhardt, 1972). Treated CAH, then, has been used as a model "experiment of nature" in which the effects of abnormal prenatal hormone exposure on postnatal sex-dimorphic behavior can be observed. Accordingly, research on this disorder is reviewed here in some detail.

Initial studies indicated that girls with CAH were more masculine and/or less feminine than control girls in their gender role behavior (Ehrhardt & Baker, 1974; Ehrhardt, Epstein, & Money, 1968). This was measured with several common behavioral markers, such as peer preference, toy preference, and fantasy play.

Although these studies have been subject to some methodological criticisms, such as the reliance on interview measures and raters' knowledge of the subjects' status (probands vs. controls) (for a review, see Berenbaum, 1990), subsequent studies have revealed similar findings using additional measurement approaches, including observation of overt behavior and the use of psychometrically sound questionnaires (e.g., Berenbaum & Hines, 1992; Berenbaum & Snyder, 1995; Dittmann, 1989, 1992; Dittmann, Kappes, Kappes, Borger, Meyer-Bahlburg, et al., 1990; Dittmann, Kappes, Kappes, Borger, Stegner, et al., 1990; Hines & Kaufman, 1994; Hurtig & Rosenthal, 1987; Müller, Kraus-Orlitta, Dirlich-Wilhelm, & Förster, 1983). Berenbaum and

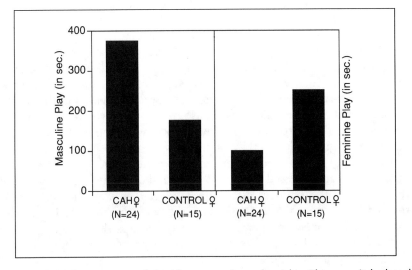

FIGURE 6.2. Time spent in play with sex-typed toys by girls with congenital adrenal hyperplasia (CAH) and control girls during 10 minutes of play (play with neutral toys not shown). Adapted from Berenbaum and Hines (1992, p. 205). Copyright 1992 by the American Psychological Society. Adapted by permission.

Hines (1992), for example, assessed the sex-typed play behavior of CAH girls and compared them with unaffected sisters or first cousins (some were relatives of CAH boys, who were also studied) in a free-play situation. The children were given the opportunity to play with stereotypical masculine, feminine, or neutral toys. Figure 6.2 shows that the CAH girls were more likely to play with the masculine toys and less likely to play with the feminine toys than were the controls; however, the two groups did not differ in their play with neutral toys. Compared to control boys, the CAH girls played about as much with the masculine toys and somewhat more with the feminine toys.

What about gender identity in girls with CAH? Ehrhardt and Baker (1974) asked their youngsters whether it was better to be a girl or a boy. Of 17 girls with CAH, 6 (35%) indicated that they were undecided or thought that they might have chosen to be a boy if such a choice had been possible. In contrast, only 1 of 11 sisters gave a similar response. Ehrhardt and Baker commented, however, that "none of the [CAH] girls had a conflict with her female gender identity or was unhappy about being a girl" (p. 43).

Although clinical experience with CAH girls regarding gender identity is consistent with Ehrhardt and Baker's (1974) impression (Meyer-Bahlburg, 1993a; Money, 1968, 1991), the percentage of CAH girls who develop formal gender identity problems and wind up living in the male social role is considerably higher than would be expected, given the base rate of gender dysphoria in the general population of genetic females (Zucker, 1994). In any case, it would be important to conduct more formal studies, including systematic interviews both with the youngsters themselves and with their parents. Ehrhardt and Baker's single item is difficult to interpret without knowing more about why the ambivalent girls felt as they did. Moreover, the data obtained by Ehrhardt and Baker were complicated by the broad age range of the girls who were assessed (4.3–19.9 years). For example, it is possible that some of the younger girls expressed gender ambivalence because they had not yet achieved gender constancy (Slaby & Frey, 1975); they may have reasoned preoperationally that perhaps they should be boys because they liked boys' toys, and so on. Older girls may have felt gender-ambivalent for different reasons.

The sexual orientation of women with CAH has been reported on in eight studies with sample sizes of at least 10 patients. Table 6.3 summarizes these reports. In considering these studies, several methodological issues require consideration. First, the age range was broad, with subjects as young as 11 years of age included. Second, the rigor in which sexual orientation was assessed varied considerably, with some authors providing only vague information regarding their methods (e.g., Lev-Ran, 1974; Slijper et al., 1992). In addition, some studies assessed sexual orientation only in behavior, not fantasy. Third, two studies examined women who did not receive cortisone-replacement treatment until late in life (mean age = 26 years, range = 8–47 years), in part because they had been born prior to its availability (Ehrhardt, Evers, & Money, 1968; Lev-Ran, 1974). Thus, these late-treated women experienced considerable postnatal virilization; for example, in the Ehrhardt, Evers, and Money (1968) report, it was noted that 18 of the women had received a clitorectomy, presumably for cosmetic purposes (i.e., correction of a phallic-like clitoris). Fourth, only three studies (Dittmann, Kappes, & Kappes, 1992; Money, Schwartz, & Lewis, 1984; Zucker, Bradley, Oliver, et al., 1992) employed concurrent controls.

The Ehrhardt, Evers, and Money (1968) study of late-treated women with CAH suggested a high incidence of bisexual fantasy and behavior, which would be consistent with an influence of excessive prenatal androgen exposure in shifting sexual orientation from an exclusively "feminine" (i.e., heterosexual) pattern. The percentage of women who reported no interpersonal sexual experiences of any kind also ap-

TABLE 6.3. Sexual Orientation in Women with Congenital Adrenal Hyperplasia

Study	Age (in years)			Country	Measure	Sexual orientation (%)			Comment
	n	M	Range			HT	BS/HS	No data[a]	
Ehrhardt, Evers, & Money (1968)	23	33	19–55	United States	Fantasy Behavior	39.1 52.2	43.5 17.4	17.4 30.4	
Lev-Ran (1974)	18	26	13–43	Soviet Union	Fantasy Behavior	77.7 38.8	0.0 0.0	23.3 62.2	Fantasy based on dreams only
Ehrhardt (1979)	13	16	11–24	United States	Fantasy/behavior	?	15.3	?	Classification as HT vs. no data not clear
Money et al. (1984)	30	21[b]	17–26	United States	Fantasy	40.0	37.0	23.0	
Mulaikal et al. (1987)	80	30	18–69	United States	Behavior	57.5	5.0	37.5	
Dittmann et al. (1992)	34	—	11–41	Germany	Fantasy/behavior	73.6	26.4	0.0	
Slijper et al. (1992)	10	21[c]	16–33	Netherlands	Fantasy Behavior	? 20.0	? 0.0	? 80.0	All said to be "heterosexual"
Zucker, Bradley, Oliver, et al. (1992)	31	24	18–36	Canada	Fantasy Behavior	70.0 73.3	23.3 0.0	6.7 26.7	Ratings for the year prior to the interview

Note. HT, heterosexual; BS/HS, bisexual or homosexual.
[a]Indicates that the subject either refused to provide information or reported no fantasies or interpersonal sexual experiences.
[b]Mean age provided by J. Money (personal communication, April 7, 1993).
[c]Median age.

peared high. However, it was recognized that the effects of excessive postnatal androgens and social influences in response to phenotypic masculinization on sexual orientation development could not be ruled out. The only other study on late-treated women with CAH was conducted by Lev-Ran (1974) in the former Soviet Union. Unlike Ehrhardt, Evers, and Money (1968), Lev-Ran reported no evidence of a bisexual/homosexual orientation in fantasy, although a large percentage of his subjects apparently had had no interpersonal sexual experiences. Unfortunately, the assessment methods were poorly described, and Lev-Ran speculated that the absence of bisexual/homosexual fantasy might have been underreported because of cultural factors.

The first methodologically adequate study of sexual orientation in early-treated CAH women was reported by Money et al. (1984), who found a high rate of bisexual/homosexual fantasy compared to a control group of women with either 46 XY androgen-insensitivity syndrome (reared as females) or the Rokitansky syndrome (vaginal atresia). These findings have been replicated by Dittmann et al. (1992) and ourselves (Zucker, Bradley, Oliver, et al., 1992); both studies employed unaffected sisters and cousins as controls. All three of these studies pointed to a higher rate of bisexual fantasy and lower rates of interpersonal sexual experiences of any kind, the latter finding also being observed by Mulaikal, Migeon, and Rock (1987).

The Mulaikal et al. (1987) study was also the first to divide their patients into two groups—those with the salt-wasting (SW) form of the disorder (n = 40) and those with "simple" virilization (SV) (n = 40). This distinction was deemed important for at least two reasons: first, the SW patients required more complex medical treatment (i.e., treatment directed at the salt wasting as well as the virilization); second, there is some evidence that SW patients are also more severely masculinized physically (Verkauf & Jones, 1970).

Regarding physical status, Mulaikal et al. (1987) found that the SW subjects were shorter and were more likely than the SV subjects to have an inadequate introitus. The two groups did not differ with regard to extent of hirsutism and regularity of the menstrual cycle. The physical differences probably reflected the greater virilization of the SW group.

Apart from sexual orientation in behavior (discussed above), Mulaikal et al. found that 50% of the SV group had been married for over 4 years at the time of the study, compared to only 13% of the SW. Fifteen of the SV subjects had conceived a child, in contrast to only one of the SW subjects.

Mulaikal et al.'s study was informative in several respects. It is clear that the psychosexuality of their CAH women was impaired, as inferred from the low rate of marriage and the absence of interpersonal sexual experience. Moreover, the study revealed important distinctions between the SV and SW groups with regard to physical status and differential conception rates. We (Zucker, Bradley, Oliver, et al., 1992) also found that our SW subjects were less likely than the SV subjects to be cohabitating or married, and they were also less likely to have had interpersonal sexual experiences with men.

Discussion of the CAH Findings

On the whole, the data on CAH might be interpreted as continuous with data on animals in which experimental manipulation of the prenatal hormonal milieu alters the patterning of sex-dimorphic behavior. This interpretation has not, however, been universally accepted. Critics have appealed to alternative explanations of the CAH data, such as parental response to the ambiguous genitalia (which are sometimes not corrected until toddlerhood or later), expectancy effects for a child of ambiguous sex, and medication side effects (e.g., Birke, 1981; Bleier, 1984, pp. 97–101; Doell & Longino, 1988; Fausto-Sterling, 1985, pp. 133–138; Kaplan, 1980; Kessler, 1990; Quadagno, Briscoe, & Quadagno, 1977; Rogers & Walsh, 1982; Unger & Crawford, 1992, pp. 211–214; van den Wijngaard, 1991a, 1991b). In our view, these explanations have tended to reject *in toto* the possibility that the prenatal androgen milieu affects, in Money's (1988) terminology, the "threshold" for the development and expression of sex-dimorphic patterns of behavior.

The behavioral sequelae (increased male-typical behavior and/or decreased female-typical behavior) are consistent with a large body of animal data in which prenatal androgens have been varied experimentally. The CAH data are also consistent with animal studies that have examined the effects of diethylstilbestrol (DES), a nonsteroidal estrogen in which testosterone is aromatized to estradiol and estrogen receptors. Pre- or perinatal exposure to DES masculinizes both sexual and nonsexual sex-dimorphic behavior in lower animals (see, e.g., Meyer-Bahlburg & Ehrhardt, 1986).

In humans, the opportunity to study the effects of exposure to DES on sex-dimorphic behavior arose because of its widespread use to treat at-risk pregnancies—a practice that was halted because of adverse physical effects on the offspring (e.g., Herbst, Ulfelder, & Poskanzer, 1971). Several studies on DES-exposed females have revealed some evidence for a shift to male-typical behavior, including gender role, cognitive abilities, and sexual orientation in fantasy (e.g., Ehrhardt et al.,

1985, 1989; Hines & Shipley, 1984; Meyer-Bahlburg, Ehrhardt, et al., 1985; Meyer-Bahlburg et al., 1995; for no effects, see Lish et al., 1991; Lish, Meyer-Bahlburg, Ehrhardt, Travis, & Veridiano, 1992). The effects, however, appear weaker, perhaps because DES is a less potent masculinizing agent than the androgen effect in CAH. But the DES data are important in another respect: The genitalia are not masculinized in female offspring, which would rule out one commonly hypothesized influence on socialization.

Nonetheless, it should be recognized that important individual differences in the psychosexual differentiation of CAH females have not as yet been fully accounted for. Apart from "error variance" (e.g., underreporting of bisexual or homosexual feelings because of social stigma), how might individual differences be explained? One possibility is that variation in exposure to prenatal androgens is associated with atypical psychosexual sequelae. This is hinted at in the SW-SV differences that have been found (e.g., Dittmann, Kappes, Kappes, Borger, Meyer-Bahlburg, et al., 1990; Dittman et al., 1992; Mulaikal et al., 1987; Slijper, 1984; Zucker, Bradley, Oliver, et al., 1992). But even within the more affected SW subgroup, there are individual differences. Another possibility, then, is that social effects intensify or attenuate the presumed biological predisposition toward a male-typical bias in behavior. Unfortunately, little empirical work has assessed social influences directly. There is some indirect evidence that speaks against social influences. For example, Berenbaum and Hines (1992; see also Berenbaum, 1990) found no relation between measures of physical masculinization (e.g., clitoral length) and degree of behavioral masculinity (cf. Dittmann, Kappes, Kappes, Borger, Stegner, et al., 1990b). Nevertheless, it would be important to design future studies that focus more directly on social variables, to test for variations that augment or reduce the likely biological predisposition toward culturally defined masculinity in CAH girls and women. Other than anecdotal accounts or case report studies (e.g., Money, 1991; Money & Lewis, 1987), it is surprising how little work has been done to determine how CAH youngsters themselves understand their condition and what impact this has on their psychosexual development.[4]

Although the study of psychosexual differentiation in persons with intersex conditions has been informative, some researchers have questioned the extension of the conclusions drawn from this work to humans without intersex conditions (e.g., Hoenig, 1985b). As several researchers have noted, gross intersex conditions rarely co-occur with gender identity disorder in children and adults or with homosexuality. If any of these psychosexual conditions are influenced by prenatal hormonal factors, then other markers need to be identified that would implicate such an influence. Over the past couple of decades, several lines of research have addressed this issue.

The Positive Estrogen Feedback Effect

In contemporary sexology, the so-called *positive estrogen feedback effect* (PEFE) or *Hohlweg effect* (Dörner, 1976) has been particularly influential in debates pertaining to prenatal hormonal effects on both sexual orientation and gender identity disorder (transsexualism) in adults and, indirectly, on gender identity disorder in children.[5]

In the human female, rising estrogen levels during the follicular phase of the menstrual cycle elicit a transient decrease in luteinizing hormone (LH) secretion (negative feedback), which is then followed by a surge in LH—the so-called PEFE—that results in ovulation. This phenomenon is believed to be the consequence of (prenatal) hormone-mediated sexual differentiation. A similar effect can be demonstrated experimentally by the exogenous administration of estrogen preparations, such as Premarin. In the human male, exogenous administration of estrogen does not yield a corresponding PEFE, at least to the same extent that it does in women (e.g., Dörner, Rohde, & Schnorr, 1975).

Experimental studies on rats have demonstrated a similar sex dimorphism with regard to the PEFE (for reviews, see Dörner, 1976, 1988; Meyer-Bahlburg, 1982, 1984). The PEFE is substantially diminished in female rats that have been neonatally androgenized. It cannot, however, be strongly elicited (if at all) in male rats that have been castrated in adulthood and then administered estrogen. Dörner (1988) has also noted that the effect is not found in castrated males of other species, including hamsters, pigs, sheep, and rhesus macaques. These experimental studies suggested a prenatal and/or perinatal hormonal organizational influence on the sex-dimorphic PEFE.

Dörner and his group in the former German Democratic Republic reasoned that if the rat model could be applied to humans, one might expect that homosexuals and transsexuals would show a sex-atypical PEFE on the presumption that they had been exposed to atypical prenatal hormonal events.[6] To test this hypothesis, Dörner, Rohde, Stahl, Krell, and Masius (1975; see also Dörner, Rohde, & Krell, 1972) studied 20 heterosexual men, 21 homosexual men, and 5 bisexual men. The participants were injected with 20 mg of an estrogen preparation (Presomen), and changes in LH levels from baseline were measured. Although there were individual differences, it can be seen in Figure 6.3 that the homosexual men showed a greater PEFE than did the heterosexual and bisexual men combined. According to Dörner, Rohde, Stahl,

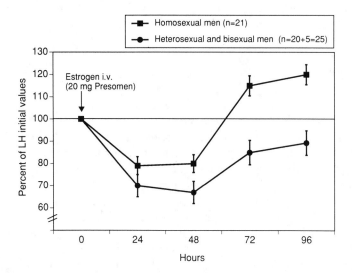

FIGURE 6.3. Plasma LH responses to an intravenous estrogen injection, expressed as percentages of the mean initial LH values in homosexual and hetero- or bisexual men (means ± *SEM*). Adapted from Dörner, Rohde, Stahl, Krell, and Masius (1975, p. 5). Copyright 1975 by Plenum Publishing Corporation. Adapted by permission.

et al. (1975), their data suggested that homosexual men "may possess, at least in part, a predominantly female-differentiated brain" (p. 2)—what Dörner (1976) characterized elsewhere as "central nervous [system] pseudohermaphroditism, possibly caused by an absolute or relative androgen deficiency during the critical hypothalamic organizational phase in prenatal life" (p. 6).

In light of the growing body of evidence that failed to yield sexual orientation effects for systemic hormones (as described earlier), Dörner, Rohde, Stahl, et al.'s (1975) study was of significance in shifting the focus of research to prenatal hormonal influences, particularly along the hypothalamic–pituitary–gonadal axis, and in identifying a neuroendocrine marker that differentiated homosexual and heterosexual men who were free of any gross intersex condition affecting the genitalia.

Dörner's group then reported a similar effect in transsexual men, but a suppression of the PEFE in transsexual women (Dörner, Rohde, Seidel, Haas, & Schoft, 1976). A suppression effect in transsexual women was subsequently reported by a second research team (Seyler, Canalis, Spare, & Reichlin, 1978). (Livingstone, Sagel, Distiller, Morley, & Katz, 1978, did not find a PEFE in heterosexual vs. homosexual men. However, their experimental procedure differed so strongly from that of Dörner, Rohde, Stahl, et al., 1975, including only very brief postinfusion time lines, that it cannot be considered a legitimate replication; in fact, Livingstone et al. did not even refer to the Dörner et al. study. See also Halbreich, Segal, & Chowers, 1978.)

Gladue, Green, and Hellman (1984) reported the results of a replication of the Dörner, Rohde, Stahl, et al. (1975) experiment in a study of 17 heterosexual men, 14 homosexual men, and 12 heterosexual women in the United States. Although Dörner and colleagues had stated that the PEFE was less pronounced in homosexual men than in the (presumably heterosexual) women studied by Van de Wiele et al. (1970), they had not included women in their own experimental design. Gladue et al. found that in response to an injection of 25 mg of Premarin, homosexual men showed an LH surge intermediate between that of heterosexual men and women (Figure 6.4).

Given the complexity of the experimental procedure, this replication effort was an important empirical step in verifying the status of Dörner, Rohde, Stahl, et al.'s (1975) original claim that the PEFE might be a neuroendocrine marker of sexual orientation. At about the same time as Gladue et al. (1984), Dörner, Rohde, Schott, and Schnabl (1983) reported evidence for the PEFE in transsexual men with a homosexual orientation, but not in transsexual men with a heterosexual or bisexual sexual orientation. Their data suggested that among transsexuals, the PEFE is more strongly related to sexual orientation than to a gender identity anomaly per se, or that it is restricted to adult gender dysphoria associated with childhood cross-gender identification (see also Rohde, Uebelhack, & Dörner, 1986).

Critiques of the PEFE

Over the past 10 years, however, the validity of the PEFE as a neuroendocrine marker of sexual orientation or anomalous gender identity has been the subject of intense empirical, methodological, and theoretical debate.

On the empirical front, Gooren (1986a, 1986b) and colleagues (Gooren, Rao, van Kessel, & Harmsen-Louman, 1984) reported a failure to replicate the PEFE in homosexual men, transsexual men, and transsexual women, and Hendricks, Graber, and Rodriguez-Sierra (1989) reported a similar failure to replicate in homosexual men. Several other studies using different experimental procedures have also been conducted with samples of transsexual men and women. Some have reported results in line with the Dörner and colleagues' original findings (e.g., Boyar & Aiman, 1982; Kula, Dulko, Pawlikowski, Imielinski, & Slowikowska, 1986; Kula & Pawlikowski, 1986), whereas others have not (e.g., Goodman et al., 1985; Spijkstra, Spinder, & Gooren, 1988;

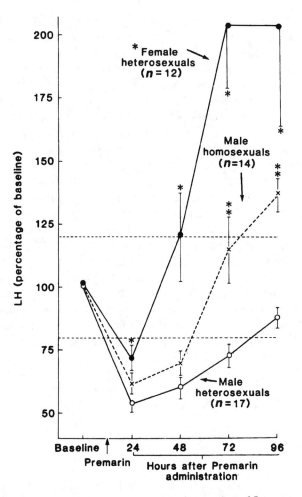

FIGURE 6.4. Changes in LH in response to a single injection of Premarin. Values are means ± *SE* (vertical bars). Dashed lines indicate the 95% confidence interval for baseline values for all groups. Group comparisons: *Female heterosexuals significantly different from male heterosexuals and homosexuals at all times ($p < .05$); **male homosexuals significantly different from male heterosexuals at 72 and 96 hours ($p < .05$). All groups showed a decrease from baseline at 24 hours. From Gladue, Green, and Hellman (1984, p. 1496). Copyright 1984 by the American Association for the Advancement of Science. Reprinted by permission.

Spinder, Spijkstra, Gooren, & Burger, 1989; Wiesen & Futterweit, 1983).

In our view, the debate regarding the validity of the PEFE vis-à-vis sexual orientation or transsexualism has not been advanced by the multiple replication efforts. This state of affairs contrasts sharply with the results obtained from the multitude of studies leading to the conclusion that systemic hormones do not distinguish homosexual and heterosexual men and women.

Both methodological and conceptual issues have made the interpretation of the putative PEFE reported by Dörner, Rohde, Stahl, et al. (1975) and Gladue et al. (1984) even more complicated. From a methodological standpoint, for example, the Hendricks et al. (1989) study has been criticized as having an insufficient sample size to achieve adequate statistical power (3–5 men per dosage level). Similarly, the number of subjects in Gooren's (1986a) study of transsexuals never exceeded six. Moreover, in Gooren's (1986a) study of transsexual men, both homosexual and nonhomosexual patients were probably included. If the PEFE is more germane to sexual orientation (and/or childhood cross-gender identity), then the inclusion of nonhomosexual transsexuals is problematic, since they could, in principle, cancel out the PEFE in the homosexual transsexuals. Indeed, if the Dörner, Rohde, et al. (1983) study could be confirmed (see above), this would further weaken the merit of Gooren's study. Regarding Gooren's (1986a) study with homosexual men, it has also been argued that the procedure was not an exact replication of either Dörner, Rohde, Stahl, et al. (1975) or Gladue et al. (1984).

The conceptual and interpretive criticisms point to even more difficult issues. In this regard, there have been a number of important observations:

1. Some researchers have argued that the PEFE is not sex-dimorphic in all nonhuman primates (e.g., Hodges, 1980), and hence they question the conceptual underpinnings of the model as it has been applied to humans. But this argument is not completely persuasive: The PEFE is clearly sex-dimorphic in gonadally intact heterosexual men and women, and if a within-sex difference in sexual orientation exists, then this needs to be explained in its own right.

2. It has also been argued that the LH surge in homosexual or transsexual men does not meet the clinical criterion for a true PEFE (Gooren, 1986a). But this argument is not entirely satisfactory, since the significant quantitative effects would still need to be explained; moreover, neither Dörner, Rohde, Stahl, et al. (1975) nor Gladue et al. (1984) predicted that the PEFE in homosexual men would perfectly mimic the PEFE observed in heterosexual women.

3. Perhaps the most important argument advanced has been that the PEFE is dependent largely on the concurrent hormonal status of the individual, not on any putative sex-dimorphic prenatal influence. Thus, in male monkeys the PEFE can be observed after gonadectomy, suggesting that the rise in LH is not preordained by prenatal hormonal events. Gooren (1986b) demonstrated, for example, that transsexual men showed the PEFE only after treatment with female sex hormones had been initiated. On the other hand, Leyendecker, Wardlaw, Leffek, and Nocke (1971) indicated that a PEFE could be induced among women of various menstrual statuses (normally menstruating, oligomenorrheic, amenorrheic, and postmenopausal). Nevertheless, the possibility of a PEFE in males or of a negative feedback effect in females receiving cross-gender hormones has led to other interpretations of the data. For example, unlike the results obtained by Dörner, Rohde, Stahl, et al. (1975), the administration of Premarin by Gladue et al. (1984) resulted in a marked reduction in testosterone levels in both heterosexual and homosexual men (but not in women), and the testosterone levels took longer to rise to baseline in the homosexual men. Baum, Carroll, Erskine, and Tobet (1985) noted that in some nonhuman primates the absence of LH secretion in normal males might be related to "the potent inhibitory action of a testicular hormone on the responsiveness of the neuroendocrine axis to estrogen" (p. 961), and suggested that a similar mechanism might be operative in human males. The origin of this putative testicular factor is unclear (cf. Gladue, 1985). Gooren (1990a) took the position that the depressed testosterone levels could be caused by such environmental factors as recreational drug use, testicular infection, or other health-related causes. Although Gladue et al. (1984) reported that their subjects were drug-free and in good health, Gooren's (1990a) argument seems to be that the depressed testosterone levels were artificially inducing a putative PEFE and had nothing to do with prenatal hormonal events.

Meyer-Bahlburg (1993b) noted that as a result of the current AIDS epidemic, many homosexual men may well have compromised endocrine systems, making further study of the PEFE problematic. As it turns out, some of the homosexual men in Gladue et al.'s (1984) study were retrospectively determined to have HIV, but post hoc analyses showed no differences between HIV+ and HIV− men (B. A. Gladue, personal communication, June 29, 1993). In any case, the methodological, empirical, and conceptual ambiguities regarding the PEFE led Money (1988, p. 113) to conclude that the issue was at an "impasse." Our reading of the literature suggests that no current efforts are being made to study the PEFE in homosexual and transsexual men and women. It could be argued that additional empirical studies might clarify whether there is a phenomenon to be explained; on the other hand, the conceptual criticisms seem to have led some researchers to conclude that even if sexual orientation effects exist, they are probably unrelated to prenatal psychosexual differentiation.

Conclusion

So what can the literature on prenatal hormonal influences in nonhuman animals, in humans with intersex conditions, and in human adults with either a homosexual orientation or an anomalous gender identity tell us about similar mechanisms among children with gender identity disorder?

Invariably, youngsters with gender identity disorder show no signs of physical hermaphroditism, including hormonal anomaly. On its own this is a remarkable finding, since, as many experienced clinicians will attest, many of these youngsters show a profound cross-gender identification. Recent research developments, however, clearly open the possibility of prenatal hormonal influences that leave external genital reproductive structures intact. The work on nonhuman primates may be particularly instructive.

In female rhesus macaques (*Macaca mulatta*), Goy, Bercovitch, and McBrair (1988) were able to induce behavioral masculinization in the absence of genital hermaphroditism by varying the timing of exogenous injections of testosterone propionate during the pregnancy. It should be noted that the male analogue of this experiment has not yet been conducted. From an interpretive point of view, this methodology is of interest because it eliminates a confound—the possibility that the masculinized behavior is in part a function of how the social group reacts to the anomalous genitalia of the female offspring.

As partly depicted in Figure 6.5, early-exposed females, which were genitally virilized, showed increased rates of mounting their mothers and peers (male-typical behaviors) and lowered rates of grooming of their own mothers (a female-typical behavior) compared to normal females but did not differ from normal females in their rates of rough play. In contrast, late-exposed females, which were not genitally virilized, showed increased rates of rough play and of mounting their peers, but did not differ from normal females in their rates of mounting their mothers. The mothers of the early-exposed females were more likely to inspect their offspring's genitalia than were the mothers of normal females, but the mothers of the late-exposed females were not. Goy et al. (1988) concluded that "the individual behavior traits that are components of the juvenile male role are independently

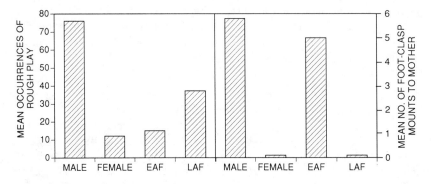

FIGURE 6.5. Mean occurrences of rough play (left panel) and foot-clasp mounts to mother (right panel) in normal male, normal female, early-androgenized female (EAF), and late-androgenized female (LAF) rhesus macaques. Adapted from Goy, Bercovitch, and McBrair (1988, pp. 559, 565). Copyright 1988 by Academic Press. Adapted by permission.

regulated by the organizing actions of androgen and have separable critical periods" (p. 552).

The association between prenatal androgen exposure and increased rates of some male-typical behaviors, despite the absence of genital masculinization, suggests that there can be a separation of morphological and behavioral effects in nonhuman primates. This clearly opens the possibility that similar mechanisms operate in humans.

As noted earlier, gross intersex conditions are usually not associated with a homosexual orientation. Dörner's (1976) notion of "central nervous [system] pseudohermaphroditism" suggests, however, more subtle variations in fetal masculinization or defeminization, including the possibility of some type of "defect" in androgen receptors.

Macke et al. (1993) recently reported an effort to test this idea, at least indirectly, by searching for anomalous DNA sequence variations in the androgen receptor gene in homosexual and presumably heterosexual men. Some of the homosexual men were participants in the Hamer et al. (1993a) study. Three approaches were used: the degree of concordance of androgen receptor alleles in 36 pairs of homosexual brothers; the lengths of polyglutamine and polyglycine tracts in the amino-terminal domain of the androgen receptor in homosexual and heterosexual men; and screening of the entire androgen receptor coding region for sequence variation in homosexual men with brothers or relatives who were also homosexual. Macke et al. (1993) found that none of these approaches resulted in any evidence for sequence variation. They suggested that it would be of interest to test "additional components involved in the action of gonadal steroids to determine whether inherited variations at other points in the system [influence] sexual orientation" (p. 851).

PRENATAL MATERNAL STRESS

Animal Research

In pregnant rats, maternal stress can be induced exogenously by aversive means (e.g., frequent exposure to floodlights and restraint). Increased plasma levels of corticosterone in both the mother and male offspring indicate the effectiveness of the manipulation (Ward & Weisz, 1980, 1984). If such stress occurs during a specific period of the pregnancy, it alters fetal testicular enzyme activity, resulting first in a brief rise in androgens and then in a permanent androgen deficiency (see Figure 6.6). Although external reproductive morphological structures remain intact, exposure to stress alters the size of the sexually dimorphic nucleus of the preoptic area (Ward, 1992). These changes appear to have an anomalous effect on postnatal sex-dimorphic behavior in the male offspring (Figure 6.7), including demasculinized (e.g., reduced initiation of copulation) and feminized (e.g., lordosis) sexual behavior, as well as nonsexual but sex-typical behavior (e.g., rough-and-tumble

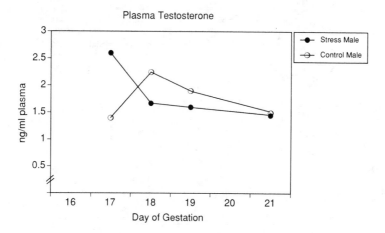

FIGURE 6.6. Mean concentration of testosterone in plasma samples obtained from male rat fetuses between day 17 of gestation and day 21 (2 days prior to birth). Stressed and control groups were significantly different ($p < .05$) from each other on days 17 and 18 of gestation. Adapted from Ward and Weisz (1980, p. 328). Copyright 1980 by the American Association for the Advancement of Science. Adapted by permission.

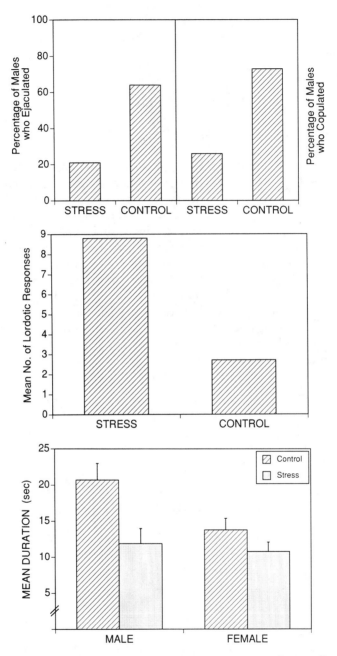

FIGURE 6.7. Effects of exogenously induced stress in pregnant Sprague–Dawley rats on male-typical sexual behavior (top panel), female-typical sexual behavior (middle panel), and male-typical, nonsexual but sex-dimorphic behavior (rough-and-tumble play) (bottom panel) in male offspring (all three panels) and female offspring (bottom panel). Adapted from Ward (1972, p. 83, and 1992, pp. 166, 173). Copyright 1972 by the American Association for the Advancement of Science and 1992 by Plenum Publishing Corporation. Adapted by permission.

play) (Ward, 1972, 1984, 1992). As noted by Ward (1992), similar neuroanatomic and behavioral effects in female offspring have been less consistent.

More recently, several researchers have shown comparable effects by exposing pregnant rats to ethanol. In both male and female off-spring, Meyer and Riley (1986) observed inverted proclivities toward play fighting and, in male offspring, shifts toward female-typical sexual behavior (Dahlgren, Matuszczyk, & Hård, 1991; Ward, Ward, Winn, & Bielawski, 1994; Watabe & Endo, 1994). In another study, ethanol exposure suppressed the normal surge in fetal testosterone observed in unexposed male rats (McGivern, Raum, Salido, & Redei, 1988).

Although mechanisms in rodents have been used to consider the possibility that comparable mechanisms exist in humans (Everitt & Bancroft, 1991), data on nonhuman primates may well be of greater utility in predicting generalizability to humans. Unfortunately, studies concerning the effects of prenatal maternal stress on the sex-dimorphic behavior of nonhuman primate offspring have not been conducted.

There is, however, some evidence that "mild" prenatal maternal stress in nonhuman primates affects aspects of the offspring's physical status and behavioral functioning. For example, Schneider (1992) showed that prenatal maternal stress in rhesus monkeys (*Macaca mulatta*), induced by brief removal from the home cage and exposure to unpredictable noise, resulted in lower birth weights, delayed self-feeding, increased distractibility, decreased activity, and poorer neuromotor maturation in the offspring. As noted by K. Wallen (personal communication, July 27, 1993), however, this form of stress induction is considerably less severe than the procedures used with rats (Ward, 1984); moreover, it is likely that for ethical reasons the use of procedures with primates analogous to those used with rats would not be permitted.

The Prenatal Stress Hypothesis and
Human Sexual Orientation

Ward's (1972) experimental procedure with rats, dubbed the *prenatal stress syndrome,* led Dörner et al. (1980) to predict that there would be an increase in the incidence of homosexuality if the risk of maternal prenatal stress were heightened. To test this hypothesis, they examined the birth year of homosexual men in the former German Democratic Republic who were being treated by physicians for sexually transmitted disease.

They reported that significantly more homosexual men (57.5 per 100,000 males) were born during World War II (1940–1945)—a period of presumed exogenous stress for pregnant women—than in the years before (1932–1939) or after (1946–1953) the war (19.3 and 35.1 per 100,000 males, respectively).

In a second study, Dörner, Schenk, Schmiedel, and Ahrens (1983) asked 100 bisexual/homosexual men and 100 heterosexual men about maternal stressful events that might have occurred during their own prenatal lives. The subjects were asked to consult their parents for this information. It was found that the mothers of the bisexual and homosexual men recalled more "moderate" and "severe" stress during the pregnancy than did the mothers of the heterosexual men. In this study, it was noted that the influence of war and unwanted pregnancies accounted for most of the putative maternal stress. This led Dörner, Schenk, et al. (1983) to the bold conclusion that "prevention of war and undesired pregnancies may render possible a partial prevention of the development of sexual deviations" (p. 87).

The results of these studies were consistent with a previous observation by Allen (1949), a psychiatrist, who commented that "it is commonly noticed that there tends to be a wave of homosexuality following wars. This was very evident in Germany after the First World War and probably will recur after the recent one" (p. 128). Unfortunately, Allen did not indicate the basis for this remark.

The studies by Dörner and colleagues have been subjected to several methodological criticisms (e.g., Bailey, 1989), including absence of reliability checks for the independent (maternal stress) and dependent (sexual orientation) variables, demand characteristics, and alternative interpretations, such as the higher rate of fathers' absence during wartime (Allen, 1962). Moreover, it should be recognized that the presumed mechanism of influence—induction of temporary androgen deficiency in the human male fetus—has not been directly documented.[7,8]

Mechanisms of influence aside, there have been several efforts to replicate the hypothesized association between recalled prenatal maternal stress and sexual orientation. Ellis, Ames, Peckham, and Burke (1988) asked mothers of heterosexual, bisexual, and homosexual men and mothers of heterosexual and homosexual women to complete a questionnaire that included information on the number and severity of stressful life events during the year prior to the pregnancy and during the pregnancy. Because the second trimester of pregnancy is considered a sensitive period for sexual differentiation of the brain (Money, 1988), stress during the pregnancy was rated separately by trimester. Ellis et al. (1988) found that the mothers of homosexual men had a higher stress severity score during the year *prior* to the pregnancy, but not during pregnancy, than that of the mothers of bisexual and heterosexual men. When the data were analyzed by trimester, it was found that 9–12 months *before* the pregnancy and during the second trimester, the mothers of homosexual men recalled having experienced more severe stress than that recalled by the mothers of heterosexual men. The mothers of heterosexual and homosexual women did not differ significantly in their recollection of stress.

Unfortunately, Ellis et al.'s (1988) statistical analyses were flawed, including an inflated Type I error rate. Descriptively, the most consistent aspect of the Ellis et al. data was that the mothers of homosexual men recalled more severe stress than did the mothers of heterosexual men both *before* and *during* the pregnancy up until the third trimester, when the pattern of means inverted. Although recalled maternal stress was not limited to the second trimester, the pattern of the results was not inconsistent with the importance of stress during this period of fetal development.

It could be argued that social desirability would influence maternal reports of prenatal stress. Research guided by attribution theory has shown that people externalize responsibility for negative outcomes (Weiner, 1993). Thus, to avoid self-blame for their offspring's homosexuality, mothers could easily externalize its cause by overreporting stressful life events during their pregnancies (one would presume that the average mother might intuitively guess the hypothesis under study). But given that Ellis et al. (1988) did not find differences between the mothers of homosexual and heterosexual women, this interpretation is not entirely persuasive.

Perhaps the best methodological study on the hypothesized connection between maternal stress and sexual orientation was conducted by Bailey, Willerman, and Parks (1991). Recalled maternal stress during each of the three trimesters correlated close to zero with Kinsey et al. (1948) ratings of sexual orientation in fantasy and of self- and maternal-report measures of childhood cross-gender behavior in heterosexual and homosexual men (absolute r's ranged from .00 to .11). Interestingly, however, Bailey et al. (1991) found that maternal "stress-proneness" was modestly correlated with degree of boyhood effeminacy recalled by both the men themselves and their mothers, which is somewhat consistent with the interpretation offered above regarding the Ellis et al. (1988) data set. One could argue that the stress reported by the mothers in Bailey et al. (1991), who were from the United States, was less severe than the putative stress experienced by the mothers during wartime in the studies conducted by Dörner and colleagues.

Null findings have also been reported by Wille, Borchers, and Schultz (1987) and Schmidt and Clement (1990), although these two studies were less solid methodologically than the Bailey et al. (1991) report. For example, Wille et al.'s (1987) sample size probably lacked statistical power adequate to detect significant effects. Perhaps other co-horts of homosexual men who grew up in countries racked by war could be studied to examine the maternal stress hypothesis further.

Conclusion

Although maternal prenatal stress in humans has been associated with several problems in offspring (see, e.g., Levin & DeFrank, 1988; Lobel, 1994; Ward, 1991), no empirical work has examined its association with gender identity disorder or, more generally, with patterns of cross-gender behavior that would fall below the threshold for a formal diagnosis. Given Bailey et al.'s (1991) retrospective findings, we doubt that such a study of mothers of children with gender identity disorder would yield positive findings. However, the more recent findings on ethanol effects on sex-dimorphic behavior in rats tempts one to wonder about comparable effects in humans, especially in light of one pilot study in which five pregnant women who were heavy users of alcohol had male fetuses with suppressed amniotic fluid levels of 4-androstenedione and testosterone (Westney et al., 1991). It would seem that a controlled, prospective study of sex-dimorphic behavior in children born to alcoholic mothers would be feasible to execute. It is conceivable, however, that the presence of severe maternal stress during the pregnancy would have nonspecific effects that might function as a nonspecific risk factor.

COGNITIVE ABILITIES, NEUROPSYCHOLOGICAL FUNCTION, AND NEUROANATOMIC STRUCTURES

A great deal of research has focused on normative sex differences (and similarities) in cognitive abilities, neuropsychological functioning, and neuroanatomic structures—research that has guided studies of persons with atypical psychosexual differentiation (see note 1). In this section, we review the status of the research in these areas.

Cognitive Abilities

The basic empirical question of whether the two sexes differ in their verbal and nonverbal (e.g., spatial, mathematical) cognitive abilities has received an enormous amount of attention. It is well beyond the scope of this volume to provide a detailed consideration of this literature. But, as a working assumption, let us accept as fact the view that, on average, women perform better than men in certain verbal areas (e.g., on tests of verbal fluency), whereas men perform better than women in certain nonverbal areas (e.g., on tests of spatial ability). In attempts to account for these sex differences, various biological and psychosocial explanations have been proposed. A reading of this dense literature indicates clearly that no one factor is adequate in accounting for sex differences, and both biological and psychosocial explanations have received some empirical support (e.g., Baenninger & Newcombe, 1989; Casey & Brabeck, 1990; Fairweather, 1976; Feingold, 1988, 1993; Halpern, 1992; Harris, 1978; Hyde, 1981; Hyde & Linn, 1988; Krekling & Nordvik, 1992; Liben, 1991; Linn & Petersen, 1985, 1986; Mann, Sasanuma, Sakuma, & Masaki, 1990; Masters & Sanders, 1993; Nyborg, 1983; Pascual-Leone & Morra, 1991; Sherman, 1978; Signorella & Jamison, 1986; Thomas & Turner, 1991; Vasta, Lightfoot, & Cox, 1993; Wittig & Petersen, 1979). We have made the arbitrary decision to place this area of research in the section on biology, mainly because the majority of the researchers of the empirical studies to be reviewed appeared to be inclined to approach the problem from a biological perspective.

Intersex Conditions

The literature on cognitive abilities and intersex conditions (along with the literature on individuals exposed to exogenously induced atypical hormonal environments) has been reviewed in detail many times (e.g., Collaer & Hines, 1995; Hines, 1982; Hines & Collaer, 1993; Nyborg, 1984; Reinisch & Sanders, 1992; Reinisch, Ziemba-Davis, & Sanders, 1991), so this task is not repeated here. It will suffice to note that many quasi-experimental studies have supported the hypothesis that the prenatal hormonal milieu is associated with sex-related patterns of cognitive ability. For example, Resnick, Berenbaum, Gottesman, and Bouchard (1986) found that women with CAH showed performance superior to that of unaffected female relatives on several tests of spatial ability. In another study, Hier and Crowley (1982) reported that men with idiopathic hypogonadotropic hypogonadism had impaired spatial ability, but not verbal ability, compared to normal controls.

Sexual Orientation

Eleven studies have examined the cognitive abilities of heterosexual and homosexual men and women, employing measures that, on average, have yielded significant sex differences. Unlike the work on inter-sex conditions, this research has not been systematically reviewed, so we do so here. Table 6.4 provides information on sample sizes, sex, sexual orientation, measures, and a summary of the results.

The research questions under consideration have been rather straightforward. It was hypothesized that homosexual men and hetero-sexual women would outperform heterosexual men on verbal tests, whereas heterosexual men would outperform homosexual men and heterosexual women on certain spatial tests. For homosexual women, the inverse of such patterns was expected.

Regarding men, two studies used selected subtests from the Wechsler Adult Intelligence Scale (WAIS) to test these hypotheses. Willmott and Brierly (1984) found that homosexual men outperformed heterosexual men on the Verbal subtests, but underperformed on the Performance (i.e., spatial) subtests. However, Tuttle and Pillard's (1991) results were more equivocal; in fact, on selected Performance subtests, the homosexual men tended to perform better than the heterosexual men.

Both studies contained participants who were generally quite intelligent, suggesting that the samples were unusually skewed for this trait. From Willmott (1975), it could be determined that 60% of the participants had a prorated Verbal and/or Performance IQ $\geq$ 130! Another methodological issue concerns measurement selection. In a review of the WAIS literature, Snow and Weinstock (1990) concluded that there was little evidence for sex differences in Verbal IQ or Performance IQ. Similarly, sex differences on specific subtests, when they occurred, were of small effect size. Thus, the use of WAIS subtests may not be the best strategy to test for within-sex sexual orientation differences in cognitive function (Halpern, 1992).

Four studies used other tests of verbal ability in comparing homosexual and heterosexual men. Gladue, Beatty, Larson, and Staton (1990), McCormick and Witelson (1991), and Moose (1993) found no significant differences, whereas Tkachuk and Zucker (1991) found that heterosexual men outperformed homosexual men on the Peabody Picture Vocabulary Test—Revised (PPVT-R), a test of receptive word knowledge. In this last study, however, the homosexual men were significantly older and slightly less well educated, which may have contributed to the difference.

Using spatial tests that show reasonably strong sex differences favoring males, seven studies found that heterosexual men outperformed homosexual men on at least one measure (Gladue et al., 1990; Hall & Kimura, 1995; McCormick & Witelson, 1991; Sanders & Ross-Field, 1986a, Exps. 1–2; Sanders & Wright, 1993; Tkachuk & Zucker,

1991). In all of these studies, the heterosexual men also outperformed the heterosexual women on the tests that yielded the within-sex sexual orientation effect. In one other study (Tuttle & Pillard, 1991), the homosexual men performed midway between the heterosexual men and heterosexual women, although in the other studies, the homosexual men generally performed at a level comparable to that of the heterosexual women (for one exception on one measure, see Gladue et al., 1990). In the study by McCormick and Witelson (1991), there were also complicated and inconsistent interaction effects with handedness.

The two most recent studies on spatial ability by Moose (1993) and Gladue and Bailey (1995) have, however, thrown a monkey wrench into these previous findings. Both studies failed to find significant within-sex sexual orientation effects for homosexual and heterosexual men, even though the Gladue and Bailey study had a larger sample size than any of the previous investigations. The statistical methods were rigorous, and the recruitment technique did not appear notably different from those used in the previous investigations.

Regarding women, five studies all found no sexual orientation effects in verbal ability (Gladue et al., 1990; McCormick, 1990; Moose, 1993; Tkachuk & Zucker, 1991; Tuttle & Pillard, 1991). On tests of spatial ability, four studies found no significant differences (Gladue & Bailey, 1995; McCormick, 1990; Tkachuk & Zucker, 1991; Tuttle & Pillard, 1991). In two other studies, the results were negative or inconsistent. On the Mental Rotations Test (MRT), both Gladue et al. (1990) and Moose (1993) found no significant differences; on the Water Jar Test (WJT), Gladue et al. found that the heterosexual women performed better than the homosexual women, whereas Moose found the opposite! Lastly, Hall and Kimura (1995) found a trend for homosexual women to outperform heterosexual women on a targeted throwing task.

To sum up, the results of studies to date examining the relation between putatively sex-dimorphic cognitive abilities and sexual orientation have yielded largely negative findings for females. For males, significant effects have been almost entirely in the domain of spatial ability, but there are now two recent negative exceptions (Gladue & Bailey, 1995; Moose, 1993).

Can the pattern of results be placed in a broader perspective, and what lines of inquiry might be best pursued? If anything, the data so far suggest sexual orientation effects for males in the area of spatial ability, not verbal ability. Perhaps this is the case because the sex difference in effect size is stronger for spatial ability than it is for verbal ability (Halperin, 1992). Alternatively, it is possible that researchers have not employed the most potent verbal tests that have yielded sex differences.

TABLE 6.4. Cognitive Abilities and Sexual Orientation (SO)

Study	n	SO-Sex	Measures	Results
Willmott & Brierly (1984)	20 20 18	HS-M HT-M HT-F[a]	WAIS Verbal and Performance subtests	Verbal: HS-M > HT-M HT-F = HS-M,HT-M Performance: HT-M > HT-F = HS-M
Sanders & Ross-Field (1986a, Exp. 1)	8 8 8	HS-M HT-M HT-F	WJT	WJT: HT-M > HT-F = HS-M
Sanders & Ross-Field (1986b, Exp. 2)	13 13 13	HS-M HT-M HT-F	WJT Vincent Mechanical Diagrams (VMD)	WJT: HT-M > HT-F = HS-M VMD: HT-M > HT-F = HS-M
Gladue et al. (1990)	16 16 15 15	HS-M HT-M HS-F HT-F	MRT WJT Fargo Map Test, revised (FMT) Everyday Spatial Activities Test (EAST) Verbal ability (SH and oral word association)	Verbal ability: no differences MRT: HT-M > HS-M; HT-F = HS-F WJT: HT > HS for average deviation from horizontal; no differences for number of correct responses FMT: M > F EAST: M > F (trend) for mechanical drawing; F > M (trend) for arranging objects
McCormick (1990)	31 31 31	HS-F HT-F HT-M	Verbal ability (WAIS Digit Symbol, Animal Naming) WJT Spatial Relations subtest of the PMA Spatial Relations subtest of the DAT	Verbal ability: no differences WJT: HT-M > HT-F = HS-F PMA: HT-M > HT-F = HS-F DAT: HT-M > HT-F = HS-F
McCormick & Witelson (1991)	38 38 38	HS-M HT-M HT-F	Verbal ability (WAIS Digit Symbol, Animal Naming) WJT Spatial Relations subtest of the PMA Spatial Relations subtest of the DAT	Verbal ability: no differences WJT: HT-M > HS-M = HT-F PMA: HT-M > HS-M = HT-F DAT: HT-M > HS-M = HT-F

164

Study	Groups	N	Tests	Results
Tkachuk & Zucker (1991)	HS-M HT-M HS-F HT-F	24 26 21 30	MRT WJT PPVT-R	MRT: HT-M > HS-M = HT-F = HS-F (trend) WJT: no differences PPVT: HT-M > HS-M; HS-F > HT-F
Tuttle & Pillard (1991)	HS-M HT-M HS-F HT-F	49 47 34 34	WAIS Verbal and Performance subtests Spatial Relations subtest of the PMA	Verbal: HS-M > HT-M (trend) Performance: HS-M > HT-M (trend) Spatial Relations: HT-M > HT-F No differences between HS-F and HT-F on any measure
Moose (1993)	HS-M BS-M HT-M HT-F BS-F HT-F	15 15 15 16 17 17	MRT WJT SH	MRT: BS > HT; BS = HS; HS = HT WJT: HT-M = BS-M = HS-F = BS-F > HT-F; HS-M = HT-F SH: BS > HT; BS = HS; HS = HT
Sanders & Wright (1993)	HS-M HT-M HT-F	15 15 15	Throw Task ("male biased") Purdue Pegboard ("female-biased")	Throw Task: HT-M > HS-M, HT-F Purdue Pegboard: HT-F = HS-M > HT-M
Gladue & Bailey (1995)	HS-M HT-M HS-F HT-F	72 76 68 73	MRT WJT	MRT: M > F WJT: M > F
Hall & Kimura (1995)	HS-M HT-M HS-F HT-F	34 28 12 20	Throw Task ("male-biased") Purdue Pegboard ("female-biased")	Throw Task: HT-M > HS-M; HT-M > HT-F; HS-F > HT-F, HS-M > HS-M (trends) Purdue Pegboard: F > M

Note. HS, homosexual; BS, bisexual; HT, heterosexual. WAIS, Wechsler Adult Intelligence Scale; WJT, Water Jar Test; MRT, Mental Rotations Test; SH, Shipley–Hartford; PMA, Primary Mental Abilities Test; DAT, Differential Aptitudes Test; PPVT, Peabody Picture Vocabulary Test—Revised.

[a] Two homosexual women were also included in the sample of women.

Future empirical inquiry should also attempt to clarify individual differences in cognitive ability patterns within sexual orientation groups. For example, apart from any putative biological influence, there may be important experiential factors that affect sex-dimorphic cognitive function. There is some evidence, for instance, that childhood gender identity patterns are associated with spatial ability in adults (Krasnoff, Walker, & Howard, 1989). Only one of the studies reviewed above (Tkachuk & Zucker, 1991) attempted to examine such a relation, with largely negative results, but the sample size was small. Ideally, it would be informative to develop purer subgroups of homosexual men and women—those with versus those without a clear childhood history of cross-gender identification—and then to examine linkages with adult patterns of cognitive ability.

Transsexualism

Little attention has been given to patterns of cognitive ability in transsexuals who are biological males, and still less to such patterns in those who are biological females. On the WAIS, evidence for differential cognitive performance on the Verbal and Performance subtests has been equivocal (Hunt, Carr, & Hampson, 1981; Kenna & Hoenig, 1978, 1979; Money & Epstein, 1967).

La Torre, Gossmann, and Piper (1976) studied 8 preoperative male-to-female transsexuals and 26 presumably heterosexual controls (12 men, 14 women) who were comparable in age and education. They were administered tests of "cognitive style" (field independence–dependence) and spatial ability. On the Embedded Figures Test, the control males performed better than the transsexuals and the females, respectively. The transsexuals took longer to complete the Porteus Maze Test than did the two control groups, which did not differ from each other. On the O'Connor Finger Dexterity Test, the transsexuals also performed less well than the control groups, which differed from each other in the predicted direction only on the first half of the task.

Cohen-Kettenis, Doorn, and Gooren (1992) studied 29 right-handed male-to-female and 8 right-handed female-to-male transsexuals, who were matched with controls for age, sex, and education. All of the transsexuals were attracted sexually to members of their original biological sex. On a mental rotations test, the male-to-female transsexuals performed less well than male controls, whereas the reverse was found for female-to-male transsexuals, but in both instances the differences fell short of statistical significance. On a verbal memory test, the male-to-female transsexuals performed better than male controls, whereas the reverse was found for female-to-male transsexuals; however, the difference was significant only for the male transsexuals.

Unfortunately, these studies have a number of methodological problems. Money and Epstein (1967), Kenna and Hoenig (1979), and Hunt et al. (1981) all combined homosexual and nonhomosexual transsexuals, which probably weakened the likelihood of detecting sex-atypical cognitive ability patterns. The study by Hunt et al. (1981) clearly contained a biased subgroup of gender-dysphoric adults, since these authors tested only about 10% of their referrals. None of these studies employed concurrent controls. Cohen-Kettenis et al.'s (1992) study suggests that the relative deficit in spatial ability shown in some of the studies of homosexual men may also be present in transsexual men with a homosexual orientation.

Gender Identity Disorder in Children

Money and Epstein (1967) administered the Wechsler Intelligence Scale for Children (WISC) or the WAIS to 19 "effeminate" boys and adolescents (mean age = 11.25 years; range = 5–19 years). Verbal IQ (M = 114.5) was significantly higher than Performance IQ (M = 106.9), and the Verbal Comprehension factor score was significantly higher than the Perceptual Organization factor score.

Our group has also studied in a limited way the cognitive functioning of children with gender identity disorder (Finegan, Zucker, Bradley, & Doering, 1982; Grimshaw, Zucker, Bradley, Lowry, & Mitchell, 1991; and our own unpublished data). In 164 boys (mean age = 7.1 years; SD = 2.4 years), the range in IQ was 48–139 with a mean of 108.0, which falls at the high end of the average range. In contrast to Money and Epstein (1967), we found no significant difference between Verbal IQ and Performance IQ or between the Verbal Comprehension and Perceptual Organization factor scores.

In 25 girls (mean age = 8.0 years; SD = 3.0 years), the mean IQ was 106.8 with a range of 53–144; there were no significant differences between Verbal IQ and Performance IQ or between the two factor scores.

To study more specific sex-related aspects of verbal and spatial ability, we examined certain subtests from the WISC-R and the Wechsler Preschool and Primary Scale of Intelligence (WPPSI) (or their revised editions, the WISC-III and WPPSI-R). Vocabulary and Comprehension were selected as narrower markers of verbal ability, in part because of their very high factor loadings on the Verbal Comprehension factor score (Kaufman, 1975); Block Design and Object Assembly (or Geometric Design) were used as narrower markers of spatial ability, in part because they most closely index the construct of "spatial visualization" as discussed in the literature on sex differences (Kerns & Berenbaum, 1991; Linn & Petersen, 1985).

Boys with gender identity disorder performed significantly better on the verbal ability subtests than on the spatial ability subtests, t (149) = 2.1, p = .037, two-tailed (Figure 6.8).[9] Additional analyses showed that these differences held for boys who met the complete DSM criteria for gender identity disorder and for boys who did not.

Some of these boys were also compared with clinical and normal control boys who had served as research participants in several studies conducted in our clinic. The boys with gender identity disorder were pair-matched with the clinical and normal controls with regard to age and parents' social class and marital status. When possible, they were also pair-matched in advance with the clinical controls with regard to Full Scale IQ. In both comparisons, the boys with gender identity disorder did not differ from the controls on the verbal ability subtests (both t's < 1); however, they performed significantly more poorly on the spatial ability subtests (respective p's = .017 and .001) (Figures 6.9 and 6.10). Thus, the boys with gender identity disorder appeared, on average, to have a relative deficit on tasks that measured an aspect of the narrower cognitive domain of visuospatial ability. There did not appear to be a "compensation" of superior verbal ability, as judged by the comparisons with the controls.

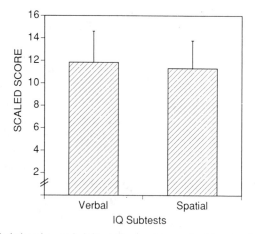

FIGURE 6.8. Verbal and spatial ability in boys with gender identity disorder (n = 150).

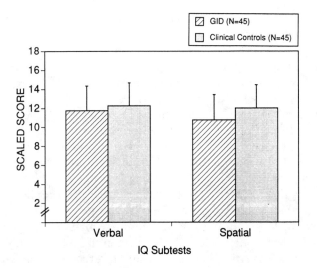

FIGURE 6.9. Verbal and spatial ability in boys with gender identity disorder and pair-matched clinical controls.

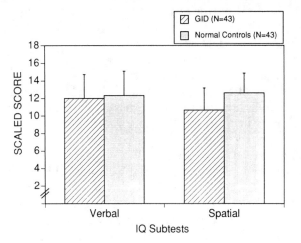

FIGURE 6.10. Verbal and spatial ability in boys with gender identity disorder and pair-matched normal controls.

For the girls with gender identity disorder, it was possible to compare only their functioning on the Verbal and Performance subtests. The difference was not significant ($t < 1$).

Coates and Friedman (1988) tested 25 boys with gender identity disorder, of whom 16 were matched to normal boys with regard to age, ethnicity, social class, and parents' marital status. The two groups did not differ in Full Scale IQ. On the Block Design subtest, the two groups also did not differ. For the subgroup of boys to whom the WISC-R was administered, the two groups did not differ on the Perceptual Organization factor (information on the Verbal Comprehension factor was not reported).

Coates and Friedman's study was an attempt to replicate our initial report, which included only 13 boys with gender identity disorder (Finegan et al., 1982). In both of our samples (including the much larger, updated one reported here), the Perceptual Organization factor score did not detect either between-group differences (Coates & Friedman, 1988) or within-group differences when compared to the Verbal Comprehension factor (our data); the latter finding differed from Money and Epstein's (1967) data. In the Finegan et al. (1982) paper, we reported a significant difference between Vocabulary and Block Design, favoring the former, in our sample of boys with gender identity disorder; there was also a relative deficit on Block Design when these boys were compared with either male siblings or clinical controls. Our much larger sample has enhanced our confidence in the validity of these findings. It is therefore possible that Coates and Friedman's (1988) failure to replicate them reflected unknown differences in sample characteristics or poor statistical power resulting from the relatively small sample size.

Assuming that our data are veridical, how might the relative deficit in spatial ability be understood? As noted earlier, the absence of a gross intersex condition in boys with gender identity disorder leaves open only the possibility of a hormonal influence limited to neural structures mediating cognitive functioning (cf. Hines & Collaer, 1993). Unfortunately, it will be difficult to test this notion directly.

Regarding psychological (experiential) influences, many researchers have argued that differential socialization of boys and girls contributes to the sex difference in spatial ability (this mechanism has also been viewed as explaining within-sex variations). One line of reasoning has held that exposure to, or encouragement in, stereotypical masculine activities should be associated with better spatial ability, and there is some support for this contention in both boys and girls (e.g., Connor & Serbin, 1977; Serbin & Connor, 1979; Serbin, Zelkowitz, Doyle, Gold, & Wheaton, 1990).

It is reasonable to presume that markedly feminine boys have less experience in activities that putatively enhance spatial ability. An indirect test of this hypothesis would be to show that the spatial deficit increases with age, since the relative uninvolvement in masculine activities would be expected to exert a stronger effect over time. To test this idea, we computed a correlation between age and the difference score between the Verbal and Performance subtests. Because social class was negatively correlated with age and marital status was correlated with both variables, they were both partialed out. The correlation was −.12, which was not in the predicted direction and not significant.

Another experiential hypothesis is that the deficit in spatial ability would correlate positively with degree of behavioral femininity (or negatively with degree of behavioral masculinity). To test this hypothesis, we calculated correlations between the Verbal–Performance subtest difference score and several of our parent and child measures of sex-typed behavior (see Table 4.8). Because the demographic variables of age, social class, and marital status were correlated with at least some of these measures, they were partialed out. Of 18 correlations, only one was statistically significant at ($p < .05$, one-tailed) and was opposite to our prediction; three other correlations were significant at $p < .10$ (one-tailed), of which two were in the predicted direction.

In summary, these data show that the relative deficit in spatial ability is a characteristic of boys with gender identity disorder that is unrelated to age (at least the age range under consideration). There were only a few significant correlations with sex-typed behavior, and the direction was inconsistent. Nevertheless, the relative spatial ability deficit appears to be a between-group characteristic and worthy of further exploration.

Neuropsychological Markers of Functional Cerebral Asymmetry

Handedness

Functional cerebral asymmetry refers to the differential processing of language and nonverbal (or spatial) abilities in the left and right hemispheres, respectively. An individual's preference for using the right or left hand in manual activities has long been viewed as an indirect index of functional cerebral asymmetry (e.g., whether language is represented in the right or left hemisphere). Men appear to show greater functional cerebral aysmmetry than women (McGlone, 1980), although the strength of the sex difference is modest (Hiscock, Inch, Jacek, Hiscock-Kalil, & Kalil, 1994).

Quite recently, there has been an interest in the relation between handedness and psychosexual differentiation, particularly sexual orientation. This interest was stimulated in part by Geschwind and Galaburda's (1985a, 1985b, 1985c) model of the origins of cerebral lateralization and anecdotal data: "Several homosexuals have written to us suggesting that there is a high rate of [left-handedness] in this population but no study of this has yet been reported" (Geschwind & Galaburda, 1985b, p. 546).

A central feature of the model posited that prenatal testosterone levels are related to the development of cerebral lateralization. More specifically, it was hypothesized that high levels of fetal testosterone during embryogenesis slow the development of the normally dominant left hemisphere, allowing the right hemisphere to become predominant and hence causing handedness and language lateralization to shift from the left hemisphere to the right hemisphere. It was deduced that the sex difference in the fetal production of testosterone explains why males are more likely than females to be left-handed, and also why males are more likely to suffer from developmental learning disorders involving language. (Hereafter in this subsection, LH is used as an abbreviation for both *left-handed* and *left-handedness,* and RH for both *right-handed* and *right-handedness.*)

In females, the hypothesis regarding handedness and sexual orientation is straightforward: An overexposure to testosterone, as predicted by the prenatal hormone theory (described earlier), predisposes to homosexuality and, as predicted by the Geschwind and Galaburda model, to LH. Thus, the synthesized model for females predicts a shift to more male-typical behavior—that is, increased LH and sexual attraction to females. In males, however, there have been two versions of the model's predictions. If homosexuality in men is the result of an underexposure to testosterone, as predicted by the prenatal hormone theory, then there should be a higher rate of RH (Lindesay, 1987), which thus predicts a shift to more female-typical behavior—that is, increased RH and sexual attraction to males. But Geschwind and Galaburda (1985b) modified this prediction because of Ward's studies of prenatally stressed pregnant rats (reviewed earlier), in which the male fetus responded with an initial rise, followed by a permanent drop, in testosterone and then more postnatal "homosexual" behavior—that is, increased lordosis. They then referred to Dörner and colleagues' work on the putative prenatal stress experienced by the mothers of homosexual men (also reviewed earlier). Citing these observations, James (1989) concluded that "it seems reasonable to suggest that prenatal stress is associated with both high and low levels of [fetal] testosterone (at different stages of pregnancy) and thus . . . with both left-handedness and homosexuality in the same individual" (p. 179).

Several researchers have examined empirically the relation between handedness and sexual orientation. Before these studies are reviewed, two comments are in order regarding the basis of these two interrelated hypotheses. First, although it is true that LH is somewhat more common in males than in females (see, e.g., Perelle & Ehrman, 1994), the evidence linking testosterone and handedness is largely indirect. In normal males, for example, it has not been formally demonstrated that variations in prenatal testosterone are associated with handedness (Grimshaw, 1993). Three studies of females with atypical prenatal hormonal environments have yielded mixed results. Nass et al. (1987) found that girls with CAH showed an LH shift compared to their unaffected sisters, although this difference was not significant when their entire sample of CAH girls was compared with the entire sample of sisters (some of whom were siblings of CAH boys). Helleday, Siwers, Ritzen, and Hugdahl (1994) reported no handedness differences between young women with CAH and age-matched normal controls. However, Schachter (1994) found an LH shift in women exposed prenatally to DES compared to control women attending a gynecological clinic. Second, the relation between prenatal stress and sexual orientation in humans, if our earlier review of the data is accurate, is far from certain. Nevertheless, it appears that if a relation was to be established between handedness and sexual orientation, then some neurobiological explanation would be required, since it is unlikely that psychosocial phenomena would provide a plausible alternative account.

Five studies have examined the relation between handedness and sexual orientation in women, and 14 studies have examined the relation in men. Table 6.5 provides information on sample sizes, control groups, measures, and a summary of the results. One additional study reported no handedness effects for sexual orientation in both men and women, but did not provide adequate information for inclusion here (Ellis & Peckham, 1991).

The data on women are reviewed first. McCormick, Witelson, and Kingstone (1990) classified subjects as consistently RH (CRH) if the right hand was used to perform all 12 unimanual or bimanual skills or as nonconsistently RH (non-CRH) if the left hand was used for at least one skill. The prevalence of CRH and non-CRH subjects was compared with data from Annett's (1970) study of 1,692 British men and women. They reported that 69% of the homosexual women were non-CRH, compared to 35% in Annett's study—a significant difference.

Tkachuk and Zucker (1991) assessed handedness with a continuous measure. Because males were also studied, the data were analyzed in a 2 (sex) × 2 (sexual orientation) analysis of variance; this yielded a main effect for sexual orientation at a trend level of significance ($p = .073$), indicating that the homosexual participants were less strongly

TABLE 6.5. Handedness and Sexual Orientation

Study	Homo-sexuals	Concurrent controls[a]	Referent norms	Handedness measure	Results[b]
			Females		
McCormick et al. (1990)	32	—	1,692 (M + F)	Annett (1970)	HS > referent norms
Tkachuk & Zucker (1991)	21	31	—	Oldfield (1971)	HS > controls[c]
Moose (1993)	16	17	—	Writing hand	No differences
Holtzen (1994)[d]	56	178	—	Self-categorization	HS > controls
Gladue & Bailey (1995)	68	73	—	Annett (1970)	No differences
			Males		
Willmott (1975)	17	17 (M) 16 (F)	—	Willmott (1975)	No differences
Lindesay (1987)	94	100	—	Annett (1970)	HS > controls
Rosenstein & Bigler (1987)	7	29	—	Oldfield (1971)	HS > controls (see reanalysis by Daniel & Yeo, 1993)
McCormick et al. (1990) and McCormick & Witelson (1991)	56	—	1,692 (M+ F)	Annett (1970)	HS > referent norms
Marchant-Haycox et al. (1991)	378	287 (M) 109 (F)	—	McManus et al. (1990)	No differences[e]
Satz et al. (1991)	993	—	ND[f]	Modified Annett (1970)	No differences[g]
Tkachuk & Zucker (1991)	26	24	—	Oldfield (1971)	HS > controls[h]
Becker et al. (1992)	1,612	—	845 (M)	Modified Annett (1970)	HS > referent norms
Götestam et al. (1992)	394	—	380 (M)	Modiefied Oldfield (1971)	HS > referent norms
Moose (1993)[i]	15	15	—	Writing hand	No differences
Halpern & Cass (1994)	149	149	—	Preferred hand use for four activities	HS > controls
Holtzen (1994)[d]	85	82	—	Self-categorization	HS > controls

(continued)

TABLE 6.5. *(Continued)*

Study	Homo-sexuals	Concurrent controls[a]	Referent norms	Handedness measure	Results[b]
Gladue & Bailey (1995)	72	76	—	Annett (1970)	No differences
Bogaert & Blanchard (in press)	843	3,600	—	Gebhard & Johnson (1979)	No differences

Note. As this volume went to press, Pattatucci, Patterson, Benjamin, and Hamer (1995) completed another study on handedness and sexual orientation. Handedness was self-rated for four behavioral tasks. Homosexual women ($n = 478$) were significantly more left-handed than heterosexual women ($n = 276$). Unlike any other study, homosexual men ($n = 273$) were significantly more right-handed than heterosexual men ($n = 246$).

[a]Same-sex controls unless indicated otherwise. M, male controls; F, female controls.

[b]HS (homosexuals) > controls or referent norms indicates that the probands were more likely to be left-handed or nonconsistently right-handed.

[c]Statistical test conducted simultaneously with data for males.

[d]Homosexual group included a small number of bisexuals.

[e]See text for our reanalysis.

[f]ND, no data (sample size not reported).

[g]Statistical tests not reported.

[h]Statistical test conducted simultaneously with data for females.

[i]Also studied bisexual males and females (see Table 6.4).

RH than the heterosexual participants. On the basis of self-report, Holtzen (1994) classified handedness as ranging from exclusively LH to exclusively RH and found that a smaller percentage of homosexual women than heterosexual women were nonexclusively RH (60.7% vs. 77.0%, respectively).

Gladue and Bailey (1995) used both continuous and dichotomous measures of handedness and found no significant differences between the probands and concurrent controls. Moose (1993) assessed only writing hand and found no effects.

Of the four studies of men with relatively small samples, but with concurrent controls, the results were nonsignificant (Moose, 1993; Willmott, 1975) or marginal (Rosenstein & Bigler, 1987; Tkachuk & Zucker, 1991).

Of the six studies with larger samples and concurrent controls, three found no differences (Bogaert & Blanchard, in press; Gladue & Bailey, 1995; Marchant-Haycox, McManus, & Wilson, 1991) and three found an LH shift in homosexual men (Halpern & Cass, 1994; Holtzen, 1994; Lindesay, 1987). However, we reanalyzed Marchant-Haycox et al.'s (1991) nominal measure and found that 11.6% of the homosexual men, 7.7% of the heterosexual men, and 6.4% of the heterosexual women could be classified as LH (homosexual men vs. heterosexual men and women combined), $\chi^2 = 4.21, p < .05$.

Of the four studies that utilized referent norms, three reported significant differences (Becker et al., 1992; Götestam, Coates, & Ekstrand, 1992; McCormick & Witelson, 1991) indicating more LH in homosexual men, and one study did not (Satz et al., 1991). Satz et al. did not report any statistical tests of their data.

Two studies have also examined handedness in transsexuals. Watson (1991) assessed 32 male-to-female transsexuals and 160 control males matched for age. On a dichotomous measure, 40.6% of the transsexuals were LH, compared to 11.9% of the controls—a significant difference. The continuous measure also differentiated the two groups. Watson and Coren (1992) subsequently reported additional data: The sample of transsexuals was now 45, of whom 37% were classified as heterosexual, 28% as homosexual, 19% as bisexual, and 16% as asexual. The control sample consisted of 225 males (five for every proband) matched for age, who were randomly selected from a larger sample of more than 10,000 subjects. In this article, however, a different handedness inventory was described. The percentages of LH in the two groups were 35.6% and 11.6%, respectively. Among the transsexuals, the percentage of LH was reported not to differ by sexual orientation.

Orlebeke, Boomsma, Gooren, Verschoor, and van den Bree (1992) assessed 93 male-to-female and 44 female-to-male transsexuals from the Netherlands. A trichotomous handedness classification did not distinguish the male and female transsexuals; however, compared to age-matched subjects from the general population of the Netherlands ($n = 4,769$; Van den Brekel, 1986), the proportion of LH transsexuals was significantly higher (19% vs. 11.2%, respectively).

To sum up, the data on handedness and sexual orientation appear equivocal, and the acceptance in the literature that there is an empirical phenomenon to be explained seems premature (cf. Bancroft, 1994; Coren, 1992, pp. 199–202; Halpern & Coren, 1993, p. 239). Let us consider some of the methodological ambiguities of the extant studies.

1. How handedness was operationalized varied considerably across studies. For example, McCormick et al. (1990) and McCormick and Witelson (1991) classified subjects as non-CRH if at least one task was performed with the left hand. In contrast, Satz et al. (1991) classified subjects as mixed-handed or LH according to more conservative criteria; this could explain why the two groups reached different conclusions. The different classification rules also account for the highly divergent percentage of subjects classified as non-CRH (about 45% vs. about 13–16%).

There are different views regarding the most valid way to classify handedness patterns. Steenhuis, Bryden, Schwartz, and Lawson (1990) noted that the stability of handedness classification is weakest among mixed-handers, so placing reliance on single responses, as was done by McCormick et al. (1990), could contribute to measurement error.

2. Some studies relied primarily on writing hand to classify handedness (e.g., Bogaert & Blanchard, in press; Moose, 1993), whereas others used more diverse measures. In McCormick et al. (1990), the use of the writing hand alone yielded no significant effects, but there were significant differences when other manual tasks were used to classify subjects as CRH or non-CRH.

3. Four studies of men and one study of women did not employ concurrent controls, but relied on putative norms taken from general population studies of handedness. There are risks in the latter approach. There is some evidence that handedness is associated with demographic variables, such as age and intelligence (e.g., Dellatolas et al., 1991; Gilbert & Wysocki, 1992); if variables of this kind are not controlled for, they will introduce important confounds. Becker et al.'s (1992) data are an example of this. LH was overrepresented among both the highly educated and poorly educated homosexual men, yet the reference group data were used without regard to education and associated demographics (Lansky, Feinstein, & Peterson, 1988).

4. It should be recalled that an underlying assumption of the handedness research is the existence of a sex difference in LH. But it should be recognized that this difference is rather small. Although no formal study has examined effect sizes for sex differences in handedness, J. M. Bailey (personal communication, September 1, 1994) suggests that it is "small" by Cohen's (1988) criteria. Thus, to detect within-sex sexual orientation effects, one would need rather large samples to achieve adequate statistical power. Unfortunately, the studies with the largest sample sizes (see Table 6.5) did not always assess handedness in the manner suggested by McCormick et al. (1990), which these authors suggest has better external validity.

5. Watson and Coren's (1992) study showed dramatic differences between transsexuals and controls. Unfortunately, they described their control group poorly; different assessment measures were reported in their two articles; and it is unclear whether the transsexuals represented a biased subsample of the subject pool. A clinical control group should be included in future research, since there is evidence that diagnostic groups of psychiatric patients other than transsexuals also show an increased prevalence of LH (see, e.g., Levine, 1980; Fleminger, Dalton, & Standage, 1977; Taylor, Dalton, Fleminger, & Lishman, 1982). Because diagnostic comorbidity is common among transsexuals (e.g., Levine, 1980; Lothstein, 1983; Meyer, 1982), it is unclear whether the appar-

ent increase in LH is diagnostically specific to transsexualism per se. Orlebeke et al.'s (1992) study of transsexuals is uninterpretable, since it defined handedness differently in the probands than in the general population reference group.

Watson and Coren (1992) reported no effects of sexual orientation on handedness among their sample; Orlebeke et al. (1992) did not test for sexual orientation effects. Because there is good evidence that, in etiological research, groups of heterosexual, bisexual, and asexual transsexuals should be collapsed and compared with homosexual transsexuals (see Blanchard, 1985a, 1989; Blanchard et al., 1987; Zucker, 1993), it would be important to examine this variable further in future research, since one might predict that only the homosexual transsexuals would show an increased incidence of LH.

In light of the initial studies on handedness, we began collecting such data on children and adolescents with gender identity disorder. As of this writing, we have collected data on 74 boys with gender identity disorder. Each boy was asked to perform 12 behavioral tasks (e.g., drawing a circle, throwing a ball, opening a jar) that were taken from Bryden, MacRae, and Steenhuis's (1991) questionnaire designed to assess handedness in children. For each task, the examiner recorded whether the right or left hand was used. Using different criteria of non-RH, preliminary analyses showed no evidence that the percentage of non-RH boys was disproportionately high as compared to the percentages obtained in normative studies of handedness in children assessed by questionnaire (Bryden et al., 1991). Before a definitive conclusion can be reached, it will be necessary to collect data on concurrent controls performing the same behavioral tasks. The comparisons with the extant normative data, however, suggest that the likelihood of detecting significant differences is low (G. M. Grimshaw, personal communication, October 6, 1993).

Neuropsychological Tests

Neuropsychological tests are also used to document functional cerebral asymmetries, which have long been noted to detect sex differences (e.g., Bryden, 1979; Kimura & Harshman, 1984; Levy & Heller, 1992; McGlone, 1980).

Sanders and Ross-Field (1986b) administered a dot detection task to the participants studied in Sanders and Ross-Field (1986a). The heterosexual men showed an advantage in the left visual field, whereas the homosexual men and heterosexual women did not.

McCormick and Witelson (1994) used a dichotic listening test to derive a laterality quotient (LQ) in both heterosexual and homosexual men and women, the same subjects who participated in the handedness studies described earlier. Because handedness is known to affect LQ, the data were analyzed as a function of sex, sexual orientation, and handedness. The results showed a sexual orientation × handedness interaction. CRH heterosexual subjects were more lateralized than non-CRH heterosexual subjects, whereas CRH and non-CRH homosexual subjects were not.

Cohen-Kettenis et al. (1992) also administered a dichotic listening test to their transsexual participants (see above). The RH male-to-female and female-to-male transsexuals were significantly less lateralized than the controls (but see Herman, Grabowska, & Dulko, 1993).

Given that the number of studies is small, it is premature to conclude that this line of research has identified a neuropsychological correlate of sexual orientation and, perhaps, of an inverted gender identity. When McCormick (1990) analyzed the data on LQ separately for homosexual men and women, there were no significant effects involving sexual orientation for women. In any case, the next step should be to establish the consistency of the findings in new and larger samples, with handedness carefully controlled for.

Neuroanatomic Structures and Anthropometrics

As with other putative neurobiological correlates of psychosexual differentiation, the possibility of neuroanatomic sex differences has long been controversial (Swaab & Hofman, 1984). In this section, we review some of the studies pertinent to atypical psychosexuality.

The Preoptic Area of the Hypothalamus

Swaab and Fliers (1985) studied the preoptic area (POA) of 13 men and 18 women (age range = 10–93 years). Morphometric analysis showed a sexually dimorphic cell group (termed the *sexually dimorphic nucleus* [SDN]) that was 2.5 times as large in men as in women and contained 2.2 times as many cells (see also Hofman & Swaab, 1989). This finding was consistent with Gorski, Gordon, Shryne, and Southam's (1978) original observation of a sex difference in the medial POA of the rat: "A cell group within this area revealed such a clear cytoarchitectonic sex difference that it could even be seen with the naked eye" (Swaab & Fliers, 1985, p. 1112). Swaab and Fliers were cautious in their conclusion, commenting that the "function of the [SDN]-POA . . . is unknown both in the rat and in humans" (p. 1114).

In a subsequent study, Swaab and Hofman (1990) examined the SDN in 10 nondemented homosexual men who died of AIDS, 6 nondemented heterosexuals (4 men, 2 women) who also died of AIDS, and 18 other male controls. The volume and cell number of the SDN did not distinguish the homosexual men from the heterosexual men. On the other hand, the volume of the suprachiasmatic nucleus (SCN), another cell group in the hypothalamus, was 1.7 times as large in the homosexual group as in the male control group and contained 2.1 times as many cells.

Swaab and Hofman (1990; see also Swaab, Gooren, & Hofman, 1992a, 1992b) were cognizant of the implications of their findings for the prenatal hormonal theory of sexual orientation development (described earlier): "The fact that no difference in SDN cell number was observed between homo- and heterosexual men . . . refutes the most global formulation of Dörner's hypothesis that male homosexuals have 'a female brain'" (p. 145). On the other hand, Swaab and Hofman wondered whether the SCN finding could be related to prenatal sex hormones on the basis of animal studies, although the SCN is apparently not sex-dimorphic (Hofman, Fliers, Goudsmit, & Swaab, 1988; Swaab, Fliers, & Partiman, 1985).

Interstitial Nuclei of the Anterior Hypothalamus

Allen, Hines, Shryne, and Gorski (1989) commented that because the POA shows the greatest number of reported sex dimorphisms in lower mammals, it would be a likely candidate for a similar effect in humans. Allen et al. noted that because some anatomists consider the POA to be the anterior region of the anterior hypothalamus, they selected the preoptic–anterior hypothalamic area (PO-AHA) for quantitative study. The normal autopsied brains of 11 males and 11 females (mean age = 48 years, range = 5–81 years) were selected from a brain bank of about 100 hypothalami.

Allen et al. (1989) were unable to identify any cell group "clearly homologous to a sexually dimorphic nucleus of another species" (p. 498). Accordingly, they chose for analysis four relatively discrete cell groups within the PO-AHA that stained darkly with thionin, which were named the interstitial nuclei of the anterior hypothalamus (INAH) and numbered from INAH-1 to INAH-4.

For each cell group, the dependent measure was its absolute volume. Males had significantly larger cell volumes than females for INAH-2 and INAH-3—differences that remained significant with brain weight covaried (Table 6.6). Allen et al. argued that INAH-1 probably

TABLE 6.6. Cell Volume (mm³) of Four Interstitial Nuclei of the Anterior Hypothalamus (INAH) in Human Males and Females

	Males (n = 11)		Females (n = 11)	
	M	*SEM*	*M*	*SEM*
INAH-1	.366	.024	.299	.030
INAH-2	.044	.006	.022	.005
INAH-3	.132	.019	.047	.010
INAH-4	.086	.017	.056	.012

Note. Data from Allen, Hines, Shrine, and Gorski (1989, Table 1).

corresponded to what Swaab and Fliers (1985) had named the SDN-POA, and they considered methodological differences between the two studies that might have accounted for the larger sex difference found in the Swaab and Fliers study than in their own. Although cautious about the functional significance of the observed sex differences, Allen et al. (1989) commented:

> It is interesting to speculate that factors such as prenatal stress that both feminize and demasculinize sexual behavior . . . and decrease the volume of the SDN-POA in male rats . . . may, similarly, contribute in human males to homosexuality . . . and to a decrease in the volume of the sexually dimorphic INAH; moreover, the INAH are located in a region of the brain influencing sex differences in gonadotropin secretion which may be altered in some homosexual men.[10] (p. 504)

Following Allen et al. (1989), LeVay (1991) measured the INAH in the autopsied brains of 19 homosexual men who had died of AIDS, 16 presumably heterosexual men, of whom 6 had died of AIDS, and 6 presumably heterosexual women, of whom one had died of AIDS. The age of the three groups of subjects was comparable (range = 26–59 years), although somewhat lower than that of the subjects studied by Allen et al.

As in the Allen et al. (1989) study, INAH-1 and INAH-4 were not found to be sex-dimorphic; however, INAH-2 was also not found to be sex-dimorphic. INAH-3 was found to be sex-dimorphic, thus partially replicating Allen et al. (Figure 6.11). Moreover, there was a sexual orientation effect: The cell volume of INAH-3 in the homosexual men and the heterosexual women was comparable, and both were significantly smaller than INAH-3 in the heterosexual men. Thus, LeVay (1991) re-

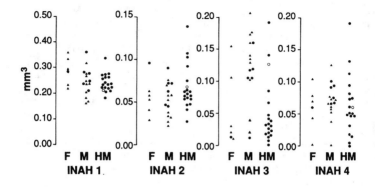

FIGURE 6.11. Volumes of the four hypothalamic nuclei studied (INAH-1, 2, 3, and 4) for the three subject groups: females (F), presumed heterosexual males (M), and homosexual males (HM). Individuals who died of complications of AIDS are represented by filled circles; individuals who died of causes other than AIDS are represented by filled triangles; and an individual who was a bisexual male and died of AIDS is represented by an open circle. For statistical purposes, this bisexual individual was included with the HM group. From LeVay (1991, p. 1036). Copyright 1991 by the American Association for the Advancement of Science. Reprinted by permission.

ported for the first time a neuroanatomic difference between heterosexual and homosexual men that also showed a sex difference.

The Anterior Commissure

In another neuroanatomic study, Allen and Gorski (1991) reported that the anterior commissure (AC), a fiber tract, was about 12% larger in women than in men. Because the AC may connect the two hemispheres, they suggested that it might underlie functional sex differences in cognitive abilities and cerebral lateralization; however, they also noted that the functional significance of the AC size difference was unknown.

Given the relation between sexual orientation and these sex-dimorphic cognitive abilities (discussed above), Allen and Gorski (1992) studied the size of the AC in the brains of 30 homosexual men, 30 presumably heterosexual men, and 30 presumably heterosexual women, selected from a larger subject pool and matched for age. A majority of the homosexual men and a small minority of the heterosexual men had died of AIDS, but histoneuropathology suggested that this did not affect the AC.

The average area of the AC at the midsagittal plane (mean ± *SEM*) for each of the three groups was as follows: 10.6 ± 0.5 mm^2 for heterosexual men, 12.0 ± 0.5 mm^2 for heterosexual women, and 14.2 ± 0.6 mm^2 for homosexual men. The AC of the homosexual men was thus 18% larger than that of the heterosexual women and 34% larger than that of the heterosexual men. The AC was 13.4% larger in the heterosexual women than in the heterosexual men, which replicated the finding of Allen and Gorski (1991). When Allen and Gorski (1992) recomputed their data after removing the results for the two homosexual men with the largest AC, the AC of the homosexual men continued to differ significantly from that of the heterosexual men but not from that of the heterosexual women. Furthermore, after adjustment for brain weight (which was the same for the homosexual and heterosexual men) the AC was 36% larger in the homosexual men than in the heterosexual men, but only 5.9% larger in the homosexual men than in the heterosexual women. Comparisons as a function of AIDS status did not alter the results.

Along with other demonstrations of neuroanatomic human sex differences related, at least in lower mammals, to sex-dimorphic behaviors (both sexual and nonsexual) (e.g., Allen & Gorski, 1990; Allen et al., 1989; Allen, Richey, Chai, & Gorski, 1991), Allen and Gorski (1992) concluded that it was likely that prenatal factors "operating early in development differentiate sexually dimorphic structures and functions of the brain in a *global* fashion" (p. 7202, italics in original).

Readers who track the sexual politics of our time will recall that LeVay's (1991) study received enormous attention in the print media (e.g., Angier, 1991a, 1991b; Begley, 1991; Gelman, 1992) and on the nightly news. LeVay made the obligatory appearance on television shows such as *Nightline* and *Donahue,* and has recently written a book describing his line of research for the educated public (LeVay, 1993). Comments by fellow scientists were both positive ("It's quite a striking observation, and as far as I know it's unprecedented" [Insel, in Angier, 1991a, p. A1]) and negative ("Nonsense" [De Cecco, in Angier, 1991b, p. A1]).

Discussion of Neuroanatomic Studies

From a scientific standpoint, LeVay's (1991) study was of significance because it opened up another line of neurobiological inquiry regarding atypical psychosexual differentiation in people without gross intersex conditions. By 1991, as noted earlier, research on the PEFE had stalled and there was no new direct biological work (the Hamer et al., 1993a, study, also described earlier, followed LeVay's work and that of Allen & Gorski, 1992).

Given the erratic history of previous biological studies of sexual orientation, several commentators have stressed the importance of independent replications (Byne & Parsons, 1993; Friedman & Downey, 1993a, 1993b, 1994; Meyer-Bahlburg, 1993b); as yet, no such replications have been reported. There has also been discussion of LeVay's (1991) methodology, some of which we comment on here. Unlike Allen et al. (1989), who had three individuals trace the INAH regions independently of one another, LeVay (1991) traced them alone. Given the apparent difficulty in identifying the borders of these regions (Friedman & Downey, 1993a), one would hope that the replication efforts will include multiple raters.

Both Byne and Parsons (1993) and Friedman and Downey (1993a) commented on the relative lack of sexual biographical information on the deceased subjects. Byne and Parsons also commented on the small sample size in LeVay's (1991) study, and Friedman and Downey (1993a) discussed the overlap in range among the three groups of subjects. In our view, these criticisms are not entirely convincing. Misclassification of subjects by sexual orientation would simply contribute to error variance and weaken the chance of finding a between-group difference. Significant differences with small samples make the results even more impressive than they would be otherwise. Overlapping scores are, of course, the rule and not the exception in behavioral research, so one should not be too critical of this drawback in neurobiological studies.

The contention that AIDS status might affect INAH cell volumes is a more interesting criticism (Byne & Parsons, 1993). Although both LeVay (1991) and Allen and Gorski (1992) reported no effects of AIDS status on their data, Byne and Parsons (1993) argued that "significant reductions of testosterone levels have been documented in end-state human immunodeficiency virus infection . . . and in some mammals, the volume of a cell group presumed to be comparable with INAH3 is dependent on adult testosterone levels" (p. 235). They speculated that the homosexual men who died of AIDS may have had a disease course different from that of the heterosexual men who died of AIDS, which may have differentially influenced the results. Ideally, the replication studies should include subjects who died of causes unrelated to neuropathies; it would be very difficult to do this, however, since sexual orientation is not routinely recorded at the time of death.

Lastly, Friedman and Downey (1993a) noted that studies of stimulation or ablation, cited by LeVay (1991), of the anterior hypothalamus and their impact on sexual behavior in nonhuman primates are of only indirect relevance for sexual orientation since these studies did not show a change in the direction of object choice per se (see Oomura, Yoshimatsu, & Aou, 1983; Perachio, Marr, & Alexander, 1979; Slimp, Hart, & Goy, 1978).

Dermatoglyphy

The most recent biophysical study of sexual orientation has turned to a research methodology familiar to physical anthropologists—namely, the study of fingerprint patterns, or *dermatoglyphy*. Hall and Kimura (1994) have noted that dermal ridges are formed by the 16th week of fetal life. The total ridge count on the fingertips is largely under genetic control, but can be affected by environmental variables, such as alcohol ingestion or maternal stress (see, e.g., Ahuja & Plato, 1990; Newell-Morris, Fahrenbruch, & Sackett, 1989). Some data on nonhuman primates suggest an influence of variations in the prenatal hormonal milieu on dermatoglyphic patterns (Jamison, Jamison, & Meier, 1994).

Kimura and Carson (1993) reported that men have a higher ridge count than women and that there is also a sex difference in dermatoglyphic asymmetry: Women are more likely than men to have more ridges on the left hand than on the right hand. Hall and Kimura (1994) subsequently studied ridge patterns in 182 heterosexual men and 66 homosexual men. The two groups did not differ in total ridge count, but the percentage who showed a leftward asymmetry (i.e., more ridges on the left hand than on the right hand) was significantly greater among homosexual men than among heterosexual men (30.3% vs. 14.2%).

Unlike the neuroanatomic studies, which are complex and difficult to execute for obvious reasons, the measurement of fingerprints appears rather easy. Thus, attempts to replicate the Hall and Kimura (1994) study should be quick in coming. Linkage to models of psychosexual differentiation, such as those pertaining to the prenatal hormonal environment, will be more complex (cf. Jamison et al., 1994); however, experimental animal studies might provide preliminary tests of the alleged association in humans.

SIBLING SEX RATIO AND BIRTH ORDER

Sibling sex ratio is the ratio of brothers to sisters collectively reported by a given group of probands. In white populations, the ratio of male live births to female live births is close to 106:100 (Chahnazarian,

1988). *Birth order* can be calculated with Slater's (1958) index—a proband's number of older siblings divided by the total number of siblings—which expresses birth order as a quantity between 0 (first-born) and 1 (last-born). Observed birth orders can be compared between groups or with the theoretical mean of .50 for samples drawn at random from the general population.

Sibling Sex Ratio

The relation between sibling sex ratio and sexual orientation, particularly in males, was first studied by several investigators between the 1930s and the early 1960s. Blanchard and Sheridan (1992) recently reviewed this literature and noted that homosexual men had been shown to come from sibships with an excess of brothers to sisters (e.g., Jensch, 1941; Kallmann, 1952b; Lang, 1940, 1960). Money (1970a) had also reviewed this pattern, but interest in the phenomenon waned, perhaps because the initial attention given to it had been guided by the inaccurate hypothesis that homosexual men were genetic females (see the beginning of this chapter).

Over the last few years, however, several studies at the Clarke Institute have taken another look at this somewhat forgotten biodemographic variable. We have examined sibling sex ratio in homosexual men (unselected for gender dysphoria), in homosexual men with gender dysphoria (transsexualism), and in boys with gender identity disorder.

Table 6.7 summarizes the studies on homosexual men. In all three studies, the sibling sex ratio did not differ significantly from the known proportion of male live births in the general population. Table 6.7 also shows the results of two studies on homosexual men with gender dysphoria. In both studies, the sibling sex ratio indicated a significant excess of brothers. Lastly, we examined the sibling sex ratio of prepubertal feminine boys (many of whom met the DSM criteria for gender identity disorder) and male effeminate homosexual and/or gender-dysphoric adolescents. Again, the sibling sex ratio indicated a significant excess of brothers (Table 6.7).

Birth Order

Regarding the birth order of homosexual men, which was also studied by some of the earlier investigators interested in sibling sex ratio, the two largest older studies found birth order indices significantly greater than the theoretical mean, indicating that homosexual men were born

TABLE 6.7. Sibling Sex Ratio (SSR): Recent Empirical Studies

Study	Number of target subjects	Number of siblings	SSR	Number of controls	Numberof siblings	SSR
Homosexual vs. heterosexual men						
Blanchard & Bogaert (in press)[a]	844	1,954	110.8:100	4,104	9,155	104.1:100
Blanchard & Bogaert (1995)	302	735	104.7:100	434	977	103.1:100
Blanchard & Zucker (1994)[b]	575	1,144	103.9:100	284	552	105.2:100
Zucker & Blanchard (1994)[c]	106	154	97.7:100	100	150	123.8:100
Gender-dysphoric homosexual vs. nonhomosexual men						
Blanchard & Sheridan (1992)	193	623	130.7:100	273	625	117.0:100
Blanchard et al. (in press)	83	246	134.3:100	53	166	112.8:100
Feminine boys/adolescents vs. clinical control boys						
Blanchard et al. (1995)	156	255	140.6:100	156	255	104.0:100

[a]Data derived from Kinsey et al. (1948) and Gebhard and Johnson (1979).
[b]Data derived from Bell et al. (1981).
[c]Data derived from Bieber et al. (1962).

later than members of the general population (Hare & Moran, 1979; Slater, 1962).

Figure 6.12 summarizes our studies of birth order. In the three studies of homosexual men, in three samples of gender-dysphoric homosexual adolescent boys or adult men, and in the study of feminine boys and adolescent males, they were all shown to be later-born.[11]

Summary

Taken together, the results from these studies suggest that sibling sex ratio is a biodemographic variable that distinguishes markedly feminine homosexual men (i.e., those with gender dysphoria) and boys with gender identity disorder from controls, whereas birth order is a biodemographic variable with an even greater generality—that is, it also distinguishes more ordinary samples of homosexual men from controls (i.e., homosexual men unselected for marked femininity).

Are there any plausible biological explanations to account for the birth order effect? MacCulloch and Waddington (1981) speculated that antibodies to testosterone, produced by a woman pregnant with a male fetus and passed through the placenta from the mother to the fetus, could reduce the hormone's biological activity and thus affect the sexual differentiation of the fetal brain (see also Ellis & Ames, 1987). Such

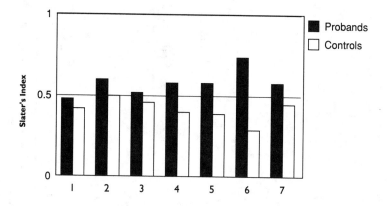

FIGURE 6.12. Mean birth order values (Slater's index) in samples of homosexual men (studies 1–3), homosexual transsexual men (studies 4–6), and boys with gender identity disorder (study 7). 1, Blanchard and Zucker (1994); 2, Zucker and Blanchard (1994); 3, Blanchard and Bogaert (in press); 4, Blanchard and Sheridan (1992); 5, Blanchard et al. (in press, Study 1); 6, Blanchard et al. (in press, Study 2); 7, Blanchard et al. (1995). Values can range from 0 (first-born) to 1 (last-born).

a maternal immune response might develop over several pregnancies (like the Rh incompatibility phenomenon), leading to a higher probability of homosexuality and/or cross-gender behavior for later-born males. This hypothesis implies that only older brothers will increase this probability, because male fetuses produce greater quantities of testosterone than female fetuses, and the testosterone produced by female fetuses does not pass across the placenta into the maternal circulation (Meulenberg & Hofman, 1991).

There are various difficulties with MacCulloch and Waddington's hypothesis, including the general nonantigenicity of steroid hormones, as well as the lack of empirical evidence that some pregnant women do in fact develop antibodies to testosterone. It is conceivable that maternal immune responses to other substances are involved, although the literature is silent on what these might be.

The data on birth order, if they do reflect some type of biological process, do serve as one concrete demonstration that genes cannot completely account for a homosexual orientation or cross-gender behavior in males, because purely genetic phenomena do not show birth order effects. The previously reviewed finding that a substantial proportion of MZ twins, who share both a genotype and a birth order, are discordant for sexual orientation shows that even the confluence of these factors falls far short of explaining sexual orientation, and that various other influences must be involved.

Regarding the data on sibling sex ratio, a biological explanation needs to account for the observation that the excess of brothers was observed only among males with marked cross-gender behavior. Biological explanations of this effect might be suggested by a review of factors already hypothesized to influence an individual couple's probability of producing male children, which does vary from couple to couple (James, 1987). Such factors might include sociobiological mechanisms, maternal–paternal blood group interactions, maternal and paternal hormone levels, and coital frequency (for discussion, see Blanchard, Zucker, Cohen-Kettenis, Gooren, & Bailey, in press). The influence of all of these factors on the human sex ratio at birth is still being debated by demographers and social biologists; thus their heuristic value for theories of psychosexual differentiation remains unclear.[12]

TEMPERAMENT DIMENSIONS: ACTIVITY
LEVEL, ROUGH-AND-TUMBLE PLAY

The complex construct of *temperament* has been sharply debated in the normative developmental literature. Typically, the markers of temperament are assumed to have a constitutional basis (although they are subject to environmental influence), to appear in infancy and show some degree of continuity, and to be objective characteristics of the individual (Bates, 1980). Over the years, various research efforts have attempted to identify dimensions of temperament in young children (for some reviews, see Hubert, Wachs, Peters-Martin, & Gandour, 1982; Kohnstamm, Bates, & Rothbart, 1989; Plomin, 1983; Prior, 1992). In this section, we review several studies that have examined two specific dimensions of temperament in children with gender identity disorder—activity level and involvement in rough-and-tumble play (hereafter abbreviated in this subsection as AL and RT play, respectively).

AL has long been recognized as an important dimension of temperament, and empirical studies have identified appropriate behavioral markers of this trait. In dealing with gender identity disorder in children, AL is a useful dimension of temperament to study because it shows a rather strong sex difference, with boys having a higher AL than girls (Eaton, 1989; Eaton & Enns, 1986; Eaton & Yu, 1989).

Bates et al. (1973) factor-analyzed a questionnaire given to mothers of boys with gender problems and normal boys. One factor, which they labeled Extraversion, included several items compatible with the concept of AL (e.g., "He jumps from heights and across ditches"), although other items on this factor were more interpersonal in nature (e.g., "He likes people"). Bates et al. found that the gender problem boys had a lower score on this factor than the normal boys. In a subsequent study (Bates et al., 1979), the gender problem boys were also found to have a lower score than a group of clinical control boys.

RT play bears some similarity to AL in that it is often characterized by high energy expenditure; however, a distinguishing feature of RT is that, by definition, it is a social-interactive behavior involving such sequences as "play fighting" and "chasing." Several studies have shown RT to be more common in boys than in girls, particularly in same-sex groups (e.g., Boulton, 1991; DiPietro, 1981; Finegan, Niccols, Zacher, & Hood, 1991; Moller, Hymel, & Rubin, 1992; Smith & Lewis, 1985; Whiting & Edwards, 1973.

Green (1976) had parents of feminine and control boys rate their sons' interest in RT play. As might be expected, the feminine boys were judged to have a lower interest in RT play than that of the control boys.

We have studied AL in both boys and girls with gender identity disorder. Items pertaining to AL and RT were taken from several other studies, including Bates et al. (1973) and Rowe and Plomin (1977), and a factor analysis identified a 17-item factor that was labeled Activity Level/Extraversion. Comparison groups consisted of sibling, clinical, and normal controls. Because the control groups did not differ on this factor, their data were collapsed. Figure 6.13 displays the results, which show a strong group × sex interaction, F (1, 468) = 45.7, $p < .001$. The boys with gender identity disorder had a lower score than that of the control boys, whereas the girls with gender identity disorder had a higher score than that of the control girls. Moreover, the score of the girls with gender identity disorder was higher than that of the boys with gender identity disorder, whereas for the controls the score of the boys was higher than that of the girls.

From these data sets, it appears that RT play and AL are important characteristics associated with gender identity disorder in both boys and girls. There are both biological and psychosocial explanations that account for this relation. Regarding biological factors, there is some evidence that AL has a genetic basis (e.g., Saudino & Eaton, 1991, 1995; Stevenson, 1992; Willerman, 1973). AL also appears to be related to hormonal factors, as judged, for example, by studies of girls with CAH (Ehrhardt & Baker, 1974; but see Hines & Kaufman, 1994, for no difference in RT play) and animal experiments that manipulate the prenatal hormonal milieu. In a study of 7,018 children from the National Collaborative Perinatal Project, Eaton, Chipperfield, and Singbeil (1989) found that early-borns were more active than later-borns, which is of interest in light of our finding that boys with gender identity disorder were, on average, later-born (Blanchard, Zucker, Bradley, & Hume, 1995). As noted by Eaton et al. (1989), the relation

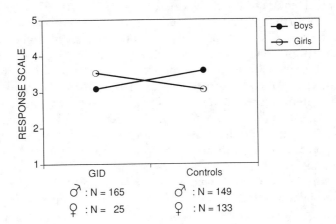

FIGURE 6.13. Maternal ratings on Activity Level/Extraversion factor. GID, gender identity disorder. Controls included siblings, clinical controls, and normal controls. Controls were participants in our own research (see text) and from Maing (1991).

between AL and birth order could be accounted for by perinatal hormone differences within a sibling line.

Regarding psychosocial influences on AL, Eaton et al. (1989) noted that changes within the family could be important; for example, older siblings are more verbally and physically aggressive than younger siblings (e.g., Abramovitch, Corter, Pepler, & Stanhope, 1986), and parents may be less tolerant of high AL when they have several children. It is also conceivable that aspects of the social environment exacerbate or attenuate the expression of AL (see, e.g., Fagot & O'Brien, 1994; Routh, Walton, & Padan-Belkin, 1978). There is, for example, some evidence that certain highly physical activities are perceived by children as more appropriate for the masculine social role (Pellett & Harrison, 1992) and that children are more active when engaged in masculine play behavior (O'Brien & Huston, 1985).

From a more clinical perspective, various hypotheses can be entertained regarding how a child's proclivity for active play and behavior could affect his or her social relations, particularly with peers. For example, a less active boy with gender identity disorder may find the typical play behavior of other boys to be incompatible with his own behavioral style, which would make it difficult for him to fit successfully into a male peer group. Similarly, avoidance of RT play may increase the likelihood that a boy will develop social affiliations with girls rather than boys, again on the grounds of behavioral compatibility (e.g., Biddle & Armstrong, 1992; Ignico, 1990; Thomas & French, 1995). Many clinicians experienced in the assessment and treatment of boys with gender identity disorder have noted their marked anxiety with regard to involvement in RT play (Coates, 1985; Green, 1974).

Unfortunately, no systematic efforts have been made to understand the specific role that AL may play in the genesis of gender identity disorder. In our own research, AL showed a negative correlation with age (see Table 4.8), which probably reflects a combination of age-related changes in AL and measurement error (the AL factor we identified contained items that were developed primarily with younger children).

One could postulate that the less active boys with gender identity disorder would be the most feminine, since they might be particularly prone to avoiding other boys as playmates and/or finding sex-typical feminine activities temperamentally compatible. To test this possibility, we correlated AL with several of our parent and child measures of sex-typed behavior (see Table 4.7). Because our demographic variables of age, IQ, social class, and marital status were in some instances significantly associated with these measures, they were partialed out. Table 6.8 displays the results. Of 17 correlations, 9 were statistically significant at $p < .05$ (one-tailed); of these, 6 were in the predicted direction.

TABLE 6.8. Correlations between Activity Level and Measures of Childhood Gender Identity/Role in Boys with Gender Identity Disorder

Measures	r	p^a	n
Parent measures			
Revised Gender Behavior Inventory for Boys			
Factor 1 (Masculinity)	.21	.004	156
Factor 2 (Femininity I)	.02	n.s.	156
Factor 3 (Femininity II)	.18	.013	156
Factor 4 (Mother's Boy)	−.01	n.s.	156
Play and Games Questionnaire			
Scale 1 (Feminine/Preschool)	.19	.009	156
Enjoyment	.21	.005	156
Scale 2 (Masculine, Nonathletic)	.15	.029	156
Enjoyment	.23	.003	156
Scale 3 (Masculine, Athletic)	.13	.055	156
Enjoyment	.15	.015	156
Gender Identity Questionnaire	.07	n.s.	108
Child measures			
Draw-a-Person (% opposite-sex persons drawn first)	.03	n.s.	163
Draw-a-Person heights (same-sex − opposite-sex)	.17	.018	161
Free play (same-sex − cross-sex)	.12	.086	145
Rorschach (same-sex − cross-sex responses)	−.13	.057	155
Gender Identity Interview			
Factor 1 (Affective Gender Confusion)	−.17	.058	93
Factor 2 (Cognitive Gender Confusion)	−.32	.002	93

[a]One-tailed.

Four other correlations were significant at $p < .10$ (one-tailed); of these, three were in the predicted direction.

In summary, there is some evidence that AL is associated with patterns of sex-typed behavior. It is obvious that a prospective design is needed to study the direction of effect more closely. Given the proband–control differences, the relatively low AL of the boys (and the relatively high AL of the girls) appears to be a very strong between-group characteristic.

PHYSICAL ATTRACTIVENESS

Variations in physical attractiveness are no doubt at least partially determined by objective, biophysical properties (Langlois & Roggman,

1990). Serendipitously, physical attractiveness was implicated as an etiological factor in one of the first clinical studies of boys with gender identity disorder (Stoller, 1968b). Maternal report of the physical beauty of their feminine sons during infancy led Stoller (1975) to remark, "We have noticed that they often have pretty faces, with fine hair, lovely complexions, graceful movements, and—especially—big, piercing, liquid eyes" (p. 43). Although Stoller (1975) placed great weight on parental influences, he also suggested that the extreme physical attractiveness of the boy served as a type of stimulus that facilitated parental feminization, particularly on their mothers' part.

Green (1987) and his colleagues (Green, Williams, & Goodman, 1985; Roberts et al., 1987) studied physical attactiveness in a larger sample of feminine boys and a male control group. At the time of assessment (mean age = 7.1 years), the parents of both groups of boys were asked to describe the faces of their infant sons. Masked ratings of interview transcripts and questionnaire responses showed that the parents of the feminine boys more often described their sons during infancy as "beautiful" and "feminine" than did the parents of the controls. There was also a trend for the parents of the feminine boys to recall more often than the parents of the control boys that strangers commented, "He would make a beautiful girl."

The extent to which Green and colleagues' data implicated objective properties of the feminine boys during infancy rather than parental retrospective distortions remains unclear. It could be argued that the sons' current femininity affected parental recall of earlier attractiveness. Recollection of the boys as feminine would provide a certain continuity to, or perhaps even an explanation of, the current behavioral pattern.

We (Zucker, Wild, Bradley, & Lowry, 1993) compared the attractiveness of 17 boys who had gender identity disorder with that of demographically matched clinical control boys. Facial and upper-torso photographs were taken at the time of clinical assessment (mean age = 8.1 years). College students who were unaware of the boys' group status rated five traits: "attractive," "beautiful," "cute," "handsome," and "pretty." With the exception of the trait "handsome," these traits were intended to be somewhat feminine in valence, in order to make them consistent with the clinical accounts of the physical appearance of boys with gender identity disorder. The boys with gender identity disorder were rated as significantly more attractive than the clinical control boys on all five traits (Figure 6.14).

These data therefore complemented and extended the parental recall data reported by Green and his colleagues. However, the extent to which the between-group difference in attractiveness was attributable

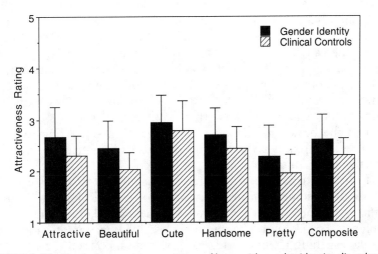

FIGURE 6.14. Physical attractiveness ratings of boys with gender identity disorder and clinical controls. Adapted from Zucker, Wild, Bradley, and Lowry (1993, p. 30). Copyright 1993 by Plenum Publishing Corporation. Adapted by permission.

to physical differences, socially shaped differences, or some combination of both remains unclear. It is conceivable, for example, that a structural analysis of the boys' faces would yield differences in the direction suggested by Hildebrandt and Fitzgerald (1979) to be associated with cuteness in infants. Along the same lines, infant photographs of boys with gender identity disorder might be analyzed to see whether similar properties could be identified. Such an analysis would be particularly intriguing from a psychosexual perspective, since recent studies have found that objective properties of infant faces, even the faces of newborns, are correlated with accurate predictions of biological sex (e.g., Gewirtz & Hernandez, 1984, 1985; Gewirtz, Weber, & Nogueras, 1990).

Regardless of the role of objective facial properties in determining attractiveness, clinical evidence suggests that the parents of some feminine boys, particularly the mothers, dress and style their sons' hair in a manner that might be construed as "cute" or unmasculine, possibly even feminine (e.g., Green, 1974). Clinical evidence also suggests that the boys themselves shape their appearance to create a softer, cuter look. This type of evidence implicates social (subjective) determinants of the attractiveness. When engineered by the boys, the heightened feminine-like attractiveness could even be interpreted as simply a symptom of the underlying cross-gender identification.

Our correlational data (Zucker, Wild, et al., 1993) on the relation between age and attractiveness appeared to implicate social influences. Age and attractiveness were substantially negatively correlated among the clinical control boys, suggesting that with age these boys were losing the features that elicited feminine-valenced attractiveness ratings. In contrast, the relation between these two variables was substantially lower in the boys with gender identity disorder, suggesting that with age these boys retained the features that elicited the feminine-valenced attractiveness ratings.

Physical attractiveness in girls with gender identity disorder has also received some clinical attention. Stoller (1972) noted that the mothers of some of these girls perceived them as relatively unattractive in infancy. For example, one mother described her infant daughter as "the ugliest thing in the world. . . . I was disappointed more that she was so ugly more than I was disappointed that she was not a boy. And then after a couple of days, naturally, these things went away" (quoted in Stoller, 1972, p. 54). However, Stoller (1972) described the "physiognomy and build" of such girls as "fine-featured and girlish. The . . . unpretty quality of the first months does not grow into a masculine look in bone structure or muscle distribution" (p. 60). Later, Stoller (1975) remarked that the premasculine infant daughter did not "*strike* the parents . . . as beautiful, graceful, or 'feminine' (whatever that would be to the parents of a newborn)" (p. 226, italics added). Thus, it appears that Stoller was more inclined to view such parental recollections as some type of retrospective distortion.

In Green et al.'s (1982) study of masculine ("tomboy") girls, their mothers indicated more frequently that other adults commented that their daughters "would make a handsome boy" than did the mothers of feminine ("nontomboy") girls. However, actual assessment of the girls' physical attractiveness was not made.

We (Fridell, Zucker, Bradley, & Maing, in press) compared the attractiveness of 12 girls with gender identity disorder with that of 22 clinical and normal control girls. College students, unaware of group status, rated five traits: "attractive," "beautiful," "cute," "pretty," and "ugly." With the exception of the trait "ugly," the girls with gender identity disorder were rated as significantly less attractive than the control girls (Figure 6.15).

In contrast to the correlational data obtained in the Zucker, Wild, et al. (1993) study, age was negatively related to the attractiveness ratings for the girls with gender identity disorder, suggesting that with age

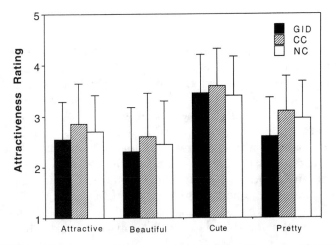

FIGURE 6.15. Physical attractiveness ratings of girls with gender identity disorder (GID), clinical controls (CC), and normal controls (NC). Adapted from Fridell, Zucker, Bradley, and Maing (in press). Copyright by Plenum Publishing Corporation. Adapted by permission.

these girls were being perceived as less attractive. In contrast, there was little relation between age and attractiveness in the controls.

SUMMARY OF BIOLOGICAL RESEARCH

In this chapter, we have reviewed the etiological (or quasi-etiological) literature across a variety of domains pertaining to biological influences on psychosexual differentiation. Only some of this work has examined children with gender identity disorder; the majority of it has sampled subjects with allied psychosexual conditions.

Regarding children with gender identity disorder, we have adduced evidence for between-group differences in the areas of cognitive abilities, sibling sex ratio, birth order, temperament (activity level and rough-and-tumble play), and physical attractiveness. In all instances, the underlying biological influences (if there are any at all) remain unclear and require further exploration.

Regarding allied psychosexual conditions, we have reviewed the evidence for contributions from behavior genetics, molecular genetics, prenatal sex hormones, maternal stress, neuropsychology, neuroanatomy, and physical anthropometry. Some of the work in these areas has just begun. For example, if we consider findings from molecular genetics and neuroanatomy, every positive result is based on only one study (or one research team), so definitive conclusions are obviously premature and the field eagerly awaits replication efforts. In other areas (e.g., handedness), the empirical returns have been mixed, complicated by methodological issues and perhaps a dubious theoretical rationale.

To conclude, it might be fair to say that we are currently in the midst of a biological *Zeitgeist* pertaining to psychosexual differentiation. Just in the past few years, we have observed novel contributions from several subspecialties within the biological and neurosciences. Because sexological research is conducted by only a small number of investigators, and is perhaps complicated by greater political pressures than those existing in other areas of research (Bullough, 1985; Gardner & Wilcox, 1993), future empirical work is likely to be slow in coming. But answers to the unresolved issues will only come from what is yet to be done.

NOTES

1. Throughout this section, it will become apparent that research on atypical psychosexual conditions has often been guided by assumptions regarding the origins of sex differences between biologically normal males and females. Why is this? The reason is largely conceptual. For example, in some quarters, homosexuality has been viewed as a kind of intersex condition—biological, psychological, or both. Ulrichs, a 19th-century gay German lawyer, was an early advocate of this point of view (see Kennedy, 1988; Ulrichs, 1864–1879/1994). Thus, the working hypothesis would be that a factor that causes a sex difference should also differentiate homosexuals from heterosexuals (in male homosexuals, toward the female heterosexual pattern; in female homosexuals, toward the male heterosexual pattern). A variant of this hypothesis focuses only on within-sex sexual orientation differences. For example, if a close father–son relationship predisposes to heterosexuality, a distant father–son relationship should predispose to homosexuality. In this case, a distant father–daughter relationship need not be posited for female heterosexuality or a close father–daughter relationship for female homosexuality.

2. As is well known, the study of genetic influences on behavior has a complex sociopolitical history. In a remarkably blatant form of character assassination, Ellis (1963), a prominent psychologist, remarked that advocates of the genetic hypothesis "turn out themselves to be confirmed homosexuals. This may be publicly stated because these writers are either now dead or have recently in print confessed to being homosexual. What I cannot presently state because of our libel laws, but which I nonetheless know to be a fact, is that many of the other most vociferous upholders of the view that homosexuality is . . . inborn

are also themselves sex deviants" (p. 176). Have times changed? Several years ago, a prominent child psychiatrist from the United States, whom we know, was asked to comment on the recent studies that we review here. The psychiatrist commented that this work was conducted by homosexuals with an axe to grind. From another vantage point, other critics of this research have expressed concern about its eugenic implications, recalling the Nazis' position on eliminating "these congenital defectives . . . for the sake of the master race" (D'Emilio, 1992, p. A14).

3. *Shared environment* refers to environmental similarities between children in the same family; *nonshared environment* refers to environmental differences between children in the same family (see Plomin & Daniels, 1987).

4. Earlier, Baum's (1979) comments on the distinction between behavioral masculinization and defeminization in higher mammals have been quoted. Application of these concepts to human psychosexual differentiation can be considered in light of the data on CAH females. Consider first sex-typed play behavior. The data suggest that the girls' play behavior is both masculinized and defeminized (Berenbaum & Hines, 1992; Ehrhardt & Baker, 1974). But caution is required because the assessment methods do not adequately permit an independent evaluation of masculine and feminine behavior; for example, in Berenbaum and Hines's (1992) study, if the girl was playing with a feminine toy, she could not be playing with a masculine toy. A better procedure would pit masculine toys against neutral toys and feminine toys against neutral toys (cf. Doering et al., 1989). The data on sexual orientation in fantasy suggest that there is both masculinization and defeminization; however, the data on sexual orientation in behavior suggest that there is primarily defeminization (e.g., reduced rates of heterosexual dating and sexual experiences), although this may be more a result of social pressure (e.g., homophobia) than of a distinct biological process. It is clear that further work, at both the biological and behavioral levels, will be required to test the applicability of the distinction between masculinization and defeminization in humans.

5. The material discussed in this section has benefited greatly from overviews of the PEFE by Dörner (1976, 1988), Friedman and Downey (1993a), Gladue (1988, 1990), Gooren (1988, 1990a, 1990b), Meyer-Bahlburg (1982, 1984, 1993b), and symposia at the 1986 and 1993 meetings of the International Academy of Sex Research.

6. Some critics (e.g., De Cecco, 1987) object to the use of descriptors like "deficiency" or "abnormal" in the discourse on the PEFE, since it would implicate an endocrine pathology in explaining a homosexual orientation. In respect of this concern, we have chosen to use the descriptor "sex-atypical." We leave the question of equating difference with pathology to others; however, we have not altered the descriptors that were employed in the relevant studies.

7. This refers to the controversial PEFE, discussed earlier.

8. One eager supporter of the theory (James, 1989) noted that "there is strong (though admittedly selected) evidence that Mary Queen of Scots (mother of James I of England) and Mme. Proust (mother of the novelist) both underwent extreme psychological stress during pregnancies which produced sons destined

to become homosexual" (p. 178; see also Weyl, 1987). For psychologists and psychiatrists, who have long been criticized by biological colleagues for relying on soft data, it is somewhat comforting to note that James, a biologist, published these remarks in the *Journal of Theoretical Biology*!

9. For these analyses, we excluded seven boys for whom English was not the primary language spoken at home and three boys who had either a Verbal IQ, a Performance IQ, or a Full Scale IQ in the intellectually deficient range. Data were also not available for three 3-year-old boys, who had been administered other IQ tests.

10. This refers to the controversial PEFE, discussed earlier.

11. As this volume went to press, Blanchard and Bogaert (1995) completed another study, which also found a late birth order in homosexual men compared to heterosexual men.

12. In part, we have included our data on sibling sex ratio and birth order in the section on biological research for reasons of historical continuity. Psychosocial explanations of these two phenomena have been largely post hoc. If one turns to the normative literature on psychosexual development, one could ask whether or not boys or men with an excess of brothers or who are later-born are more likely to be feminine. For birth order, the answer would be no. For sibling sex composition, the data are inconsistent: Studies of young boys suggest that having a brother increases the likelihood of masculine behavior, although one study of college students found that younger males were less masculine than older males in two-brother sibships (for a review, see Blanchard et al., in press).

CHAPTER 7

Etiology: Psychosocial Research

In Chapter 5, some consideration has been given to the putative role of nonspecific parental and familial psychopathology in the genesis of gender identity disorder. In this chapter, consideration is given to psychological variables that have been viewed as influencing individual differences in sex-dimorphic behavior. Throughout this chapter, it will become apparent that the bulk of the empirical research has been on boys with gender identity disorder. At the end of this chapter, however, we summarize our own clinical experience with girls with gender identity disorder, and discuss the similarities to and differences from boys regarding the psychosocial mechanisms that are reviewed here.

Because much of the material in this section will concern parental influences, let us begin with a comment on the "politics" of studying such influences on child psychopathology. In some quarters, the study of parental influences is seen as a form of "blaming" (e.g., Caplan & Hall-McCorquodale, 1985a, 1985b), which results in, among other things, unnecessary parental guilt. Regarding boys with gender identity disorder in particular, Zuger (1980) has written:

> When . . . the parents of an effeminate . . . boy ask the physician, as they often do, "What did we do wrong, doctor?", he should have no hesitation in saying, "You did nothing wrong. [This is a condition] for which we do not have [an answer]. What you did or did not do is most probably not one of the answers." (p. 56)

From a scientific perspective, it is, of course, important to evaluate the nature of the available evidence to determine whether parental factors are involved in the development and maintenance of child problems. Across many areas of child psychopathology research, the relative contribution of environmental and organismic factors remains open to intense debate. But even if one establishes unequivocal evidence for the importance of parental variables, this should not be construed as blaming. As any good clinician knows, blaming is poor practice and is helpful to no one. Rather, from a clinical point of view, one is interested in understanding. Kohut (1984) has articulated this perspective, and it is a view that we endorse:

> [T]he self psychologically informed psychoanalyst blames no one, neither the patient nor his parents. He identifies causal sequences, he shows the patient that his feelings and reactions are explained by his experiences in early life, and he points out that, ultimately, his parents are not to blame since they were what they were because of the backgrounds that determined their own personalities. . . . we must ask whether the parents were able to fill the specific or excessive needs of certain children, and, if not, why they were unable to do so and how specifically they failed. . . . in the case of any selfobject failure . . . we [do] not judge the selfobject's shortcomings from a *moral* point of view. . . . it [is] . . . completely out of keeping with the approach of the scientist whose aim is neither to blame nor exculpate but to establish causal-motivation chains that explain the . . . psychological data." (pp. 25, 33, italics added)

SEX ASSIGNMENT

That the physical markers of biological sex are psychologically salient is apparent in the moments following parturition, when someone invariably asks, "Is it a boy or a girl?" The configuration of the external genitalia usually makes it a simple task to announce the sex assignment of a newborn. In one study of parental behavior shortly after the birth of a newborn, Woollett, White, and Lyon (1982) observed that the majority of the comments pertained to the infant's sex.

Following sex assignment, parents often select a name for their newborn that has a stereotypical masculine or feminine connotation. Many books are available to help parents in these selections; the popular press routinely reports on the most common given names of boys and girls; and there are scholars (e.g., from the American Name Society) who actually study the psychology and sociology of naming (Lieberson & Bell, 1992). With the development of such techniques as amniocentesis and ultrasound, the fetus's sex can be identified and some parents select a name prior to the infant's birth.

It is common for parents to dress male and female infants in sex-stereotypical ways. Paoletti (1983, 1987) has reviewed the history of children's fashion in North America, including differences in how boys and girls were dressed. Throughout the 19th century and the early part of this century, it was common for infant boys and girls to be clad in long white dresses until they were capable of upright locomotion. As toddlers, both boys and girls continued to be clad in dresses, but male styles differed from female styles (e.g., in color, material, trim, and even in the placement of buttons—in the front for boys, in the back for girls). Paoletti (1987) noted that the practice of putting little boys in skirts has never been adequately explained, although one possibility is that it was related to the pragmatics of changing diapers. The placement of the buttons apparently took the direction of urinary flow into consideration!

In the 1920s, the tradition of sex-dimorphic "color coding" in pink or blue began (Paoletti & Thompson, 1987). Shakin, Shakin, and Sternglanz (1985) observed infants at a shopping mall in Long Island, New York, and found that about 75% of the females had at least some pink in their clothing (compared to 0% of the males) and that 79% of the males had at least some blue in their clothing (compared to only 8% of the females).

Sex assignment and subsequent rearing as a boy or girl have long been viewed as powerful socialization influences that account for sex differences in psychosexual differentiation. But because sex assignment and rearing of an infant as male or female are usually perfectly confounded with biological sex, researchers have long made the point that it is difficult to disentangle the relative contribution of biological and psychosocial influences. This is often forgotten by socialization theorists who adhere to one-factor models (Ehrhardt, 1985). Thorne (1993), for example, has recently commented:

> While many still see gender as the expression of natural differences, the women's movement of the 1970s and 1980s launched a powerful alternative perspective: notions of femininity and masculinity, the gender divisions one sees on school playgrounds . . . the idea of gender itself—*all* are social constructions. . . . Parents dress infant girls in pink and boys in blue, give them gender-differentiated names and toys, and expect them to act differently. . . . peer groups . . . also perpetuate gender-typed play and interaction. In short, if boys and girls are different, they are not born, but *made* that way. (p. 2, italics in original)

To be fair, theorists with a biological bent also emphasize single-factor influences. For example, Swaab, Gooren, and Hofman (1992b) assert-

ed that gender identity is very difficult to change, "probably because
. . . [it is] fixed in the brain" (p. 52).

The Research of Money and Colleagues

In contemporary sexology, Money and colleagues' work on children
with intersex conditions (hermaphroditism), beginning in the 1950s,
offered a novel methodology that could separate biological from psychosocial influences to some extent (Hampson, 1955; Money, 1952,
1955; Money, Hampson, & Hampson, 1955a, 1955b, 1956, 1957).
The genital ambiguity of some newborns with intersex conditions high-
lighted the salience of sex assignment. To which sex should an infant be
assigned? Indeed, it has been written that uncertainty about sex assignment is a "medical emergency" (Pagon, 1987) requiring immediate attention and resolution.

Money et al. (1957) observed that since hermaphrodites are "neither exclusively male or female, [they] are likely to grow up with con-
tradictions existing between the sex of assignment and rearing, on the
one hand, and various physical sexual variables, singly or in combination, on the other" (p. 333). Money et al. asked "whether the gender
role and orientation that a hermaphrodite establishes during the course
of growing up is concordant with the sex of assignment and rearing, or
whether it is predominantly concordant with one or another of the . . .
physical sexual variables" (p. 333).

From their study of 105 hermaphrodites, Money et al. (1957) concluded that "the sex of assignment and rearing is consistently and con-
spicuously a more reliable prognosticator of a hermaphrodite's gender
role and orientation than is the chromosomal sex, the gonadal sex, the
hormonal sex, the accessory internal reproductive morphology, or the
ambiguous morphology of the external genitalia" (p. 333). Only 5 of
105 patients had a "gender role and orientation" that "was ambiguous
and deviant from the sex of assignment and rearing." Money et al. noted further that the

> clinching piece of evidence concerning the psychologic importance
> of the sex of assignment and rearing is provided when, among per-
> sons of identical physical diagnosis, some are reared as boys, some
> as girls. It is indeed startling to see, for example, two children with
> female hyperadrenocorticism [CAH] in the company of one another
> in a hospital playroom, one of them entirely feminine in behavior
> and conduct, the other entirely masculine, each according to up-
> bringing. (1957, p. 334)

Money and colleagues' original clinical research led to an important conclusion: An infant with an intersex condition could be assigned to either the male or female sex and develop a sense of gender identity consistent with that assignment, despite having some biological attributes more typical of the opposite sex. Thus, it was found that the vast majority of genetic females with CAH (see Chapter 6 for a discussion of this disorder) developed a female gender identity after being assigned to the female sex, and presumably reared accordingly. Genetic females with CAH assigned to the male sex developed a male gender identity (see, e.g., Money, 1970b; Money & Dalery, 1976). This conclusion echoed that of Ellis (1945), who had previously reviewed the extant literature on 84 cases of hermaphroditism:

> The hermaphrodite assumes a heterosexual libido and sex role that accords primarily not with his or her internal and external somatic characteristics, but rather with his or her masculine or feminine upbringing. . . . heterosexuality and homosexuality in hermaphrodites are primarily caused not by directly hormonal or other physiological factors but by environmental ones. (p. 120)

Money et al. (1957) also emphasized the importance of an early decision about sex assignment (see also Money, 1965, 1987b). They recommended that the decision be made when the child is no more than 18–30 months old, and noted that "uncompromising adherence to the decision is desirable" (p. 334). Otherwise, it was claimed that the child would be vulnerable to "psychologic nonhealthiness" (p. 334), presumably related to a more conflicted or ambiguous gender identity (cf. Stoller, 1964a, 1964b, 1965, 1968a). In part, Money et al.'s (1957) recommendation of an early sex assignment was based on the observation that among intersex children who experienced a sex reassignment after the neonatal period, 11 of 14 children adjusted to the change without complications if the reassignment occurred prior to 27 months, in contrast to only 1 of 4 children who adjusted to the change without complications if it occurred after 27 months (Fisher's exact test, $p = .0379$, one-tailed; our analysis). Money et al. (1957) attributed this age effect both to the chronic ambivalence on the part of significant others (such as the parents) about the child's true sex, and to what they characterized as a "sensitive period" for the differentiation of gender identity (see also Stoller, 1964a). They saw this period as analogous to the period in which one's native language is established, and they referred to the nascent ethological literature on imprinting. More recently, Money, Devore, and Norman (1986) commented on the implications of delayed surgical correction of the genitalia for the child's self-perception.

Regarding the intersex youngster with ambiguous genitalia who is reared as a girl, Money et al. (1986) observed:

> She becomes subject not only to stigmatization by others, but also to self-stigmatization. In a world dichotomized by sex, if she does not look completely like a girl, then the only other alternative is that she must look like a boy, or a half-boy, half girl. Self-stigmatization leads the way to a self-generated development of a gender transposition . . . (p. 179)

Money et al. (1955b) theorized that "in place of a theory of instinctive masculinity or femininity which is innate, the evidence of hermaphroditism lends support to a conception that, psychologically, sexuality is undifferentiated at birth and that it becomes differentiated as masculine or feminine in the course of the various experiences of growing up" (p. 308). Diamond (1965, 1968) later characterized this as a theory of psychosexual "neutrality at birth."

If this theory is taken to its logical conclusion, then one could posit that a child with perfectly "normal" biological attributes could be successfully assigned and reared as a member of the opposite sex. Of course, an ideal test of this hypothesis would be to divide randomly a series of biologically normal newborns into two groups: One group would be assigned and reared in a manner congruent with their biological sex; the other group would be assigned and reared in a manner incongruent with their biological sex. For practical and ethical reasons, however, it is unlikely that such an "experiment of nurture" will ever be conducted. Thus, tests of this hypothesis have had to rely on special cases.

Money's (1975) report of a pair of identical male twins is perhaps one of the better-known examples of a situation in which this was done. At age 7 months, one of the twins was accidentally penectomized during a circumcision. By 17 months, the decision was made to reassign and rear the youngster as a female. Money (1975) reported that at 9 years, the child had adapted well to a female gender identity and gender role, although she had "many tomboyish traits, such as abundant physical energy, a high level of activity . . . and being often the dominant one in a girls' group" (p. 70). (However, this child's subsequent adjustment was less positive, as we note later.) Stoller (1975, Chap. 17) also reported on an 8-year-old-boy who was, for all practical purposes, being raised as a girl; unfortunately, long-term follow-up was unavailable (H. P. von Hahn, personal communication, March 2, 1983).

Challenges to Money's Hypotheses

Four decades later, what can we say about the status of the original observations about sex assignment and rearing offered by Money and his colleagues?

First, the notion of psychosexual neutrality at birth is probably incorrect. It is not clear that Money ever actually accepted this notion. Historically, his emphasis on the importance of psychosocial influences on psychosexual differentiation was probably intended to counter a biological reductionism that existed in some quarters of the medical profession. Moreover, he has long been associated with an interactionist perspective, expressed, for example, in his notion of a "nature–critical period–nurture" paradigm (for useful overviews, see Money, 1986a, 1991, 1993; Money & Ehrhardt, 1972).

But it is likely that Money underestimated biological influences on psychosexual differentiation to some extent. If, for example, we reconsider the data on genetic females with CAH (who constituted a majority of the patients in the original series studied by Money and colleagues during the 1950s), it is clear that their psychosexual differentiation does not perfectly mimic that of biologically normal females.

Second, the sensitive-period hypothesis has been questioned by reports of successful reversal in gender identity after toddlerhood (Diamond, 1965; Hoenig, 1985b; Zuger, 1970a). Perhaps the best-known example of such a putative reversal was the series of genetic male patients with an inherited form of pseudohermaphroditism known as 5-alpha-reductase deficiency (5-ARD) from affected families living in small villages in the Dominican Republic (Imperato-McGinley, Peterson, Gautier, & Sturla, 1979a, 1979b, 1979c, 1985).

Male infants with 5-ARD are born with marked ambiguity of the external genitalia; in the absence of a proper work-up, their genital configuration would be judged as female. During fetal development, an impairment of steroid 5-alpha reductase activity leads to an underproduction in plasma dihydrotestosterone, which causes the incomplete masculinization of the external genitalia. However, because testosterone production is unaffected, masculinization of the internal reproductive structures is normal. Moreover, at puberty there is relatively normal physical masculinization—both primary and secondary sex characteristics develop along male lines (e.g., the phallus enlarges to become, in some instances, a functional penis; the testes descend, if they have not done so already; the voice deepens; and there is an increase in muscle mass).

From a psychosexual point of view, 5-ARD attracted a great deal of attention. According to Imperato-McGinley, Guerrero, Gautier, and Peterson (1974), the newborns affected by this condition were often assigned to the female sex at birth and "raised as girls." The physical masculinization of these "girls" at puberty was so striking that they became known locally as *guevedoces*—"penis at 12 [years of age]." Imperato-McGinley et al. commented that after puberty "psychosexual orientation" was male in all of the 18 patients who had been reared as females (i.e., the patients perceived themselves as male, adopted a masculine gender role, and were sexually attracted to females). Imperato-McGinley et al. (1974) concluded that the "male sex drive appears to be testosterone related and not dihydrotestosterone related . . . and the sex of rearing as females . . . appears to have a lesser role in the presence of two masculinizing events—testosterone exposure in utero and again at puberty with the development of a male phenotype" (p. 1215).

As with Diamond's (1965) and Zuger's (1970a) reinterpretation of existing data (largely case reports), Imperato-McGinley et al. (1974) argued that their data represented a strong challenge to the sex-of-rearing hypothesis that Money and his colleagues had advocated. Perhaps because their data were based on a new group of intersex patients, it might be said that they generated a "crisis"; after all, they were putting one of sexology's cherished notions on the line. Moreover, as Ehrhardt (1985) noted subsequently, the Imperato-McGinley et al. (1974) study had practical ramifications:

> Many clinicians have become insecure and now seriously suggest assigning genetic males with 5-alpha-reductase deficiency to the male sex, despite the fact that they will grow up severely demasculinized and with ambiguous genitalia. Such clinicians believe that by puberty everything will be all right. The alternative suggested by some clinicians, to raise these children first as females and then switch them in adulthood to males, is equally naive and simple-minded. (p. 87)

Money (1976b) offered a swift counterstrike. This rebuttal centered on the psychological significance of the "folk prognosis" of *guevedoces*. Money argued that since the parents rapidly became aware of the impending physical masculinization at puberty, they

> could not confidently assign a newborn hermaphroditic baby as a girl. Even if the birth certificate was assigned female, the parents would know they were rearing a guevedoce who would not look feminine after childhood. Even in the first generation in which hermaphrodites appeared in two families in the family tree . . . before they could be defined as guevedoces, parents would rear their child

as one of ambiguous sex, not knowing what to expect at puberty. (p. 872)

In short, Money (1976b) was critical of Imperato-McGinley et al.'s (1974) assumption that these children were reared unambiguously as females: "[Imperato-McGinley et al.] provide no data on the procedures . . . used to evaluate either the parental–child relationship with respect to ostensible sex of rearing, or the gender identity of the hermaphroditic offspring (three of whom were deceased) when they were grown up" (p. 872). Quite directly, Money (1976b) challenged the competence of the psychological evaluation: "Endocrinologists should consult with their behavioral colleagues before entering into unfamiliar territory, including the territory of gender-identity differentation" (p. 872).

Imperato-McGinley, Peterson, and Gautier (1976) responded:

> Money obviously does not know how the parents raised these children. Our interviews with some of the affected males and their parents indicate that in the first generation, the affected subjects . . . were raised as girls and there was no ambiguity on the part of the parents as to the sex of the child at birth or in early childhood. They believed they were raising a little girl. (p. 872)

Imperato-McGinley et al. (1976) concluded by arguing that their data might shed light on the "relative importance of the sex of rearing, testosterone imprinting of the brain in utero, and the thrust of a definite male puberty on the determination of gender identity in man" (p. 872).

Imperato-McGinley et al. (1979a) provided a more detailed account of their patients than that provided in the 1974 report, including a description of the community's social life, the community's behavioral expectations for children, and the gender role tasks of the community's adults. They interviewed affected individuals and significant others (e.g., parents, siblings, neighbors) "to discern any sexual ambiguity in the rearing of subjects raised as girls and to determine in these subjects the validity of the change to a male-gender identity and male-gender role" (pp. 1233–1234). Their account stated that of 18 patients "unambiguously raised as girls . . . 17 of 18 changed to a male-gender identity and 16 of 18 to a male-gender role [during or after puberty]" (p. 1233). They summarized their data as follows:

> The 17 subjects who changed to a male-gender identity began to realize that they were different from other girls in the village between

seven and 12 years of age, when they did not develop breasts, when their bodies began to change in a masculine direction and when masses were noted in the inguinal canal or scrotum. These subjects showed self-concern over their true gender. A male-gender identity gradually evolved over several years as the subjects passed through stages of no longer feeling like girls, to feeling like men and, finally, to the conscious awareness that they were indeed men. (p. 1234)

Interestingly, Imperato-McGinley et al. (1979a) also observed that because the condition had become better recognized, the

villagers now either raise the subjects as boys from birth, rear them as boys as soon as the problem is recognized in childhood or raise them ambiguously as girls. Now that the villagers are familiar with the condition, the affected children and adults are sometimes objects of ridicule and are referred to as *guevedoce, guevote* (penis at 12 years of age) or *machihembra* (first woman, then man). (p. 1235)

Imperato-McGinley et al. (1979a) maintained their view that "environmental or sociocultural factors are not solely responsible for the formation of a male-gender identity. Androgens make a strong and definite contribution" (p. 1236).

As it turns out, two other forms of male pseudohermaphroditism (3-beta- and 17-beta-hydroxysteroid dehydrogenase deficiency) have an endocrinological natural history very similar to that of 5-ARD, and several reports have described the same type of psychosexual change at puberty as apparently occurs in 5-ARD (e.g., Imperato-McGinley, Peterson, Stoller, & Goodwin, 1979; Mendonica et al., 1987; Rösler & Kohn, 1983; see also Gross et al., 1986).

And on another front, Diamond's (1982, 1993b, 1994) account of the penectomized identical male twin mentioned earlier (Money, 1975) revealed that this youngster developed severe gender dysphoria by early adolescence and, as an adult, reverted to living as a male and was sexually attracted to females.

Conclusions

Can any light be shed on this extremely intense and important debate? It is our view that a better recognition of the differences between *sex of assignment* and *sex of rearing* would be helpful in resolving the controversy.

Sex of assignment is a relatively simple construct: By and large, one is assigned to either the male sex or the female sex. In contrast, *sex of rearing* is a much more complex construct. What does it actually mean to rear a child consistently and without ambiguity as a boy or as a girl? A central criticism of Imperato-McGinley et al.'s interpretation of their data sets (and of similar data sets) is that sex of rearing was ambiguous, not consistent (Ehrhardt, 1985; Ehrhardt & Meyer-Bahlburg, 1981; Herdt, 1990b; Herdt & Davidson, 1988; Meyer-Bahlburg, 1982; Money, 1976b, 1979; Rubin, Reinisch, & Haskett, 1981; Sagarin, 1975). Thus, given the relatively masculine sexual biology and ambiguous rearing of people with 5-ARD, it can be better understood why the reversal (if it can be called this) in gender identity occurred. The same argument can be advanced with regard to Diamond's analysis of the life history of the identical twin. We simply do not know enough about the patient's life circumstances to rule out fully the compounding role of social influences. Unless investigators can reach agreement on what constitutes consistent sex of rearing, this issue will never be satisfactorily resolved. For example, Diamond (1965) cited an example of a successful change of sex from female to male in a youngster with hypospadias who was allegedly "dressed and treated in every way as a girl" (Dicks & Childers, 1934, p. 508; see also Dicks & Childers, 1944). But our rereading of this case report suggests to us that the situation was not so clear-cut. Post hoc analysis, however, is far from satisfactory in re-examining this very complicated controversy.

Regarding the Imperato-McGinley et al. data in particular, a more refined analysis must be provided. It will be recalled that Imperato-McGinley and colleagues wondered about the possible importance of prenatal testosterone in gender identity formation. It should be noted that in their original report, the putative effects of prenatal testosterone were confounded with those of pubertal testosterone production and, possibly, ambiguous sex of rearing. A more precise test of the effects of prenatal testosterone on gender identity would involve patients who are surgically modified to look as phenotypically female as possible, whose gonads are removed, who are hormonally feminized at puberty, and who are reared unambiguously as girls (a situation reminiscent of the usual course of surgical, hormonal, and psychosocial events for girls with CAH). Unfortunately, little is known about the psychosexual development of 5-ARD patients treated in this manner. Money (1979) anecdotally described one patient so treated, who as a teenager was "consistently female in gender identity/role" (p. 771). Hurtig (1992) described the psychosexual development of two sisters with 5-ARD, both of whom received urogenital surgery and the maintenance of estrogen therapy. One girl apparently made a "satisfactory adjustment to her status as a female," but the other girl "rejected her female identity and has taken on the identity of a male, including sexual attraction and orientation to women" (p. 24).

Thus, from an interactionist perspective, one might posit that individuals with certain forms of hermaphroditism have a sexual biology that makes them more labile to psychosocial rearing conditions than biologically normal individuals are. Depending on psychosocial factors and the manner in which the abnormal sexual biology is treated medically, psychosexual differentiation will be, on average, more likely to move in one direction rather than the other.

Is sex of assignment important in understanding the etiology of gender identity disorder in children and adults? We think not. Sex of assignment is invariably in accordance with the external markers of biological sex. Are individuals with gender identity disorder, therefore, the exceptions that prove the rule (cf. Money, 1969)? In our view, the answer to this question depends not on the variable of sex assignment, but on sex-differentiated socialization influences (rearing). What is the evidence, then, that children with gender identity disorder are reared in a manner congruent with their biological sex and sex assignment?

Sex-related socialization is clearly a very complicated psychological process, and scholars of developmental psychology have looked closely at the evidence for differences in how boys and girls are raised. Below, we review some of the research pertaining to sex-related socialization, particularly with regard to parental attitudes, social reinforcement processes, and self-socialization variables. In other words, we attempt to decompose the construct of rearing into more specific components.

PRENATAL SEX PREFERENCE

It is not unusual for parents to express a prenatal sex preference; witness, for example, the recent explosion in "sex selection" clinics. Williamson (1976, 1983) has noted that parents tend to prefer that their first-born child be male, and it is also common that they prefer the next-born child to be female.

Other things being equal, parents will have a child of the nonpreferred sex about 50% of the time. Does this outcome predict atypical or nonoptimal behavioral sequelae in the child? In a descriptive clinical report, Sloman (1948) noted that of 62 "planned" children with emotional problems seen in a child guidance clinic, 9 (14.5%) had been "rejected" by their parents because of "not being of the hoped-for sex" (p. 528, italics omitted). Sears, Maccoby, and Levin (1957, pp. 57–58, 514) found that mothers were "relatively cold" toward newborn sons if their previous children were male. Stattin and Klackenberg-Larsson (1991) followed a Swedish cohort of children from birth to maturity, and reported that there was somewhat more parent–child conflict in families with a child whose sex was not consistent with the parents' prenatal preference. None of these studies, however, specifically addressed the issue of subsequent gender development in the children.

One might ask, then, whether parents of children with gender identity disorder had desired a child of the opposite sex. Although several clinical case reports of boys with gender identity disorder noted that their mothers had desired daughters (e.g., Charatan & Galef, 1965), only two controlled studies have investigated this question systematically.

Zuger (1970b, 1974) reported that of 21 feminine boys 38% of their mothers had wanted a girl (four other mothers simply reported that they had not wanted to have a child). A comparable percentage of clinical control mothers had also wanted a girl, but the specific percentage was not reported.

Roberts et al. (1987) found that mothers of feminine boys ($n = 52$) had not expressed a prenatal wish for a daughter significantly more than had mothers of control boys ($n = 52$). In fact, the percentage of mothers who had wished for a girl was low in both groups (26.9% and 19.2%, respectively).

In a third sample of 103 boys with gender identity disorder seen in our clinic (Zucker et al., 1994), 43.7% of the mothers had wished for a daughter. This percentage was significantly higher than the percentage reported by Roberts et al. (1987); however, a comparison group was not available.

Further analyses of Roberts et al.'s (1987) data and our own data showed that the maternal wish for a girl was significantly associated with the sex composition and birth order of the sibship (Zucker et al., 1994; see Table 7.1). Among the probands with older siblings who were only male, the percentage of mothers who recalled a desire for a daughter was significantly higher than among the probands with other kinds of sibship combinations (e.g., the probands who had at least one older sister). This pattern was also observed in Roberts et al.'s control group.

Although the wish for a daughter per se is probably not of etiological importance in explaining the genesis of gender identity disorder, maternal reactions to bearing a child of the nonpreferred sex may be. In our clinical experience, we have observed several quite striking examples of maternal disappointment. One mother cross-dressed her second-born son in infancy and took photographs of him in hair curlers and pink baby clothes. Another mother took 2 months to name her second-born son and then chose a variant of the preselected girl's name (Zucker, Bradley, & Ipp, 1993). During her teenage years, a third mother had given up an infant daughter for adoption. She was very disappointed

TABLE 7.1. Maternal Gender Preference as a Function of Sibling Sex Composition and Birth Order

Sibship categories	Boy	No preference	Girl	No data
1. Older brother(s)	2 (6.8)	4 (13.8)	23 (79.3)	8 (21.6)
2. Older sister(s)	10 (43.5)	7 (30.4)	6 (26.1)	15 (39.5)
3. Singleton	5 (41.7)	1 (8.3)	6 (50.0)	6 (33.3)
4. Younger brother(s) and/or sister(s)	12 (30.8)	17 (43.6)	10 (25.6)	7 (15.2)
Categories 2–4	27 (36.5)	25 (33.8)	22 (29.7)	28 (27.5)

Note. Values outside parentheses are number of cases. Values in parentheses are percentages. For the "No data" column, values in parentheses are percentages of missing cases for each sibship category. Data from Zucker et al. (1994)

when her second-born son was not a girl. She commented wistfully that she still "hoped" to "get a daughter" someday, and that she was quite jealous of friends who had had girls. A fourth mother wondered whether her feminine son was the "reincarnation" of a daughter who had died in infancy from multiple congenital abnormalities. Since she had longed for a daughter when pregnant with the proband, this mother acknowledged how deeply depressed she had been after her son was born. The depression continued unabated until about her son's third month, when a "look" in his eyes suggested to her that he understood what she was feeling. Considerable clinical work with this mother indicated that she interpreted her infant son's "gaze" as meaning that he now understood her need for a daughter. Lastly, a fifth mother kept a detailed diary during her pregnancy with her third-born son, which included repeated entries of prayer to God for a daughter. Similar entries occurred during her pregnancy with her fourth-born son. At this time, the third-born son began to show signs of cross-gender behavior, which increased notably after the birth of the fourth baby. The parents then placed their names with an adoption agency, requesting a 3-year-old girl.

In a review of our clinical cases to document such reactions, we found that they occurred—with one exception—only if the mother had wanted a daughter and had had only older sons. The one exception was a sibship with older boys and one older daughter (the "reincarnation" case noted above). The daughter was quite "tomboyish" and never behaved in a way consistent with the mother's ideals.

The reactions appear extreme, perhaps representing a form of pathological mourning (Parkes, 1975). They point to the importance of exploring with parents the possible meanings that underlie their gender preferences. In the family demography literature (e.g., Williamson, 1976), several variables associated with prenatal sex preferences have been considered, but these variables tend to be macrosocial in nature (e.g., economic, religious, ethnic), rather than psychological characteristics of individuals. In our clinical experience, the most common psychological trait that underlies the strong wish for a daughter is the need to nurture and be nurtured by a female child, which often reflects compensatory needs originating in childhood. For example, one mother commented that she wanted very much to dress a daughter in "frilly" clothes and to brush a daughter's long hair in ways that she had never experienced from her own mother. For complex psychological and cultural reasons, it is unlikely that such compensatory fantasies can be acted out with a male child. Unfortunately, no empirical study has formally assessed the reactions of mothers of boys with gender identity disorder, to see whether they differ in any systematic way from those of mothers of control boys. It would be particularly important to see whether these two groups of mothers react differently to the birth of a child of the nonpreferred sex.

SOCIAL REINFORCEMENT

Since the appearance of Mischel's (1966) seminal, largely theoretical essay almost 30 years ago, a reinforcement account of sex-typed behavior has been given much attention. In some respects, the notion that sex-typed behavior is socially shaped has great intuitive appeal, perhaps because of its commonsense, parsimonious nature. Yet it has been repeatedly pointed out that empirical confirmation of social reinforcement explanations of such behavior has been slow in coming; this view was advanced most forcefully in Maccoby and Jacklin's (1974) tour de force on the normative sex difference literature.

At least five overarching questions can be considered: (1) What is the evidence that parents (and others), on average, respond in sex-specific ways to sex-typed behavior in boys and girls? (2) Are certain specific domains of behavior responded to more than others? (3) Are there particular age periods in which differential parental responses occur? (4) Do parents (and others) actually shape sex-dimorphic behavior, or do they simply respond to differences between boys and girls that are already present? (5) Do parental responses actually affect the subsequent behavior of children?

Normative Studies of 2- to 4-Year-Olds

Because the behavioral signs of gender identity disorder usually first appear between the ages of 2 and 4 years (see Chapter 2), normative research on this age range has the most important bearing on etiological issues. Such signs most typically include toy, dress-up, and role play; thus, parental responses to these kinds of sex-dimorphic behaviors are of particular import.

Work by Fagot and colleagues has focused on the microsocial parent–child interactions vis-à-vis such behaviors. For example, Fagot (1978) conducted home observations of 24 boy and girl toddlers (mean age = 22.8 months) and categorized parental responses as positive, neutral, or negative to specific child sex-preferred behaviors—that is, behaviors engaged in significantly more frequently by boys or by girls (e.g., for boys, use of transportation toys, play with blocks; for girls, play with dolls or soft toys, dress-up play). Parents responded differentially as a function of the child's sex to four of seven sex-preferred behaviors. For example, they responded more positively to block play when it was engaged in by boys rather than by girls, whereas they responded to doll play more positively when it was engaged in by girls and more negatively when it was engaged in by boys (cf. Caldera, Huston, & O'Brien, 1989; Eisenberg, Wolchik, Hernandez, & Pasternack, 1985; Jacklin, DiPietro, & Maccoby, 1984).

Fagot's (1978) study (see also Fagot & Hagan, 1991) did not, however, address these key questions: Were the behavioral sex differences present prior to the initiation of the differential parental reactions, or were they shaped by these reactions (cf. Snow, Jacklin, & Maccoby, 1983)? Do parental reactions affect the child's subsequent behavior (cf. Smith & Daglish, 1977)?

Fagot and Leinbach (1989) have provided evidence that parental attention to (putatively) sex-dimorphic behavior affects the pace at which children develop patterns of sex-differentiated behavior. Toddlers and their parents were studied at 18 and 27 months. At 18 months, none of the toddlers were able to "pass" a gender-labeling task (Leinbach & Fagot, 1986), but at 27 months 48% passed ("early labelers") and 52% failed ("late labelers"). At 18 months, future early and late labelers did not differ in their degree of sex- typed behavior; in fact, both groups showed little evidence of sex-differentiated behavior. At 27 months, however, early labelers showed patterns of sex-differentiated behavior stronger than those of late labelers; for example, the boys who were early labelers played more with masculine toys than did the other three groups, whereas the girls who were early labelers played more with feminine toys than did the other three groups (cf. Fagot, Leinbach, & Hagan, 1986).

Parent–child observation at 18 months revealed that the parents of future early labelers were more likely than were the parents of future late labelers to emit *both* positive and negative responses to masculine *and* feminine behavior in their toddlers; however, the two groups of parents did not differ in their rates of "instructional" behavior (e.g., directive, verbal interaction) in response to their toddlers' sex-typed play.

These findings do not provide unequivocal support for the social learning account of sex-typed behavior, since early labelers received more negative *and* positive feedback about their masculine and feminine behavior than did late labelers. This led Fagot and Leinbach (1989) to emphasize the importance of affect per se in sensitizing toddlers to the salience of gender. The scenario becomes complicated, however, because by 27 months the parents of both groups were much more likely to give their toddlers positive feedback for same-sex play than for cross-sex play, and (except for the fathers of girls) more likely to give them negative feedback for cross-sex play than for same-sex play. By age 4, both groups of toddlers showed similarly conventional sex role preference scores, although the former early labelers had a more sharply developed awareness of sex role stereotypes than did the former late labelers.

Case Reports and Studies of Clinical Populatons

Do studies of this genre contribute to our understanding of parental responses to the early sex-dimorphic behavior of children with gender identity disorder? Our own and others' clinical experience with gender identity disorder suggests that the parental response to early cross-gender behavior is typically neutrality (tolerance) or positive encouragement. Consider, for example, McDevitt's (1985) remarks regarding maternal shaping of sex-typed behavior, which were made in a case report describing a psychoanalytic treatment carried out for 4 years (four sessions per week) of a 4-year-old boy, Billy, who showed all the characteristic signs of a youngster with gender identity disorder:

> The mother had wanted a daughter. . . . [She] never thought of baby boy or baby girl, just baby. . . . It soon became apparent that Billy preferred to play with girls, liked the colors pink and purple, liked jewelry, and liked the touch of fabrics such as velvet. When he wanted a pink bracelet he saw in a store . . . the mother thought it was in-

appropriate. Yet, she could not be firm. It was difficult for her to say
no to Billy. She let him play with an old white straw handbag of
hers, thinking this was cute. . . . [The mother commented,] "I must
have identified with this child, from 2 to 3, without knowing it—because he did have a lot of me in him, and possibly I encouraged him
to be artistic and gentle as a mother might do with a daughter." (pp.
2–3, 6–7)

In discussing the case, McDevitt (1985) concluded that the mother had
"selectively responded to, mirrored, and attuned to those aspects of Billy's behavior that would contribute later to feminine behavior. . . . The
mother could not tolerate Billy's aggression. Billy became less aggressive. The mother could not tolerate Billy's masculinity" (p. 18).

Parental recall of such responses, taken from clinical and structured interviews, was systematically studied by Green (1974, 1987).
From seminal observations of boys with gender identity disorder, Green
(1974) provisionally concluded that "what comes closest so far to being a *necessary* variable is that, as any feminine behavior begins to
emerge, there is *no* discouragement of that behavior by the child's principal caretaker" (p. 238, italics in original). In a subsequent report
(Roberts et al., 1987), ratings of recalled parental reactions to the boy's
initial feminine behaviors were shown, on average, to be in the neutral-
to-positive range. For the mothers, initial approval of feminine behaviors was significantly correlated with a composite measure of the boy's
femininity at the time of the actual assessment (see also Green, 1987).

In our clinic, Mitchell (1991) also attempted to measure maternal
reactions to both feminine and masculine behaviors in boys with gender identity disorder (n = 24), clinical controls (n = 13), and normal
controls (n = 24). Green's (1987) structured interview schedule was
used to rate maternal responses for two time periods: within 6–12
months of the probands' assessment (and that of the controls), and
when the boys were 2–4 years of age. In Mitchell's study, the ages of the
boys averaged 6 years (range = 3–12 years), so the period of time that
had elapsed from the time for which recall was requested varied considerably. For the very young boys in the study (i.e., ≤ 4 years), current responses were requested for the past 6 months, in order to better separate those responses from the initial ones. Mothers were asked about
their responses to specific masculine and feminine behaviors (e.g., peer
preferences, toy play, and dress-up play), and Green's (1987) 6-point
rating scale was used to classify those responses. The response categories ranged from "highly positive (encouraging)" to "highly negative
(discouraging)." After the maternal responses to specific behaviors
were reviewed, global ratings were made for masculine and feminine
behaviors, respectively.

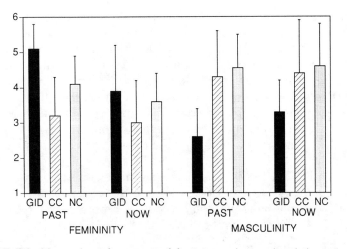

FIGURE 7.1. Maternal reinforcement of feminine and masculine behavior as rated from structured interview. GID, gender identity disorder; CC, clinical controls; NC, normal controls. Adapted from Mitchell (1991). Copyright 1991 by J. N. Mitchell. Adapted by permission.

Reliability ratings were made in two ways. For the probands, the primary rating was made by the clinician conducting the assessment. A second rater reviewed the typed clinical history or listened to an audiotape of the interview. For the control mothers, a second rater scored 14 of the maternal interviews from audiotape. For this group, Mitchell (1991) reported interrater correlations of .54 ($p < .05$) for ratings of feminine behavior and .67 ($p < .001$) for masculine behavior.

The results are shown in Figure 7.1. At both time periods, the mothers of the boys with gender identity disorder were more encouraging of feminine behavior than the mothers in the clinical control group; they also differed significantly from the mothers of the normal control group for the past rating. For both periods, the mothers of the boys with gender identity disorder were significantly less encouraging of masculine behavior than the mothers in the two control groups.

The empirical studies by Green (1987; Roberts et al., 1987) and Mitchell (1991) are consistent with the clinical case report literature regarding maternal responses to feminine and masculine behaviors in boys with gender identity disorder. However, the limitations of both studies, including reliance on interview data, should be recognized. From the standpoint of demand characteristics, one aspect of these data deserves special comment. As we have previously noted, clinicians of diverse theoretical persuasions have observed the apparent tolerance, or even encouragement, of feminine behavior shown by parents of boys with gender identity disorder. However, the fact that these parents have sought out a clinical assessment usually means that they are now concerned about their children's gender identity development (although there are instances of parental ambivalence, discussed in Chapter 4). From the standpoint of attribution theory (Weiner, 1993), one might predict that parents would minimize their encouragement or tolerance of cross-gender behavior, since it has such an obvious bearing on "causality." Yet a majority of the parents whom we have assessed do not recall systematic efforts to limit their children's cross-gender behavior.

Green (1974, 1987) has provided some examples of parental responses to sex-typed behavior in boys with gender identity disorder. Consider the following maternal responses reported by Green (1974, pp. 213–214), which might be classified as neutral:

INTERVIEWER (I): Does he play with dolls?
MOTHER (M): Yes.
I: Exactly what does he do with them?
M: He dresses them up, and he undresses them, and he puts the clothes right back on again.
I: Are these boy dolls or girl dolls?
M: Girl dolls.
I: And how often does he do this?
M: Every chance he gets to get hold of a doll.
I: And how do you feel about the doll playing?
M: I don't mind it. I don't see anything wrong with it.
I: When did you first notice his interest in doll playing?
M: Since he was very little, very little. About three.
I: Is your son aware of how you feel about the doll playing?
M: I think he knows *there's nothing wrong with it* . . . [italics added].
I: Does he play house or mother–father games?
M: He plays house a lot.
I: Do you know what role he takes?
M: He takes the mother. He gets a doll, or a stuffed animal, and pretends he's the mother. He spanks it if it's mean, or if it's bad, or he says, "You know Mommy doesn't like for you to do that" or "Mommy doesn't like that."
I: And what's your feeling about this?
M: I don't see nothing wrong with it.

Green (1974) noted that "neutrality" was the initial attitude in about 80% of his cases. Interestingly, he also noted that when parental concern did develop, mothers were more concerned than fathers in about 80% of the families.

Our clinical experience has been very similar, and the following vignette is an example of the responses of parents to sex-typed behavior as they report it during clinical assessment.

CASE EXAMPLE 7.1

Timmy was almost 4 years old with an IQ of 103. He lived with his lower-middle-class parents and an older brother. He was referred after the parents consulted with the family physician.

During an intake telephone interview, Timmy's mother commented that he "blatantly wishes he was a girl." She then described behaviors consistent with the diagnostic criteria for gender identity disorder. These behaviors included a preference for girls as playmates, role playing as a female, a preference for stereotypical feminine toys, pervasive cross-dressing, and an avoidance of stereotypical masculine activities. Timmy did not, however, manifest persistent signs of anatomic dysphoria. His mother could recall only one instance in which he expressed a wish "not to have a dink [penis]." In retrospect, she noted that the first sign of his cross-gender behavior occurred prior to his first birthday, when he developed a strong attachment to her silky underwear—an attachment that had continued to the present.

During the assessment, the parents differed dramatically in their interpersonal style. Timmy's mother was a very intense, emotionally labile woman, who spoke with great force; in contrast, his father was "laid-back" and relatively quiet. The assessment process was particularly stressful for the mother. For example, on the day that Timmy was seen for psychological testing, his mother was interviewed individually. She found it difficult to be apart from Timmy and, at breaks, raced to see her son in the waiting room. She commented that it was harder for her to be away from him than it was for him to be away from her.

The initial family interview was somewhat chaotic. The parents began by requesting that their sons, Timmy and Jimmy, answer questions. Jimmy was enthusiastic about this, but his parents quickly became annoyed with him because he was so dominating. Timmy and Jimmy were restless throughout the interview and had difficulty settling into play activities. Timmy frequently interrupted his parents, especially his mother, and often demanded that she do things for him. Both boys whined frequently, and Timmy groaned and moaned as he attempted to engage in some pretend play under one of the tables. When Jimmy was misbehaving, his mother spoke to him sharply; in contrast, when Timmy was demanding, she spoke to him in a "sugary" tone.

Regarding Timmy's cross-gender behavior, the mother said that she was having "trouble with it" in the sense that she did not know what her response to it should be. For example, she commented, "I don't feel there's a whole lot wrong with a boy in the kitchen." She expressed concern that she would be "brainwashing" him if she tried to shift his behavior.

When asked about their specific reactions to Timmy's cross-gender behavior, his parents stated that they had been positive and encouraging. For example, they said that Timmy would get "fussed over" when he "paraded around in his dresses." The father commented that they viewed such behavior as "funny." Throughout the assessment process, the parents stated that they did not wish to make an unnecessary issue out of the situation. In terms of long-term issues, Timmy's mother expressed two points of view regarding the likelihood of an eventual homosexual orientation—an outcome that she anticipated. On the one hand, she stated, "I don't care one way or another. I love him." Her best friend was a gay man, who had told her, "Whatever will be, will be." On the other hand, she commented that she did not want Timmy to be homosexual "after seeing what all my gay friends have had to go through . . . being gay is not pleasant." When questioned about how she would feel if Timmy eventually sought out sex reassignment surgery, she asked rhetorically, "Can you see us going to Mary Kay parties together?"

It was our impression that Timmy's parents had been either tolerant of or encouraging toward his cross-gender behavior, and had not systematically attempted to encourage markers of stereotypical masculine behavior.

Conclusions

Overall, then, it seems that there is some evidence of continuity between normative and clinical studies of reinforcement (or tolerance) of certain core sex-typed behaviors. Lytton and Romney's (1991) recent meta-analysis of parental gender socialization in different behavioral domains led them to conclude that, with one exception, there was "little differential socialization for social behavior or abilities" (p. 267). The exception was in the domain of "encouragement of sex-typed activities and perceptions of sex-stereotyped characteristics" (p. 283), for which the mean effect sizes for mothers, fathers, and parents combined were .34, .49, and .43, respectively. Although Lytton and Romney's (1991) overall conclusion minimized the influence of parental socialization on sex-dimorphic behavior, the domain for which clear parental gender socialization effects were found is precisely the domain that encompasses many of the initial behavioral features of gender identity disorder.

Although social reinforcement appears to be an important mechanism in explaining the genesis of individual differences in sex-dimorphic behavior, it would be prudent to note the limitations of the data sets currently available, particularly as they pertain to understanding children with gender identity disorder. First, it is somewhat difficult to know how parents of "normal" children react to cross-gender behaviors, because the base rates seem to be so low. In the Fagot (1978) study, for example, toddler boys engaged in female dress-up play so infrequently that statistical comparisons with girls who engaged in such behavior could not be made. Cross-dressing is one of the first behavioral signs of gender identity disorder (Green, 1976), so it is somewhat frustrating to note how little is known about how normative populations might respond to such a behavior.

At least under conditions of observation, parents seem to give positive attention to same-sex behaviors more frequently than they give negative attention to cross-sex behaviors (Fagot & Leinbach, 1989); thus, future studies of children with gender identity disorder might try to assess encouragement of same-sex behavior separately from discouragement of cross-sex behavior (cf. Green, 1987). When instructed to do so, mothers of boys with gender identity disorder were as adept as control mothers in encouraging masculine behavior, although they were less likely to encourage such behavior during a no-instruction condition (Doering, 1981).

Second, in normative populations the meaning of a positive parental response to a rare behavior is difficult to interpret (cf. Langlois & Downs, 1980). Roberts et al. (1987) encountered a similar problem, in that their control group of boys so rarely engaged in feminine behaviors that it was impossible to generate ratings of parental reactions to such behaviors. Thus, determining how parents of "normal" children react to consistently deviant sex-typed behavior is not an easy task. Creation of laboratory simulations is a possible solution (see Langlois & Downs, 1980), but is ecologically suspect. Perhaps interview studies conducted in order to understand the importance and meaning that parents attach to gender development would be of help (cf. Antill, 1987; Brooks-Gunn, 1986).

Third, although variations in parental behavior may affect a child's sex-typed behavior, the overall pattern of that behavior is still likely to be within the conventional range. This invokes a crucial assumption of developmental psychopathology—namely, that one is dealing with variations on a spectrum of normality and deviance (Cicchetti, 1984).

In the case of gender identity disorder, the behavior pattern is often so extreme that one would want to look for extreme environmental responses, such as persistent parental tolerance of cross-gender behavior, marked parental ambivalence regarding the child's sex, and even active promotion of cross-gender behavior. In some instances, the clinical literature provides evidence of such responses (e.g., Lothstein, 1988;

Stoller, 1975, Chap. 17; Zucker, Bradley, & Ipp, 1993). Green (1974) reported that about 15% of the sons in his sample were periodically dressed by their mothers in "girls' clothes" during infancy and toddlerhood, that 8% were occasionally cross-dressed by female siblings, and that 10% were subjected to cross-dressing by grandmothers. In our experience, overt cross-dressing by the mother or another caregiver is relatively rare, so clinicians should not expect to observe this in the average case.

It is clear, then, that the final word has not been written about the role of early reinforcement patterns. However, important lines of inquiry have been opened, particularly as a result of the detailed microsocial observation systems that developmentalists now have to examine the genesis of parent–child sex-typed interactions.

From a clinical point of view, it is also important to understand maternal motivations with regard to the selective reinforcement of sex-typed behaviors. On this point, there have been diverse observations and opinions. It is important for clinicians to explore this issue carefully, since developing an understanding of such motivations will prove useful in identifying approaches to treatment. For example, some mothers have said that they were influenced by recent trends toward rearing children in "nonsexist" ways (see, e.g., Carmichael, 1977), but that they had become concerned about their children's marked cross-gender identification. Lothstein (1983), for example, reported having received

> a number of calls from mothers who had intentionally tried to "masculinize" their 1-year-old girls (or "feminize" their 1-year-old boys) in order to prepare their children for what they viewed as radically new social roles. To their dismay, their experiments were failing. As their children reached age 4, instead of exhibiting an androgynous sex role, they were evidencing a stereotypical cross-gender role which was frightening to their parents. (p. 248)

With therapeutic support, such mothers are usually able to encourage a more psychosocially appropriate gender identification.

Other mothers, however, present with more complex dynamics. For example, Lothstein (1988) described the case of a mother who (in her own view) induced a gender identity disorder in her 4-year-old son by allowing him to overhear her delivery of antimale speeches to her feminist discussion group. One mother seen in our clinic told us with great intensity that she "hated men." Although she had longed for a son (her only child), she was incensed by her husband's concern about their son's marked cross-gender behavior, and she threatened to leave the marriage if he persisted in discussing the issue. The contradiction between her views about men and her desire for a son was striking. In the course of the assessment process, she commented that she should probably enter therapy to understand better why she was so angry with men and how this might affect her relationship with her son.[1]

As noted in Chapter 2, some boys with gender identity disorder are drawn to idealized, nurturant females in their fantasy play, whereas others are preoccupied with negative, angry female fantasy figures. Clinically, these two forms seem related to experiences within the family. For example, one 5-year-old boy had begun engaging in extensive doll play 2 years earlier, at a time when his mother had become severely depressed and withdrawn because of her own mother's impending death. She began to retreat to her bedroom for time alone, and recalled that it was at this point that her son began to play with dolls extensively in his room.

Another 5-year-old boy was preoccupied primarily with evil female characters. He would repeatedly watch films whose characters included evil women. Clinically, there was strong evidence that this preoccupation was related to his mother's chronic anger and rage, which began when he was about age 2. Prior to this, his relationship to his mother had been close (perhaps too close) and conflict-free. His mother had partial insight regarding her own conflicts, and asked rhetorically during the initial assessment, "Are those evil and angry women me?"

A third boy, age 6, and seen by one of us in individual psychotherapy for 3 years, spent much of the first year of therapy taking on the role of an extremely aggressive and controlling female (often a teacher). On one occasion he threw objects, including a chair, at the therapist, and this required intensive limit setting. Concurrent therapeutic work with the parents revealed information that had not been obtained in the initial assessment. A turning point in the therapy occurred after the boy's mother acknowledged that on the way home from a session, when she was very angry at him for misbehavior in the car, she had made him lie on the floor face down and "grovel like a pig." It turned out that for complex reasons she had often screamed at him and resorted to harsh physical discipline when he was younger ("I would spank him 12 times and I still didn't feel better"). As the boy's mother began to feel less out of control and initiated more appropriate parenting skills, his aggressive re-enactments and his general preoccupation with angry females during the therapy sessions came to an end.

From these vignettes, one could hypothesize two pure subgroups of boys with gender identity disorder. In one subgroup the familial dynamics pertain largely to maternal unavailability (e.g., due to depression), whereas in the other subgroup the familial dynamics pertain largely to maternal hostility and anger that revolve around masculinity–femininity issues. Obviously, these conjectures require rigorous empirical testing, but they suggest that different maternal influences may be at work in different cases of gender identity disorder.

THE MOTHER–SON RELATIONSHIP: QUANTITATIVE ASPECTS

Overcloseness or "Blissful Symbiosis"

In the classical clinical literature on homosexuality in men, an overly close, protective mother–son relationship was commonly but not always described (e.g., Bieber et al., 1962; Friedman, 1988). Later, Stoller (1975) extended this observation to transsexualism in men and to gender identity disorder in boys. Regarding boys with gender identity disorder, Stoller (1975) characterized the mother–son dyad as a prolonged "blissful symbiosis." Regarding one such mother–son dyad, he wrote:

> From the first . . . [the] mother felt a supreme oneness with this boy and, not surprising when one is blessed with a loving, infinitely intimate closeness with another, she did every thing possible (and necessary) never to allow that blissful feeling, created by his closeness, to be interrupted. . . . [The] mother and infant son [were] together more each day and for far more months (in fact years). This mother's intimacy with her infant contain[ed] those micro-behaviors [that are] so difficult for the outsider to see but [that] make for profound human relationships—the way two people look into each other's eyes, the intensity of their embraces, the extra moment's lingering of a touch, the soft sound, yielding muscle in cradling arms. . . . In order to keep him close . . . the mother had him with her constantly . . . he was in his mother's arms throughout a good part of the night because his sleep was broken. She carried him whenever she was standing or walking. . . . He was with her as she did the household chores, in the first year or so on her hip and later at least in the same room so that he and she could constantly link with their eyes. . . . He followed her as she went to the bathroom and was with her when she bathed or showered. (pp. 21, 24–26)

In Stoller's (1975) view, the consequence for the boy's gender identity, poignantly represented in one of his drawings (Figure 7.2), was that "he never quite learned where his mother left off and he began" (p. 25). Indeed, the clinical evidence clearly suggests that boys with gender identity disorder feel closer to, or identify more strongly with, their mothers than their fathers (Green, 1976; Zuger, 1970b).

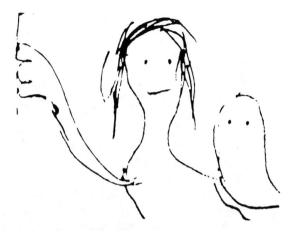

FIGURE 7.2. "Mother and Son." Title of a drawing provided spontaneously by a 5-year-old boy with gender identity disorder. From Stoller (1975, p. 20). Copyright 1975 by Hogarth Press. Reprinted by permission.

Mother–Son Shared Time

Green (1987; Roberts et al., 1987) attempted to quantify the construct of overcloseness or symbiosis by asking the mothers of feminine and control boys to indicate how much physical contact and shared time occurred in the first year of life, the second year of life, and between the ages of 3 and 5. Interestingly enough, Green's (1987; Roberts et al., 1987) data did not jibe with the overcloseness hypothesis. The two groups of mothers did not differ in their recollections of physical contact, and their recollections of shared time were opposite to the predicted results: The mothers of the feminine boys recalled spending significantly *less* time with their sons than did the mothers of the control boys.

Green (1987) also found that the feminine boys were separated from their mothers significantly more often than were the control boys, and that when such separations occurred, they were of longer duration for the feminine boys. The feminine boys were also hospitalized significantly more often and for longer periods than the controls boys. In addition, the hospitalizations of the feminine boys occurred at an earlier age. (Regarding hospitalization, Green, 1987, noted that a majority of the boys in both groups had not been hospitalized, but unfortunately he did not provide percentages.)

Given the hypothesis-testing nature of Green's (1987) study, it is apparent that the data on mother–son contact were unexpected. Green (1987, p. 376) tried to account for this. From a methodological standpoint, for example, maternal and paternal ratings of mother–son contact correlated significantly in most instances; this rules out systematic distortion of the data (e.g., in relation to demand characteristics). Green also suggested that qualitative aspects of the mother–son relationship may have been missed, or that the relative amount of time spent with mother versus father may have been more important than the absolute amount of time spent with the mother.

Another interpretation of Green's findings was suggested indirectly by Stoller (1985b, p. 41). Stoller had long made the case that the boys he studied clinically represented the most extreme form of gender identity disorder. Many of the boys in Green's sample may not have met Stoller's criteria for severity, and thus, in effect, the sample may have lumped apples and oranges.

Some clinicians (e.g., Meyer & Dupkin, 1985) have, however, questioned the accuracy of Stoller's (1975) notion of "blissful symbiosis," even among the most cross-gender-identified boys. Coates (cited in Bernstein, 1993, p. 732) has indicated that not one of the 140 boys seen in her gender identity unit fitted Stoller's "blissful symbiosis" pattern. Indeed, Coates and her colleagues have argued that such familial factors as parental psychiatric disorder, marital discord, and adverse life events appear to interfere with an optimal mother–son relationship (see Chapter 5). One could posit, therefore, that factors of this kind reduce the amount of time that mothers of boys with gender identity disorder spend with their sons. Coates et al. (1991) suggested an alternative interpretation of the recalled "blissful symbiosis" reported by the mothers whom Stoller studied:

> We were impressed that in the first few evaluation sessions many of these boys and their families seemed relatively well integrated. Often the degree of psychological suffering in the boy and a history of massive stress in the family emerged only after the family and child were in long-term treatment and knew us well enough to discuss painful realities or became able to recover dissociated memories. . . . We have noted that a subgroup of our mothers expressed a manifest wish for a blissful symbiosis. One mother said, "If I had to die, I would like for it to be with him [her son] on my shoulder. It was perfect bliss." We believe . . . that this was the expression of the mother's reparative fantasy for coping with her own conflicts about loss. . . . [Mother–son] relationships were characterized by severe, chronic stress and trauma, particularly after the first few months of life. (pp. 516–517)

Indeed, the lower amount of mother–son shared time and higher rate of separations and medical hospitalizations fit well with the hypothesis of separation anxiety resulting from maternal unavailability advanced by Coates and her colleagues (e.g., Coates & Person, 1985). From a specificity standpoint, however, the absence of a clinical control group in Green's (1987) study and in the work of Coates and colleagues deserves note. It is possible that mothers of boys with other clinical problems would, for a variety of reasons, also report relatively less shared time. The same can be said for medical hospitalization (see Douglas, 1975; Quinton & Rutter, 1976).

Conclusions

We are left with a conundrum. On the one hand, there is ample clinical evidence that boys with gender identity disorder have greater emotional closeness with their mothers than with their fathers (Green, 1976; Zuger, 1970b); on the other hand, Green's (1987) data on shared time seem inconsistent with this.

Is there a way out? Of course, Green's study represents only one data set, and it is possible that future studies would yield different results. If Stoller is correct, there may be a small subgroup of boys with gender identity disorder who have spent an inordinate amount of time with their mothers. In that case, we would find that extreme scorers ("outliers") are unique to a cohort of boys with gender identity disorder. It is also conceivable that the clinical impression of closeness is driven primarily by the boys themselves (cf. Zuger, 1970b). But, to us, this seems to be an oversimplification. Perhaps qualitative aspects of the mother–son relationship would give us a better picture of the interpersonal nuances that have been described clinically (e.g., Coates et al., 1991; Coates & Wolfe, 1995; Stoller, 1975). For example, there are techniques in the literature on facial expression in which a child is asked to "read" the nonverbal cues of the parent (e.g., Abramovitch, 1977) and vice versa. If, as some clinicians observe, boys with gender identity disorder and their mothers are so closely attuned to each other's emotional states, they would be better at this task than would control boys and their mothers.

Figure 7.3 shows the drawing of a 10-year-old boy with gender identity disorder. He drew the picture during an individual therapy session, during which he talked about how difficult it was for him to predict what mood his mother would be in each day. His mother suffered from recurrent depression, reported that she suffered from premenstrual syndrome (for which she had received a hysterectomy), and was quite irritable. It should be noted that the basis of such emotional con-

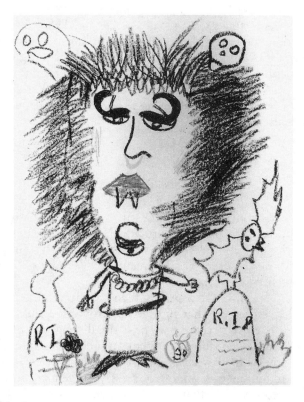

FIGURE 7.3. Drawing by a 10-year-old boy with gender identity disorder during an individual therapy session. At the time, the boy was talking about the unpredictability of his mother's moods.

nectedness may not be nonconflictual, as Stoller (1975) had conjectured. Given the psychopathology and emotional distress experienced by many mothers of boys with gender identity disorder, it may well reflect a boy's vigilance toward the mother's unpredictable emotional state or his uncertainty regarding her valuing of him as a male (cf. Bradley, 1985; Bradley & Zucker, 1990).

MATERNAL PSYCHOSEXUAL DEVELOPMENT

On the basis of several clinical cases, Stoller (1968b, 1975, 1985b) reported that the mothers of extremely feminine boys had had gender identity conflicts themselves as children, including periods of cross-dressing, competing with boys in athletics or at school, and wanting to be a boy. Stoller (1968c) characterized this childhood pattern as a kind of "bisexuality," which he defined as "a heavy proportion of sensed and observable thoughts, feelings, and behaviors reflecting both masculine and feminine identifications" (p. 112). Although these women relinquished the desire to be male at puberty, as adults they seemed somewhat uncomfortable with their femininity: "While these women have a feminine quality, inextricably woven in is this other, difficult to describe but easy to observe use of certain boyish or 'neuter' external features" (1968c, p. 298).

Stoller regarded the etiology of such a mother's own gender identity conflict as multifactorial. For example, the mother's own mother was "empty" and unable to be a model for identification; the mother's father filled this void, which led to a partial masculine identification; the family dynamics led to marked feelings of "intense penis envy" and rage.

Stoller's account of maternal psychosexual development implicates a form of familial transmission in gender identity disorder, albeit a paradoxical one: That is, a relatively masculine woman "creates" a markedly feminine son, which is a pattern inconsistent with a social learning/modeling paradigm. Stoller's observations, however, of the mother's underlying penis envy, rage, and hostility provide a clue to this paradox—namely, that the mother cannot tolerate masculinity in her son, as it evokes the sense of competitiveness and hostility present in her early childhood. Hence, she reinforces her son only when he is nonmasculine or feminine.

Aspects of Stoller's hypotheses regarding maternal psychosexual development were tested by Green and colleagues (Green, 1987; Green et al., 1985; Roberts et al., 1987), who found some support for his contentions. The mothers of the feminine boys were more likely than the mothers of the control boys to describe themselves as tomboys during childhood; on the other hand, they did not differ from the mothers of the control boys in their recalled display of specific "early girlhood sex-typed behaviors" (Green, 1987, p. 68). The two groups of mothers also did not differ in the extent of their sociosexual experiences during adolescence and young adulthood, although a within-group analysis showed that more cross-gender behavior in the feminine boys was associated with less maternal sociosexual experience.

In our own research, using a psychometrically sound measure of maternal (recalled) childhood gender identity (Mitchell & Zucker, 1991), we have identified two main factors. One of these factors pertains to a felt sense of gender identity, and the other indexes gender role preference. Table 7.2 shows our results. The mothers of boys with gen-

TABLE 7.2. Factor Scores on the Recalled Childhood Gender Identity Scale of Mothers of Boys with Gender Identity Disorder (GID), Clinical Control (CC) Boys, and Normal Control (NC) Boys

	GID ($n = 63$)	CC ($n = 13$)	NC ($n = 24$)
Factor 1			
M	2.24	2.29	2.25
SD	0.54	0.41	0.51
Factor 2			
M	2.37	2.30	2.38
SD	0.56	0.64	0.64

Note. See text for tentative factor labels. For each factor, absolute range was 1–5. A higher score indicates more cross-gender behavior or gender dysphoria. For scale's discriminant validity, see Mitchell and Zucker (1991), Tkachuk and Zucker (1991), and Zucker, Bradley, Oliver, et al. (1992).

der identity disorder had factor scores virtually identical to those of the mothers of both the clinical controls and the normal controls. Thus, we found no evidence that mothers of boys with gender identity disorder either were more unhappy about their childhood status as girls or had more masculine childhood gender role preferences than the control mothers.

There are a couple of caveats to these provisional conclusions. Stoller might argue that his observations hold only for the mothers of the most extreme of feminine boys. As noted elsewhere (Coates & Zucker, 1988; Zucker, 1982), Stoller (1968b) contended that the boys in his study were diagnostically and etiologically unique and on a developmental path toward transsexualism; thus, childhood gender identity conflict would not necessarily be expected in mothers of less markedly feminine boys. On the other hand, the evidence for the uniqueness of Stoller's group is equivocal, both diagnostically and etiologically (Coates & Zucker, 1988). We have seen too many extremely feminine boys whose mothers reported a typical childhood gender identity to be convinced that Stoller's group was unique.

Another caveat is that more in-depth analyses of the mothers' gender identity might reveal information that cannot be gleaned from self-report psychometric instruments (cf. Wolfe, 1990). On the other hand, our extensive clinical experience indicates that the vast majority of mothers of boys with gender identity disorder do not have childhood histories suggestive of psychosexual conflicts. Perhaps other aspects of the mothers' psychosexuality need to be studied, such as their current attitude toward men and their views regarding masculinity and femininity.

Despite the lack of between-group differences in recalled maternal gender identity, we examined the correlations between this variable and our other measures of maternal behavior (as described in Chapter 5)—a common strategy in the study of "at-risk" populations (cf. Garber & Hollon, 1991; McNeil & Kaij, 1979). These correlations are shown in Table 7.3. For the mothers of the probands, Factor 1 of the recall measure of childhood gender identity correlated significantly with marital status (i.e., a broken marriage), marital discord, and maternal psychopathology. It correlated negatively with the mothers' reinforcement of their sons' masculinity, both in the past and at the time of the assessment. Factor 2 also correlated with the composite measure of maternal psychopathology and with the mothers' reinforcement of their sons' femininity in the past. It correlated negatively with reinforcement of masculinity in the past. The correlations for the full sample are also shown in Table 7.3. The patterns were very similar to those for the mothers of the probands alone.

It is obvious that these correlations were not strong. Among the mothers of boys with gender identity disorder, the strongest correlations involved the mothers' failure to encourage masculinity in the past—that is, during the hypothesized sensitive period for gender identity formation. These correlations accounted for about 18% and 12% of the variance, respectively. However, the pattern was consistent with the paradoxical relationship suggested by Stoller's (1968b) clinical observations.

MATERNAL EMOTIONAL FUNCTIONING

In Chapter 5, we have presented some of our data on maternal emotional functioning and marital adjustment. We have reported that the mothers of boys with gender identity disorder were more impaired than the mothers of normal control boys. We have also reported that these mothers appeared to be as impaired as the mothers of clinical control boys, and that on some measures they appeared to be more impaired. We have shown that a composite measure of maternal psychopathology was the strongest predictor of CBCL psychopathology in the boys (see Table 5.17).

What influence, if any, does a mother's emotional state have on the genesis of gender identity disorder? If it has an influence, what is the psychosocial mechanism of transmission? Before addressing these ques-

TABLE 7.3. Correlations between Maternal Recalled Childhood Gender Identity Scale Factor Scores and Other Measures of Maternal Behavior

Measures	Factor 1		Factor 2		
	r	p^2	r	p^a	n
Mothers of boys with gender identity disorder					
Social class	−.06	n.s.	.02	n.s.	63
Marital status	.27	.018	.06	n.s.	63
Maternal psychopathology					
(composite)	.20	.054	.18	.084	63
Dyadic Adjustment Scale	−.21	.048	−.16	n.s.	61
Child-Rearing Practices Report					
Authoritarian Control	−.03	n.s.	−.08	n.s.	61
Enjoyment of Child and					
Parenting Role	.01	n.s.	−.05	n.s.	61
Autonomy	−.00	n.s.	−.03	n.s.	61
Current reinforcement of					
feminine behavior	.12	n.s.	.23	n.s.	28
Past reinforcement of					
feminine behavior	.16	n.s.	.28	.074	28
Current reinforcement of					
masculine behavior	.33	.043	.21	n.s.	28
Past reinforcement of					
masculine behavior	−.43	.012	−.35	.035	28
Combined sample					
Social class	−.08	n.s.	−.01	n.s.	100
Marital status	.16	.058	.10	n.s.	100
Maternal psychopathology					
(composite)	.18	.040	.10	n.s.	100
Dyadic Adjustment Scale	−.19	.028	−.18	.035	98
Child-Rearing Practices Report					
Authoritarian Control	−.05	n.s.	−.00	n.s.	97
Enjoyment of Child and					
Parenting Role	−.03	n.s.	−.06	n.s.	97
Autonomy	−.03	n.s.	−.13	n.s.	97
Current Reinforcement of					
feminine behavior	.08	n.s.	−.02	n.s.	65
Past reinforcement of					
feminine behavior	.08	n.s.	.10	n.s.	65
Current reinforcement of					
masculine behavior	−.21	.049	−.27	.016	65
Past reinforcement of					
masculine behavior	−.23	.035	−.32	.005	65

Note. For the reinforcement measures, 24 of the mothers of the probands were participants in Mitchell's (1991) study; reinforcement ratings were available for an additional 4 mothers; the data for the remaining mothers have not yet been cleaned and subjected to reliability checks, so they are not reported here.
[a]One-tailed.

tions, we would like to comment in somewhat more detail on the maternal data.

On the Symptom Checklist 90—Revised (SCL-90-R), the mothers of the probands had peak scores on three symptom dimensions: Obsessive–Compulsive, Depression, and Hostility (see Figure 5.4). On the Obsessive–Compulsive dimension, the probands' mothers had a significantly higher score than that of the clinical control mothers; on the other two dimensions, the scores of the two groups did not differ. Although the SCL-90-R is conceptualized as a measure of emotional state, we suspect that it also reflects more enduring patterns of emotional functioning.

The Diagnostic Interview for Borderline Patients (DIBP) was administered, in part because Marantz and Coates (1991) had reported that 4 (25%) of 16 mothers of boys with gender identity disorder met the DIBP criteria for borderline personality disorder, compared to none of 17 mothers of normal control boys. Our results were less strong. Only 2 (3.3%) of 60 mothers of boys with gender identity disorder met the DIBP criteria, compared to none of the clinical control and normal control mothers—a nonsignificant difference. On the Social Adaptation scale, however, the mothers of the two clinical groups were significantly more impaired than the mothers of the normal controls; the mothers of the boys with gender identity disorder were also significantly more impaired on the Affects scale than the mothers of the other two groups, who did not differ from each other.

Demographic variables may account for the lower rate of formal borderline pathology found in our study. The mothers in our study were from a higher social class background than the mothers in Marantz and Coates's (1991) study, and a greater percentage of them were in intact marriages. Correlational data suggest that both of these demographic variables were related to the extent of maternal psychopathology in our sample. Wolfe (1990) used the Structured Clinical Interview for DSM-III (SCID) to assess personality psychopathology in 11 mothers of boys with gender identity disorder. Although all of these mothers had at least one psychiatric disorder, none of them met the SCID criteria for borderline personality disorder. Wolfe's sample was demographically comparable to ours, which might explain why Wolfe's data showed the same discrepancy from Marantz and Coates's data, even though Wolfe's study was conducted in the same clinic as that of Marantz and Coates.

Although the vast majority of the mothers in our study did not meet the criteria for borderline personality disorder, they clearly showed difficulties in social adaptation and affect regulation, which are aspects of the borderline configuration. When we examined our DIBP data for subclinical signs of borderline personality by lowering the total cutoff score from a 7 to a 5 (in the DIBP scoring manual, a score of 5 is deemed indicative of "probable" borderline personality), 11 (18.3%) of the mothers of boys with gender identity disorder met this criterion, compared to 7.7% and 8.3% of the clinical and normal control mothers, respectively. The difference was still not significant. When we add to this percentage other mothers who had had clear signs of borderline personality functioning earlier in their lives, but were currently coping at a better level of adaptation, we estimate that about 20–25% of the mothers of boys with gender identity disorder in our sample had or formerly had borderline personality traits. Clinically, these traits appear to be most prominent in the areas of affects and interpersonal relations (e.g., idealization, devaluation, splitting) and less so in the areas of impulse action patterns (e.g., suicidality, self-mutilation) and mini-psychotic episodes. In any case, we suspect that the prevalence of borderline personality traits in our mothers of boys with gender identity disorder is considerably higher than their prevalence in the general population (Widiger & Weissman, 1991).

The data from the Diagnostic Interview Schedule (DIS) support the impression that a substantial percentage of the mothers of boys with gender identity disorder had significant psychiatric difficulties. Of the 60 mothers, 21 had no DIS disorder, 7 had one, 16 had two, 8 had three, and 8 had four or more. Thus, 32 (53.3%) of 60 mothers of boys with gender identity disorder had two or more DIS diagnoses, compared to only 3 (23.0%) of 13 clinical control mothers and 2 (8.3%) of 24 normal control mothers. On the DIS, the most common diagnoses pertained to depression, anxiety, and alcohol abuse.

In terms of involvement in therapy, 15 of the 63 mothers were or had been in outpatient treatment, and 5 were or had been in both inpatient and outpatient treatment.

One aspect of our data that surprised us concerned marital adjustment. We found no between-group difference in this domain. This was not because the normal control mothers had particularly discordant marriages; on average, their scores were within the normal range (Mitchell, 1991). When we examined our data descriptively, about 33% of the mothers of boys with gender identity disorder had scores that fell within 1 SD of the mean of divorced couples in Spanier's (1976) original study. The remaining two-thirds had marital adjustment scores within the normal range. Of the mothers with scores suggestive of discordant marriages, about half were married and about half were separated or divorced. Taken together, the data suggest that a substantial percentage of the mothers of boys with gender identity disorder were emotionally or psychiatrically impaired, and that a smaller percentage were or had been in discordant marriages.

Over the years, it has been our impression that a number of the mothers of boys with gender identity disorder were functioning particularly poorly during the period in which cross-gender behavior first emerged in their sons. But by the time of the assessment, at least some of these mothers' difficulties had lessened or been resolved. Thus, it is our opinion that the data on emotional functioning may underestimate the extent of maternal and familial psychopathology. In any case, our data suggest that the mothers of boys with gender identity disorder are, on average, at least as impaired as the mothers of clinical control boys. Thus, the central question becomes that of specificity vis-à-vis mothers of boys with other clinical problems.

Both Marantz (1984) and Wolfe (1990) conjectured that the presence of psychopathology renders mothers emotionally unavailable, which results in anxiety and insecurity in the son. As noted in Chapter 5, however, this line of reasoning is not adequate to explain the emergence of gender identity disorder as opposed to other types of clinical problems. Perhaps maternal unavailability at about the time of the hypothesized sensitive period for gender identity formation is what distinguishes boys with gender identity disorder from boys with other clinical problems, but the available data are too imprecise to permit us to evaluate this idea properly.

Even if maternal psychopathology cannot directly account for symptom onset, such psychopathology, as Wolfe (1990) noted, probably affects the capacity to be an effective parent, a capacity that includes the setting of appropriate limits to a variety of behaviors, among which are cross-gender behavior in boys. If a mother is preoccupied or burdened with her own difficulties, one might predict that she would be less mobilized to limit her son's cross-gender behavior.

We examined this idea by looking at the correlations between our maternal composite measure of psychopathology and our other maternal measures, including ratings of reinforcement of sex-typed behavior. The data are presented in Table 7.4. For the mothers of boys with gender identity disorder, maternal psychopathology was negatively correlated with social class and marital adjustment, and positively correlated with marital status (i.e., being separated, divorced, or widowed). Maternal psychopathology was also negatively correlated with enjoyment of child and encouragement of autonomy. With regard to the reinforcement of sex-typed behaviors, maternal psychopathology was most strongly related to the tolerance or encouragement of feminine behavior, and less strongly related to the encouragement of masculine behavior. The correlations for the full sample are also shown in Table 7.4.

TABLE 7.4. Correlations between Maternal Psychopathology (Composite) and Other Measures of Maternal Behavior

Measures	r	p^a	n
Mothers of boys with gender identity disorder			
Social class	−.21	.053	63
Marital status	.25	.025	63
Dyadic Adjustment Scale	−.35	.003	61
Child-Rearing Practices Report			
Authoritarian Control	.10	n.s.	61
Enjoyment of Child and Parenting Role	−.47	.000	61
Autonomy	−.32	.006	61
Current reinforcement of feminine behavior	.31	.057	28
Past reinforcement of feminine behavior	.41	.016	28
Current reinforcement of masculine behavior	−.28	.072	28
Past reinforcement of masculine behavior	−.18	n.s.	28
Combined sample			
Social class	−.21	.020	100
Marital status	.18	.034	100
Dyadic Adjustment Scale	−.34	.001	98
Child-Rearing Practices Report			
Authoritarian Control	.10	n.s.	97
Enjoyment of Child and Parenting Role	−.48	.000	97
Autonomy	−.29	.002	97
Current reinforcement of feminine behavior	.17	.087	65
Past reinforcement of feminine behavior	.24	.025	65
Current reinforcement of masculine behavior	−.16	n.s.	65
Past reinforcement of masculine behavior	−.13	n.s.	65

Note. For the reinforcement measures, 24 of the mothers of the probands were participants in Mitchell's (1991) study; reinforcement ratings were available for an additional 4 mothers; the data for the remaining mothers have not yet been cleaned and subjected to reliability checks, so they are not reported here.
[a]One-tailed.

The patterns were very similar to those for the mothers of the probands alone, although the correlations with reinforcement of feminine behavior were less strong.

It is of interest that the composite measure of maternal psychopathology was related more closely to the tolerance or encouragement of feminine behavior than to the encouragement of masculine behavior. It will be recalled that the opposite was found for the measure of childhood gender identity: This measure was related more closely to the lack of encouragement of masculine behavior than to the tolerance or encouragement of feminine behavior. Thus, there seems to be some support for the idea of a relation between maternal impairment and a difficulty in setting limits on cross-gender behavior.

We recognize that the correlations disclosed by our data are a far cry from the demonstration of a causal sequence. Clinically, we are inclined to reject the notion that tolerance of feminine behavior would lead to more maternal psychopathology. It is more likely that maternal impairment would result in a lessening of the capacity to set limits. Along this line, it should be noted that maternal impairment was associated on the Child-Rearing Practices Report with less enjoyment of the child and the parenting role and with lack of encouragement of autonomy. It is well known that emotionally impaired mothers find it more difficult to permit independent functioning in their youngsters (cf. Marantz, 1984; Wolfe, 1990).

THE FATHER–SON RELATIONSHIP: QUANTITATIVE ASPECTS

Like mothers, fathers have been afforded a central role in psychosocial accounts of psychosexual differentiation. This has been particularly true for research guided by such conceptual notions as identification, modeling, reinforcement, and internalization of parental representations (e.g., Biller, 1968; Hetherington, 1966; McCord, McCord, & Thurber, 1962; Power, 1981). Historically, there is little question that the first generation of research by developmental psychologists on psychosexual development was influenced by notions derived from psychoanalytic ideas (e.g., Biller & Borstelmann, 1967; Kagan, 1958; Lynn, 1974; Nash, 1965; Sears, Rau, & Alpert, 1965). And it is well known that the role of the father was given strong weight by psychoanalysts interested in the origins of male homosexuality. Freud (1905/1953), for example, remarked that "the absence of a strong father in childhood not infrequently favours the occurrence of inversion" (p. 146).

More recent psychoanalytic clinical work by Bieber et al. (1962) and Socarides (1982) echoed Freud's comment in implicating deficient or pathological fathering in male homosexuality. In a remark somewhat analogous to Kallmann's (1952a, 1952b) astonishing finding of 100% concordance for homosexuality among MZ twins (discussed in Chapter 6), Bieber and Bieber (1979) reported that in their evaluations of over 1,000 male homosexuals in psychoanalytically focused psychiatric assessments, they had never met "a male homosexual whose father openly loved and respected him" (p. 411).

Friedman's (1988) recent review of the literature on the quality of father–son relationships among homosexual men noted what had become a somewhat codified characterization of the prototypical family constellation: "an excessively close mother–son relationship and a distant father–son relationship" (p. 57). But Friedman's (1988) appraisal of this literature was more cautious than Bieber and Bieber's (1979), in that it reflected a greater recognition of the overlap in the types of father–son relationships recalled by homosexual and heterosexual men. For example, regarding Bieber et al.'s (1962) rating of the variable "Time spent with patient: little, very little, father absent," Friedman pointed out that while this apparently held true for 87% of the homosexual men, it also held true for 60% of the heterosexual men. In a language that would be familiar to nosologists and epidemiologists, one could say that this result had high sensitivity but low specificity (Vecchio, 1966).

The now classic study of Bell et al. (1981) also measured qualitative aspects of parental relationships in homosexual and heterosexual men. Although this may come as a surprise to some readers, the data obtained from the Bell et al. study were actually consistent with data obtained from the clinical research that preceded it. On a composite measure, for example, "detached–hostile father" was deemed relatively characteristic of 52% of white homosexual men and of 37% of white heterosexual men—a finding quite similar to the overlap in the Bieber et al. (1962) data that was emphasized by Friedman (1988; see also Bailey & Bell, 1993). In general, Bell et al. (1981) concluded that homosexual men "reported less favorable childhood and adolescent relationships with their fathers than did their heterosexual counterparts" (p. 54). But Bell et al. took their data beyond simple group comparisons. Using path analysis, it was found that the general measure "negative relationship with father" accounted for some of the variance associated with later sexual orientation. But Bell et al. were quite cautious in their interpretation of the path: "The quality of the father–son relationship . . . is not a very good predictor of a boy's eventual sexual preference. Too many other experiences must follow for it to have any effect at all" (p. 56).

Although detailed consideration of this issue is beyond the scope of this volume, we should note that the Bell et al. study will ultimately have to be understood in a broader context—that of the sexual politics of our time. When the study was in the planning stage (during the late 1960s), homosexuality per se was still considered a mental disorder (in DSM-II), and the familial pathognomonic theory was in its heyday. And Bell et al. borrowed heavily from this perspective in conducting aspects of their empirical inquiry. But by 1981, when their volume was published, homosexuality had been delisted from the DSM for 8 years.

Along with what seems to us Bell et al.'s obvious humane concern for the well-being of people with a homosexual orientation, their interpretation of their data was clearly colored by political correctness. If, in fact, aspects of their family interaction and relationship data showed a departure from an ideal of optimal functioning in homosexual men, Bell et al. (1981) were in a quandary. Thus, the tendency in their conclusion was to minimize the observed significant effects. Although this minimization was clearly in part an objective interpretation of weak effects, it was, in our view, also influenced by the *Zeitgeist*. To put it another way, Bell et al. chose to interpret their data as showing that the glass was half empty, not half full.

Sociopolitical interpretation aside, Bell et al. and others (e.g., Freund & Blanchard, 1983) recognized that the direction of effects was a more problematic aspect of their research design. Within the discipline of developmental psychology, a watershed review by R. Q. Bell (1968) had already alerted many researchers to the problems involved in interpreting retrospective and cross-sectional studies regarding the nature of causal influences. In part as a reaction to the predominant emphasis on parent-to-child effects, Bell's (1968) review noted that many developmental socialization studies could be reinterpreted as child-to-parent effects. The review—a needed antidote—stimulated researchers studying many different developmental phenomena to institute prospective, even transactional, designs that would be better able to disentangle the direction of effects (Bell & Harper, 1977; Maccoby, 1992; Sameroff, 1975). Bell et al. (1981) were cognizant of this problem when they wrote that

> familial factors commonly thought to account for homosexuality may themselves be the result of a prehomosexual son or daughter being "different" to begin with. For example, a boy who is constitutionally predisposed to be less "masculine" than other boys with regard to his temperament, his interests, or his sense of identity may be regarded with regret—if not open hostility—by a father who insists his son be as "masculine" as he. The father may respond to such a son by withdrawing emotionally or becoming openly hostile. The son, in turn, may dislike or feel bitter toward his father and become even less likely to identify with him. This example shows how an inborn predisposition toward gender nonconformity might lead to rather than proceed from the kinds of family relationships that have traditionally been held responsible for gender nonconformity. (p. 218, italics deleted)

It should be recognized that the direction-of-effects issue raised by Bell et al. (1981) will be difficult to resolve by the retrospective method of simply comparing homosexual men with heterosexual men. One's interpretation of the between-group difference becomes a matter of theoretical taste.

Pillard (1990) suggested an alternative strategy, namely to obtain information on paternal characteristics from more than one informant. Although not ideal, this strategy is an important methodological advance in interpreting recall data. In Pillard's study, both homosexual and heterosexual adult men (within and across families) were asked to rate their "closeness–distance" with regard to their fathers during childhood and adolescence. Pillard's data were consistent with previous findings: Homosexual men both within and across families rated their paternal relationships as more distant than did heterosexual men, including those who were brothers of the homosexual men. But Pillard also reported more recalled father–son distance by heterosexual brothers who had one or more homosexual brothers than by heterosexual men without homosexual brothers. This finding suggests that there was something unique about the father with at least one homosexual son that generalized to his relationship with his heterosexual son or sons.

The father's role in the development of gender identity disorder in boys and men has been considered along the same lines as those that have guided familial research on homosexuality. For example, Stoller's (1979) psychodynamic formulations identified such paternal characteristics as absence, withdrawal, and tolerance of cross-gender behavior as risk factors leading to these conditions (see also Rosen & Teague, 1974). Many of Stoller's observation were gleaned from the boys' mothers, since

> the fathers usually failed to come in for evaluation interviews. When, these completed, a conference was held and its importance emphasized for the boy's future, some fathers still did not appear. . . . when we recommended that the fathers participate in treatment, not a single one was able to cooperate. (1979, p. 844)

Eventually, Stoller (1985b) offered this pithy summation of his perspective: "the more mother and the less father, the more femininity" (p. 25).

Several characteristics of the fathers of boys with gender identity disorder have been studied empirically. We now review the results of these efforts.

Father Absence

Developmentalists have long mused about the effects of father absence on psychosexual development, particularly in boys (Stevenson & Black,

1988). Over the years, it had become increasingly clear that the term *father absence* was rather imprecise: The reasons for father absence and the age at which it occurs can vary; contact with the father can be considerable, even if the parents are no longer together; and so on. Moreover, one has to consider qualitative aspects of the father–son relationship.

Stevenson and Black (1988) conducted a meta-analysis on the relation between father absence and psychosexual development in children. They evaluated a number of variables, including the reason for father absence (e.g., divorce, military service), the nature of the sample (e.g., community vs. clinical groups), race/ethnicity, social class, publication status of each study (published vs. unpublished), and so on.

It was concluded that no simple relation could characterize the effects of father absence on gender role development. For females, virtually no effects could be attributed to father absence. There were, however, a number of effects on boys. One of the strongest effects pertained to the boy's age at the time of father absence: there was evidence for less typical gender role behavior if father absence occurred prior to age 6, which resulted in an effect size of −.52. Unfortunately, the extant database made it very difficult to evaluate interaction effects (e.g., between time of and reason for absence). Stevenson and Black pointed out that the mechanisms accounting for the age effects remained unclear. Despite their appropriate caution, it should be noted that the age effects are developmentally plausible. Given that the preschool years represent an important developmental phase for the consolidation of psychosexual identity, it makes sense that psychosocial mechanisms, whatever these might be, would have their strongest effect during this period rather than later in development.

Unfortunately, the precision that Stevenson and Black (1988) recommended be used in operationalizing father absence into its varied forms is not readily available in clinical studies of boys with gender identity disorder. The most general information pertains simply to rates of father absence, which are shown in Table 7.5. It can be seen that the mean percentage of boys from father-absent homes was 34.5%, with a range from 7.1% to 84.0%. Rekers and Swihart (1989) argued that their rate of father absence was higher than expected based on population demographics. But comparisons to general population figures are probably dubious. A better test of the hypothesis that father absence is overrepresented in families of boys with gender identity disorder would be to make case–control comparisons matched for specific demographic variables that probably co-occur with parental marital status (e.g., social class, ethnicity, etc.). For example, the high rate of father absence in Coates's (1985) sample is probably accounted for in part by such

TABLE 7.5. Rates of Father Absence (Separated, Divorced, Dead, or Never Present) in 10 Samples of Boys with Gender Identity Disorder

Study	n	Father absence
Bakwin (1968)	14	1 (7.1%)
Lebovitz (1972)	16	Not given
Bates et al. (1974)[a]	29	11 (37.9%)
Green (1976)[b]	58	14 (24.1%)
Money & Russo (1979)	11	Not given
Zuger (1984)[c]	52	12 (23.1%)
Coates (1985)	25	21 (84.0%)
Meyer & Dupkin (1985)	10	5 (50.0%)
Davenport (1986)	10	2 (20.0%)
Rekers & Swihart (1989)[d]	49	27 (55.1%)
Wolfe (1990)	12	3 (25.0%)
Arcostanzo et al. (1991)	22	Not given
Zucker & Bradley (this volume)	167	51 (30.5%)
Total	426	147 (34.5%)

Note. Only studies with at least 10 boys are cited.

[a]Inferred from descriptors "living with single parent" or "living with stepparent."

[b]In Green (1987; see also Roberts et al., 1987), where n = 66, exact percentage not reported, so this reference was used.

[c]Includes boys up to age 16 years. Data on 3 other adopted boys were excluded, since it was unclear whether they had ever lived with their fathers.

[d]Does not include data on 7 other boys who were living with adopted parents, foster parents, grandparents, or other relatives, since it was unclear whether they had ever lived with their fathers.

factors. Coates's study was conducted in the borough of Manhattan, New York; 52% of the sample was Hispanic or black, and the mean social class standing of the families was lower-middle-class (see Coates & Person, 1985). Given what is known about the rate of father absence in clinical populations (e.g., Kalter, 1977; Rembar, Novick, & Kalter, 1982; Schoettle & Cantwell, 1980; Tuckman & Regan, 1966), it is unlikely that this variable would strongly distinguish probands with gender identity disorder from other boys with clinical problems.

If father absence is truly a risk factor for femininity in boys, there remains the possibility that it would account for some of the within-group variation in measures of cross-gender behavior. Roberts et al. (1987) reported a statistically significant correlation of .24 between parents' marital status and a composite measure of femininity, which indicated more femininity in boys from father-absent families. They reported a similar correlation of .25 for their control sample.

In our own sample of boys, parents' marital status (with the dummy variables of 1 = father present and 2 = father absent) correlated .31

with the boy's age at assessment, $-.33$ with the boy's IQ, and $-.49$ with social class (all p's $< .001$). As noted in Chapter 4, we found that age correlated with a number of our measures of gender identity and role behavior (either less femininity or more masculinity with increasing age—see Table 4.8). Although these age effects may reflect in part the influence of social desirability or developmentally insensitive measurements, any assessment of the effects of father absence should take into account its covariation with other demographic variables.

To test this, we correlated parents' marital status (father present vs. father absent) with our various measures of gender identity, with age, IQ, and social class partialed out. Of 18 correlations, 6 were statistically significant at $p < .05$, one-tailed, but all were in the direction opposite of prediction (Table 7.6). Given Stevenson and Black's (1988) finding that father absence was particularly strong among preschool boys, we also analyzed our data separately for boys who were either less than or older than 6 years of age. The results were the same. How can we account for the unexpected finding that boys who came from father-absent homes were, if anything, less feminine and/or more masculine? It could represent a maternal compensation effect (cf. Biller, 1969) or a lowered threshold for initiating a clinical referral. In any case, the percentage of variance accounted for by father absence was no higher than 10% (on the free play task), and in general was considerably lower for the remaining measures.

In general, we are not persuaded that father absence per se is an important psychosocial correlate of gender identity disorder in boys. And it should be noted from the data in Table 7.5 that almost 70% of the boys with gender identity disorder in our sample had lived continuously with their fathers up until the time of their assessment.

Father–Son Shared Time

Green's (1987) study of feminine and control boys (see also Roberts et al., 1987) also examined father–son shared time. Green found that the amount of time the fathers of the feminine boys recalled spending with their sons during the second year of life, years 3 to 5, and at the time of assessment was less than the amount of time that the fathers of the controls recalled spending with their sons during the same periods. The difference in recalled shared time occurred both in two-parent families and in the families in which the parents had separated. The fathers of the feminine boys also recalled spending less time with the feminine boys than with their male siblings (when there were any) during these periods.

TABLE 7.6. Correlations between Father Presence–Absence[a] and Measures of Childhood Gender Identity/Role in Boys with Gender Identity Disorder

Measures	r	p[b]	n
Parent measures			
Revised Gender Behavior Inventory for Boys			
Factor 1 (Masculinity)	−.03	n.s.	156
Factor 2 (Femininity I)	−.04	n.s.	156
Factor 3 (Femininity II)	−.09	n.s.	156
Factor 4 (Mother's Boy)	−.06	n.s.	156
Play and Games Questionnaire			
Scale 1 (Feminine/Preschool)	.07	n.s.	156
Enjoyment	−.15	.037	156
Scale 2 (Masculine, Nonathletic)	.18	.014	156
Enjoyment	−.03	n.s.	156
Scale 3 (Masculine, Athletic)	.19	.010	156
Enjoyment	−.00	n.s.	156
Gender Identity Questionnaire	.04	n.s.	108
Child measures			
Draw-a-Person (% opposite-sex persons drawn first)	−.16	.021	163
Draw-a-Person heights (same-sex – opposite-sex)	.16	.021	161
Free play (same-sex – cross-sex)	.32	.001	145
Rorschach (same-sex – cross-sex responses)	.01	n.s.	155
Gender Identity Interview			
Factor 1 (Affective Gender Confusion)	.10	n.s.	93
Factor 2 (Cognitive Gender Confusion)	−.00	n.s.	93

[a]Dummy variables were used, where father present = 1 and father absent = 2.
[b]One-tailed.

Other Paternal Variables Studied by Green (1987)

The two groups of fathers did not differ significantly with regard to a concurrent self-rating of masculinity–femininity, recalled childhood gender identity, the wish for a daughter during their wives' pregnancies with the probands, and a self-rating of marital sexual adjustment. With respect to the division of roles between the parents, there were no differences in which parent made decisions regarding finances, which parent was responsible for child discipline, and which parent won arguments (see also Thompson, Bates, & Bentler, 1977); however, the fathers of the control boys reported that they more often took the initiative in planning family activities and in global assessments of who was the "family boss" than did the fathers of the feminine boys.

PATERNAL EMOTIONAL FUNCTIONING

Stoller's (1979) clinical account of fathers of boys with gender identity disorder suggested the presence of a great deal of character pathology among them. Unfortunately, there has been little systematic work regarding this matter. Rekers et al. (1983) reported that 45% of the fathers of 30 boys with gender identity disorder had a history of "mental health problems and/or treatment," but provided no details.

Wolfe (1990) has provided the most systematic psychiatric assessment of fathers of boys with gender identity disorder. Wolfe studied 12 fathers, who were predominantly from upper-middle-class backgrounds. On the SCID, all of these fathers received an Axis I diagnosis for either a current or a past disorder, and eight of them also received at least one Axis II diagnosis. Eight of the fathers had a current psychiatric disorder, and Wolfe reported that the remainder "were effectively being pharmacologically treated for what otherwise would have received a current diagnosis and/or described a past history of psychiatric illness" (p. 64). The most frequent diagnoses pertained to substance abuse and depression. From projective testing using the Rorschach and a systematic measurement device, Wolfe concluded that, on average, the fathers showed impairments in their object relations.

Green's (1987) and Wolfe's (1990) treatment of two paternal attributes—shared time with their feminine sons and psychiatric impairment—deserves further consideration. If shared time can be understood as reflecting the relative closeness of the father–son relationship, Green's (1987) data are consistent with previous clinical impressions that have accumulated over the years (e.g., Stoller, 1979; Zuger, 1970b). Indeed, Sherman's (1985) study of boys with gender identity disorder, using a projective measure of family relationships, indicated that their relationships with their fathers were perceived as distant, negative, and conflicted.

The within-family differences that Green (1987) reported raise an intriguing question. Why did the fathers spend less time with their feminine than with their masculine sons? Did this reflect a reaction to the boys' very different gender behavior, as a child effects model might predict? Or did it reflect some change in functioning that caused the fathers to become less available? Green (1987) reported a significant correlation between the paternal wish for a girl and less shared time in the three age periods up to age 5 years that were noted earlier (r's ranged from .26 to .32). This relation could be interpreted as the effect of a paternal characteristic (disappointment over the child's actual sex) on the fathers' motivation for involvement with their sons; however, the strength of the correlation was relatively small. Wolfe's (1990) data on psychiatric impairment could provide another plausible explanation for distance in father–son relationships.

There is, however, a fundamental problem in the study designs of both Green (1987) and Wolfe (1990). Green did not employ a clinical control group, and Wolfe had no control groups at all. One wonders whether shared time and psychiatric impairment are characteristic of fathers of clinic-referred boys in general. Thus, the specificity question looms large and remains unanswered by these two investigations.

SELF-SOCIALIZATION

The influence of parents on psychosexual socialization has been considered in previous sections. Over the years, developmental psychologists have also considered the child's own role in the acquisition of gender identity. For example, as nonverbal measurement techniques have become more sophisticated, it has been possible to demonstrate that toddlers under the age of 2, and even infants less than a year old, use socioperceptual cues to discriminate males from females (e.g., Fagot & Leinbach, 1993; Kujawski & Bower, 1993; Leinbach & Fagot, 1993; Levy & Haaf, 1994; Poulin-Dubois, Serbin, Kenyon, & Derbyshire, 1994). Eventually, young children develop a more conscious awareness of their status as male or female and begin the process of gender self-labeling. Thus, it is well known that by the age of 3, almost all children can correctly identify their own gender ("I am a girl, not a boy") (e.g., Dull et al., 1975; Leinbach & Fagot, 1986; Paluszny et al., 1973; Slaby & Frey, 1975; Thompson, 1975). Such self-labeling appears to be preceded by the cognitive capacity to correctly classify social markers associated with maleness and femaleness, such as hair length, clothing style, and body shape (e.g., Intons-Peterson, 1988; Katcher, 1955; Levin, Balistrier, & Schukit, 1972; McConaghy, 1979; Zucker & Yoannidis, 1983).

There is now some evidence that this capacity affects at least some aspects of sex-typed behavior. For example, Fagot et al. (1986) tested toddlers between the ages of 21 and 40 months on a gender-labeling task in which they were required to discriminate between pictures of boys and girls. (Because correct self-labeling precedes labeling of others [see, e.g., Eaton & Von Bargen, 1981], Fagot and colleagues assumed that toddlers who passed this task would have some awareness of their own gender status.) Over a 4-week period, these toddlers were then observed in a naturalistic play setting in which the occurrence of a number of sex-typed behaviors was assessed. It was found that the toddlers (mean age = 30 months) who "passed" the gender-labeling task spent more time playing with same-sex peers than did the toddlers (mean age = 26 months) who "failed" the task; the girls who passed the task were also less aggressive than the girls who failed it. Both behavioral differences remained significant when age was covaried. In the classical cognitive-developmental perspective of gender development (Kohlberg, 1966), correct self- labeling is viewed as an important motivational force in influencing subsequent gender role behavior: "I am a girl, and therefore I want to do girl things."

The cognitive-developmental perspective of psychosexual differentiation, which owes a great debt to Kohlberg's (1966) initial work, has been complemented and extended in recent years by theorists who employ the concept of the *gender schema* (e.g., Liben & Signorella, 1987; Martin, 1991; Martin & Halverson, 1981, 1987). Schema theorists emphasize that the young child is strongly inclined to order his or her world by classifying and categorizing information. Although these theorists differ in the weight they give to the "inevitability" of gender coding, they all agree that it exists and that it is a powerful organizing process. Once schemas have been formed and elaborated, they influence behavior and are resistant to change. Schema theorists concerned with gender equality lament the proneness of children to biases in their gender schemas (e.g., Bem, 1983, 1984; Morgan & Ayim, 1984). Gender-inconsistent information is misinterpreted (e.g., "The nurse was a female, not a male"), forgotten ("The boy wasn't playing with a doll"), or rejected ("Ladies can't be doctors") (see, e.g., Cordua, McGraw, & Drabman, 1979).

In our view, the contributions of normative empirical research on self-socialization and gender schemas are helpful in understanding the genesis and maintenance of gender identity disorder. The early appearance of gender schemas converges nicely both with Money et al.'s (1957) claim of a "sensitive period" for gender identity formation and with Stoller's (1965, 1968a) notion of a core gender identity. Coates (1992) noted that an important challenge for theory is to account for the early onset and rapid acquisition of cross-gender behavior and the pervasive effect of such behavior on the sense of self. Whereas "folk wisdom" minimized the significance of early cross-gender behavior (cf. Stoller, 1967), the self-socialization literature suggests the exact opposite—that such behavior reflects internal developments that exert an important influence on the child's gendered sense of self.

Among children with gender identity disorder, the salience of cross-sex stimuli and the attention paid to them are sometimes remarkable. One example is contained in a father's report on the reaction of his 3-year-old son with gender identity disorder to a children's movie. The only woman in the movie appeared briefly at the beginning. Yet this was the only aspect of the movie that his son subsequently talked about—what the woman said, what she wore, and so on. It was as if this was the only piece of information that the son assimilated. Clinically, one gains the impression that children with gender identity disorder have quite rigid gender schemas. In some respects, this rigidity is reminiscent of the proneness of children with aggressive behavior disorders to interpret ambiguous interpersonal situations as biased toward malevolent intent (e.g., Dodge, 1980, 1993).

From a developmental perspective, cross-gender behavior should be expected to emerge at the same time that more typical gender behavior emerges. What is novel in the work of the gender schema theorists is that it explains, in part, the internal structuring and psychological "hard-wiring" of this behavior and its eventual influence on the child's sense of gender identity.

Of course, the key question is this: What are the factors that contribute to the development of a deviant gender schema, which eventually organizes and drives the cross-gender behavior in a child with gender identity disorder? Although developmentalists have noted that normal children vary in the rigidity of their gender schemas (e.g., Carter & Levy, 1988; Levy, 1994; Signorella, 1987; Signorella, Bigler, & Liben, 1993), it is unclear whether corresponding variations in gender identity and role behaviors are outside the "normal" range and have any substantive impact on long-term psychosexual differentiation. Unfortunately, the normative literature on gender schemas has not gone very far in identifying robust correlates or predictors of individual differences (see Katz, 1987).

It is quite likely that the relation between behavior and gender schemas is reciprocal rather than unidimensional. For example, some children appear to engage in sex-typed play before developing the capacity to self-label (e.g., Blakemore, LaRue, & Olejnik, 1979; see also Eisenberg, 1983; Eisenberg, Murray, & Hite, 1982). Thus, as the ability to process sex-typed information emerges, prior interests and preferences are readily assimilated into the newly formed gender schema.

Several factors seem relevant to the development of a deviant gender schema. Some children with gender identity disorder, at least early in their development, appear to misclassify themselves as members of the opposite sex (Stoller, 1968b; Zucker, Bradley, Lowry Sullivan, et al., 1993). Why does this occur? One possible explanation pertains to their actual sex-typed behavior. A youngster with a very early onset of cross-gender behavior (say prior to age 2) may well "match" his or her self-concept with the opposite sex. A little boy who spends hours dressing in feminine apparel and playing with Barbie dolls may perceive himself to be like other children (girls) who engage in the same behaviors. Other behavioral attributes—for example, temperamental compatibility (e.g., low or high activity level)—may also play a part in causing a child to experience himself or herself as being more like an average child of the opposite sex than of his or her own sex. Physical appearance may be a second explanation. As noted earlier, many girls with gender identity disorder appear unremarkably masculine in their phenotypic appearance (e.g., hairstyle and clothing cues). Such a girl may perceive herself to be like other children (boys) who look the same way.

A third explanation pertains to the concept of gender constancy. Given that young children tend to confuse arbitrary sex-typed behaviors with identity (e.g., Eaton & Von Bargen, 1981; Emmerich et al., 1977; Marcus & Overton, 1978; Slaby & Frey, 1975), children who engage in extensive cross-gender behavior may well have difficulty in mastering the cognitive task of understanding gender invariance. In a preliminary study (Zucker et al., 1988), we found that children with gender identity disorder were delayed in achieving the putative final stage in gender constancy development. Although "antistage" researchers have shown that very young children can demonstrate competence in their understanding of gender invariance (Bem, 1989; Gelman, Collman, & Maccoby, 1986), it is unclear whether such competence would result from the everyday social life of the average child. Yet another explanation pertains to the responses that accompany marked cross-gender behavior. If, for example, parents attend primarily to such behavior, this may reinforce the child's sense that he or she is valued as being more "girl-like" or more "boy-like," as the case may be. Lastly, we might reiterate our observation that children with gender identity disorder are susceptible to internalizing disorders, including anxiety. Such anxiety may well contribute to rigidity in thinking, which might be manifested in rigidity with regard to gender schemas.

Unfortunately, apart from our studies (Zucker et al., 1988; Zucker, Bradley, Lowry Sullivan, et al., 1993) on gender self-labeling and gender constancy, no empirical work has attempted to assess formally the gender schemas of children with gender identity disorder. If such work were to show that these children do have markedly deviant gender schemas, perhaps understanding how those schemas develop would shed light on how more typical gender schemas develop in ordinary children. In this way, an investigation of deviant gender identity development could teach us something about typical gender identity development.

PSYCHOSOCIAL INFLUENCES ON GIRLS
WITH GENDER IDENTITY DISORDER

As we have noted at the beginning of this chapter, very little empirical work has focused on girls with gender identity disorder. Green and his colleagues (Green et al., 1982; Williams, Goodman, & Green, 1985; Williams, Green, & Goodman, 1979) have provided some information regarding the psychosocial correlates of gender development in "tomboy" and "nontomboy" girls. But these girls were recruited from the community, not a clinic population, and it is unclear whether the tomboys could be considered as having gender identity disorder (see Green, 1980).

In this section, we summarize our experience concerning psychosocial mechanisms in a clinic sample of 26 girls with gender identity disorder. Girls with gender identity disorder are invariably assigned to the female sex at birth. There are no indications in our data that the mothers (or fathers) of the girls in our sample disproportionately wished for a boy during the pregnancy. In terms of social reinforcement, however, it was our observation that the parents of these girls either tolerated or encouraged cross-gender behavior, much as do the parents of boys with gender identity disorder. Thus, at the least, this variable may be a perpetuating factor.

Several other parental factors have impressed us as being important in understanding gender identity disorder in girls. Maternal psychiatric impairment has been prominent. Of the 26 girls in our sample, 10 (38.4%) had mothers who were or had been in outpatient treatment, and of these mothers, two had also been inpatients (as it turned out, two other mothers were admitted as inpatients after we had assessed their daughters). According to clinical interview data, 20 (76.9%) of the mothers had histories of depression. Although many of these mothers had been depressed prior to the birth of their daughters, they were all depressed when their daughters were in their infancy and/or toddler years. Eleven of the 26 mothers showed clear evidence of Axis II character pathology. Thus, during the hypothesized sensitive period for gender identity formation, the mothers of the girls in our sample were quite vulnerable from a psychiatric point of view.

We believe that one consequence of this vulnerability was that the girls had difficulty in forming an emotional connection to their mothers. In some instances, it seemed to us that a girl either failed to identify with her mother or deidentified from her mother because she perceived her mother as weak, incompetent, or helpless. In fact, many of the mothers devalued their own efficacy and regarded the female gender role with disdain. For example, one couple, when the wife became pregnant for a second time (the proband was the couple's first-born), told us that they intended to obtain an amniocentesis and stated that they would abort the fetus if it was female, but keep it if it was male. In a smaller number of cases, it seemed that a daughter's significant medical illness or "difficult temperament" during infancy had impaired her relationship with her mother. In one other family, the proband (the youngest of three children) was sent to live with her grandmother in her infancy. The circumstances surrounding this case made it difficult to evaluate whether the girl had formed a connection with the grandmother. When she returned to her family, it was apparent that she did not have a connection with her mother (her father was unavailable for interviewing). She was a very frightened and anxious young girl who passed socially as a boy.

Six of the mothers had a history of severe and chronic sexual abuse of an incestuous nature. The femininity of these mothers had always been clouded by this experience, which rendered them quite wary about men and masculinity and created substantial dysfunction in their sexual lives. In terms of psychosocial transmission, the message to the daughters seemed to be that being female was unsafe. The mothers had a great deal of difficulty in instilling in their daughters a sense of pride and confidence about being female.

Another factor of importance is a daughter's experience of severe paternal or male sibling aggression. Such aggression had been directed at the mothers, at the girls, or at both in 12 of the 26 families. In these cases, the classic mechanism of "identification with the aggressor" seemed relevant to the girls' cross-gender identification. As noted in Chapter 2, many girls with gender identity disorder are preoccupied with power, aggression, and protection fantasies. In one family, the father's chronic anger was described by the mother as resulting in a kind of "Stockholm syndrome" (i.e., the syndrome in which the hostage identifies with the hostage taker). Another such case was that of Sammy (see Chapter 5, Case Example 5.10). The occurrence of male sibling aggression seemed important in two ways: First, it was chronic; second, the parents seemed to be incapable of modulating or buffering it. This caused the girl to feel vulnerable, and thus she developed the notion of being a boy for protective purposes.

These descriptive data obviously need confirmation from controlled studies. Another possible strategy would be to look for signs of cross-gender identity in girls who live in families in which such putative risk factors are present. For example, one might study gender identity formation in girls whose mothers had a major affective disorder during the infancy and toddler years.

Yet another possibility would be to study girls who have experienced severe physical or sexual abuse by a male. We are aware of only two studies that have adopted this approach. Maing (1991) studied 20 sexually abused girls aged 5–12 years, and 20 clinical and normal control girls. On several measures of sex-typed behavior (the Draw-a-Person test, the Rorschach test, and the Gender Identity Questionnaire), there were no between-groups differences. Because the onset of the sexual abuse occurred at a mean age of 7.2 years, the sensitive period for gender identity formation had long passed. Because the abuse lasted an average of only 6.5 months, and took place on an average of only 3.2 occasions, it may not have been severe enough to impair the girls' core sense of themselves as female.

In another study, Cosentino, Meyer-Bahlburg, Alpert, and Gaines (1993) evaluated a largely poor, Hispanic sample of 20 sexually abused girls aged 6–12 years, and 20 clinical and normal control girls. Gender identity and gender role behaviors were assessed by means of a structured interview with the girls and parent-report questionnaires. The mean age of the girls at the onset of the sexual abuse was 6.8 years; the duration of the abuse averaged 2.2 years; and in 60% of the cases, the abuse involved intercourse.

On the structured child interview measure, Cosentino et al. found considerable evidence that the sexually abused girls were more masculine and/or less feminine than the normal control girls; the clinical controls were similar to the abused girls on some measures and similar to the control girls on others. The maternal-report data yielded less consistent evidence for between-group differences. Qualitative data reported by Cosentino et al. suggested that some of the sexually abused girls were ambivalent about their female gender status and perceived it to be associated with risks. An intriguing aspect of the data was that the sexually abused girls, as compared to the controls, felt closer on average to their fathers (who were often the perpetrators) than to their mothers. Regarding this last finding, Cosentino et al. speculated that

> identification with the aggressor . . . may allow for the denial of traumatic victim roles to help defend against the feelings of vulnerability associated with abuse. Masculine gender role identification also may be related to feelings of maternal abandonment and ambivalence regarding relationships with mothers, who may have been viewed as weak, powerless, and unable to be protective. (pp. 946–947)

Devor (1994) noted that histories of physical and sexual abuse have been reported to be common in female-to-male transsexuals (Lothstein, 1983; Pauly, 1974). In Devor's own study of gender-dysphoric women, such abusive experiences were also common. Unfortunately, none of these studies employed comparison groups. The ideal study would provide information on gender identity formation both prior and subsequent to sexual or physical abuse. If such abuse is truly contributory to gender identity disorder in females, then one would predict a shift to more masculine behavior and an increase in gender dysphoria after its onset.

Lastly, it would be particularly informative to identify girls with varying numbers or combinations of the putative risk factors that we have discussed (e.g., maternal depression, maternal devaluation of femininity, paternal aggression) and to ascertain whether these factors have any type of cumulative impact on gender identity development. From our perspective, an important methodological issue would be that such factors occur during the hypothesized sensitive period for gender identity formation. We would speculate that their effects would be greatest during this period.

SUMMARY OF PSYCHOSOCIAL RESEARCH

In this chapter, we have reviewed the etiological and quasi-etiological literature across a variety of domains pertaining to psychosocial influences on psychosexual differentiation, with particular attention to gender identity formation in general and gender identity disorder in boys in particular. Our review suggests that some psychosocial factors (e.g., parents' prenatal sex preference) have little to do with the development of gender identity disorder in children. On the other hand, the evidence seems stronger for other psychosocial influences, such as social reinforcement. The role of familial psychopathology also appears important to study further, since the evidence seems to be shifting in the direction of more psychopathology in the families of children with gender identity disorder than in families of normal children. However, the problem of specificity has not been resolved, and future work will have to address this issue. As in research on biological influences, much of the variance remains unaccounted for. Models of risk need to be developed in order for us to understand better the contributions of psychosocial factors to the genesis and maintenance of gender identity disorder in children.

NOTE

1. This mother's life history interview provided some clues. An idealized relationship with her father had turned sour when he developed a severe alcohol problem and became extremely mean to her. During adolescence, she was highly

promiscuous and enjoyed the "power" that she experienced in "seducing" male partners. Her one long-term relationship prior to "picking up" her son's father in a bar was with an inept and alcoholic man. Her husband was a much more competent man, which led to many control struggles in the marriage. The parents chose to have their son seen in individual psychotherapy by a colleague, who is quite a skilled therapist (unfortunately, not all therapists are skilled). Within 6 months, her son began to give up some of his feminine behaviors and became more assertive with his mother. She panicked, withdrew her son from psychotherapy, and left her husband. Several months later, the mother chose to resume psychotherapy for her son. She also began psychotherapy for herself, with some success in understanding and resolving the ambivalence.

CHAPTER 8

A Clinical Formulation

In this chapter, we present a formulation of gender identity disorder in children—one that relies both on clinical observations and on the empirical literature that has given at least some of these observations systematic support. It is intended to provide clinicians with a framework for understanding the multiplicity of factors that appear to underlie the origins of gender identity disorder.

There have been several previous efforts to provide clinical formulations of gender identity disorder in boys. For example, Stoller's (1968c) model, which emphasized a "blissful symbiosis" between mother and infant son, has been viewed as overly narrow and inapplicable to many cases (see, e.g., Coates & Person, 1985; Meyer & Dupkin, 1985). Green's (1987) model emphasized temperamental attributes of the boys, such as avoidance of rough-and-tumble play, lack of parental discouragement of cross-gender behaviors, and parental unavailability (particularly on the father's part). However, this model did not emphasize dynamic factors. Previously, Bradley (1985) proposed an integrated model for understanding the development of gender identity disorder; more recently, Coates (1990) has proposed a "biopsychodevelopmental" model for boys. Both our own and Coates's model include biological and psychosocial variables, with concomitant consideration of several psychodynamic or interpersonal processes (see also Coates, 1992; Coates et al., 1991; Coates & Wolfe, 1995). Parts of Coates's (1990) model incorporate some of the previous observations, such as lack of discouragement of cross-gender behavior. Although we agree in large part with Coates's formulation, we feel that some aspects of this theory can be expanded to address our clinical experience more fully.

In Coates's (1990) formulation of gender identity disorder in boys, strong emphasis is placed on the importance of separation anxiety, which arises from the mother's withdrawal and rage following an adverse life event. Coates views the cross-gender behavior as a defensive fusion with the mother, the boy confusing "being Mommy" with "having Mommy" (Coates & Person, 1985). As noted in Chapter 5, however, many boys with gender identity disorder do not manifest separation anxiety. Although they appear almost uniformly to experience high levels of anxiety, we regard this anxiety as a manifestation of anxiety or insecurity about self-value or self-worth. Our model, therefore, sees the cross-gender behavior as identification with the state of being the opposite sex, which is perceived by the child as more secure, safe, or valued (Bradley, 1985). This does not suggest that there may not also be identification with the mother, but that in some circumstances the identification may be more with the state of being female (as perceived by the boy) or the state of being male (as perceived by the girl) as opposed to strict identification with either parent.

The other major point of difference in our formulation is that Coates places less emphasis on the role of the parents in limit setting for their children. In our experience, most of our families have experienced difficulties with setting limits on their children's behavior. These children respond with oppositional or avoidant behavior. This produces an intensification of the tension that exists between the children and their parents, which increases the anxiety and sense of insecurity experienced by the children. Problems with limit setting become even more important as these apply to the cross-gender behavior; they inadvertently permit its further consolidation. Coates acknowledges the importance of limit setting in her formulation of interventions, but appears to place less emphasis on it in terms of the development and perpetuation of the behavior. Coates's model stresses the importance of trauma in inducing the onset of cross-gender behavior. In our experience, what induces the cross-gender behavior is an intensification of feelings of frustration and stress within the family. This may be related to stressful or traumatic experiences, but may also develop out of intensely frustrating interactions between a child and his or her parents, related to the child's oppositional behavior or a difficult temperament.

Together with Coates (1990, 1992), we view gender identity disorder as a relatively rare disorder that requires the presence of factors within the child, the parents, and the family system to allow the development of cross-gender behavior and an identification with the opposite sex. These factors must be present at a sensitive developmental period for the child—that is, at a time when the child is developing a coherent sense of self as male or female. In agreement with Green (1987), we feel that parental tolerance of the cross-gender behavior at the time of its emergence is instrumental in allowing the behavior to develop. What has been problematic in some of the thinking about the onset of gender identity disorder is that many of the important factors occur in many children and many families with other clinical problems. What is unique in the situation with children who develop a gender identity disorder is the co-occurrence of a multitude of factors at a sensitive period in the child's development—that is, most typically in the first few years of life, the period of gender identity formation and consolidation.

In developing a clinical formulation to explain the onset and development of gender identity disorder, we believe that such a formulation must be broad enough to explain both the mild and the severe cases. This implies that each of the factors necessary for the development of the disorder may be relatively mild or severe, but that there must be a sufficient number of factors to induce a state of inner insecurity in the child, such that he or she requires a defensive solution to deal with anxiety. This must occur in a context in which the child perceives that the opposite-sex role provides a sense of safety or security. There may be many factors within the child, parent, or family system that intensify or mute the development of these behaviors, and that therefore lead to variations in its expression. We believe that *general* factors that occur in many children who develop different forms of psychopathology can set the stage for the development of a gender identity disorder. In addition, however, we believe that *specific* factors result in the unique constellation that constitutes gender identity disorder. We first describe the general factors, and then describe a way in which specific factors interact with the general factors to produce a disorder.

GENERAL FACTORS

Within the child, there appear to be two factors that make the child vulnerable to the development of a gender identity disorder: a high level of anxiety or insecurity, and a sensitivity to parental affect. The child's sense of inner anxiety or insecurity produces a situation in which he or she experiences an intense need for anxiety reduction. The child's sensitivity to parental affect makes him or her more aware of parental feelings about the child and significant others in his or her environment.

We believe that this anxiety or insecurity in the child arises in part from a constitutional vulnerability to high arousal in stressful or challenging situations. This type of reactivity, referred to as "inhibition" by Kagan (1989) and his colleagues (e.g., Kagan, Reznick, & Snidman,

1987), has been demonstrated to be heritable in monkeys by Suomi (1991). There is evidence that this vulnerability is linked to anxiety and depressive disorders; it may also be the biological factor that makes boys with gender identity disorder more avoidant of rough-and-tumble play. These individuals are more likely to have difficulties with affect regulation, especially in the context of an insecure mother–child relationship. This combination produces a child with high levels of arousal at times of stress and with poor coping strategies to regulate that distress. We believe that these are the *general* factors within the child on which the familial and other specific factors build to produce gender identity disorder. The child's sensitivity to parental affect results in an acute awareness of negative feelings in parents. Coupled with a tendency to high levels of arousal, this sensitivity may enhance the child's insecurity. Furthermore, the child may detect attitudes and feelings about gender values that the parent displays both covertly and overtly.

Parental difficulty with affect regulation constitutes another general factor predisposing to gender identity disorder, as well as to other forms of psychopathology in a child. Partly constitutionally based, this factor can explain the high prevalence of anxiety disorders, affective disorders, and substance abuse disorders in these families (Marantz & Coates, 1991; Wolfe, 1990; see also Chapters 5 and 7). As indicated above for the child, affect regulation difficulties may also result from early developmental experiences in the lives of these parents (Bradley, 1990). However such difficulties arise, they interfere with the development of a secure attachment between child and parent; thus, they produce insecurity in the child and convey messages to the child about affects, particularly discomfort with anxiety and negative affects. Such difficulties also interfere with effective problem solving between the parents, allowing tension to build and conflicts to remain unresolved. Lastly, parental difficulty with affect regulation interferes with parental limit setting and therefore leads to a lack of discouragement of cross-gender behaviors and an increase in oppositional behaviors by the child. These oppositional behaviors provoke frustration on the part of the parents, which intensifies the conflicted relationships that have begun to develop because of the earlier difficulties in the attachment relationship.

In our experience, there are often system factors that put stress on the family during the first 3 years of the child's life. These include loss of important family members, illness in parents or children, and intense parental conflict. The results of these stresses are frequently maternal withdrawal, lack of availability, depression, and maternal hostility and anger. We believe such factors act to enhance the child's uncertainty about his or her own value, and produce an inner insecurity that simply builds upon the early insecurity related to attachment difficulties. It also increases the child's sense of anger that cannot be expressed directly, given the messages about affect stemming from earlier attachment difficulties. These stresses produce a situation in which the child experiences intense anxiety and inner insecurity related to concerns about maternal affects and his or her own anger. This sets the stage for the child's desperate struggle to find a solution that relieves the anxiety.

SPECIFIC FACTORS

As noted in Chapters 2 and 6, boys with gender identity disorder are often highly avoidant of rough-and-tumble activity. In contrast, girls with gender identity disorder are often oriented toward sports and rough-and-tumble activity. Other specific factors within the boys may be that they are unusually attractive (Green, 1987; Zucker, Wild, et al., 1993) and have rather exquisite sensory sensitivities (Coates, 1990). We believe that these specific child factors act as facilitators of the child's assumption of cross-gender behaviors and of the parent's response to these behaviors.

In our experience, the mothers of boys with gender identity disorder often feel particularly intimidated or threatened by male aggression. We believe that this sense of threat leads to a discouragement of male-typical boisterous behavior and of the normative expression of aggression in their sons. Moreover, there is frequently an intense need for nurturance, which these mothers connect with femaleness. In this respect, mothers often unconsciously encourage female behaviors out of their need for nurturing. This specific revulsion toward aggression and need for nurturance may be very differently balanced in each family. In some families, the clinician sees a preponderance of desire on the mothers' part to discourage any signs of masculinity because of their fear of male aggression. In other families, the mothers' need for nurturance seems to lead to an intense encouragement of any nurturing qualities in their sons, particularly in the mother–son relationship.

With respect to the fathers of boys with gender identity disorder, what has been most striking is that they go along with the mothers' tolerance of cross-gender behaviors, despite inner discomfort with this tolerance. These men are also often easily threatened and feel inadequate themselves. These qualities appear to make it very difficult for them to connect with sons who display nonmasculine behavior. Because of their withdrawal from their feminine sons, they cannot buffer their wives' anger. They often deal with their conflicts by overwork or distancing themselves from their families, which sometimes increases the mothers' anger and sense of being abandoned.

The specific factors within the parents of girls with gender identity disorder are that the fathers particularly view females as less adequate and tend to reinforce masculine qualities in their daughters. As noted in Chapter 7, fathers may also be overtly aggressive or abusive. The mothers often feel inadequate themselves and are unable to redress this balance by standing up for their children, in the same way that they have difficulties standing up for themselves.

In our experience, other factors within the system often intensify a child's perception that being the opposite sex would make him or her feel less insecure or threatened or more safe or valued. A boy may well have a sister whom the mother appears to value more, or a sister who has been ill and requires the mother's attention. Sometimes there are family beliefs about men being unreliable or less adequate, which appear to cross generations; these may result in a multigenerational family of females who can become highly domineering, in control of, and derogating of males. In the family system of a girl, there is often parental conflict, which the child perceives as threatening; it leads to the child's perception that the mother is unable to protect herself. Such a girl frequently reports a fantasy of needing to be the mother's protector, which we regard as an identification with the aggressor. Sometimes, however, the conflict does not exist between the parents, but may take place between a patient and an older brother or other boys in the community who appear threatening to her. These situations may be perceived as intensely overwhelming by the child, who may come to feel that being male is the only way to protect herself or be safe.

SUMMARY OF THE MODEL FOR BOYS

In summary, for boys our clinical model proposes that gender identity disorder develops from a state of inner insecurity that arises out of the interaction between a boy's temperamental vulnerability to high arousal and an insecure mother–child relationship. The mother is typically in a situation in which she experiences high levels of frustration. Because of her difficulties with affect regulation, she experiences problems dealing with these feelings; she may become depressed and withdrawn, or intermittently hostile or explosive or a combination of both. The boy, who is highly sensitive to maternal signals, perceives the mother's feelings of depression and anger. Because of his own insecurity, he is all the more threatened by his mother's anger or hostility, which he perceives as directed at him. His worry about loss of his mother intensifies his conflict over his own anger, resulting in high levels of arousal or anxiety. The father's own difficulty with affect regulation and inner sense of inadequacy usually produces withdrawal rather than approach. The parents have difficulty resolving the conflicts that they experience in their own marital relationship, and fail to provide support to each other. This produces an intensified sense of conflict and hostility.

In this situation, the boy becomes increasingly unsure about his own self-value because of the mother's withdrawal or anger and the father's failure to intercede. His anxiety and insecurity intensify, as does his anger. This may result in some oppositional behaviors, which the parents again are unable to deal with because of their conflict-avoidant styles. This intensifies the conflict between parents and child, and the anxiety and insecurity mount to the point at which the child needs some anxiety relief. Given the context described above, in which there are specific factors within the child, the mother, and the system that promote such a perception, the child comes to perceive the opposite sex as being more valued or secure. When this occurs at the time that the boy is beginning to explore gender role behaviors, he appears to choose gender role behaviors that may be temperamentally compatible (with his tendency to avoid rough-and-tumble activity), but that in his mind provide the solution to the problem of feeling valued or secure.

The mother's need for nurturance and fear of aggression allow her to tolerate these behaviors, which may also be reinforced by her perception of her son as attractive; her tolerance may actually lead to a positive response to the initial cross-gender behaviors. The father is unable to intercede to discourage the cross-gender behaviors, and tends to withdraw more from his son because of his own sense of threat in this situation. The parents' ongoing difficulties in dealing with the child's cross-gender behaviors may intensify the child's anxiety and insecurity, but also permit the child to develop a fantasized but valued opposite-sex self. With development and the repeated need to use this fantasized other self, the child may be very resistant to relinquishing this defensive solution. On the other hand, the parents' valuing of their son as a male and discouragement of cross-gender behaviors allow a gradual relinquishing of the defensive solution and a building of confidence in a same-sex identity.

SUMMARY OF THE MODEL FOR GIRLS

In the girl who develops gender identity disorder, we also see a temperamentally vulnerable child who easily develops high levels of anxiety. As in the case of a boy, the mother's own difficulty with affect regulation leaves the mother prone to depression and withdrawal in a situation of marital dissatisfaction; it also leaves her uncomfortable with her child's and her own negative affects. This leaves the child feeling less secure about herself as a whole, perceiving the mother's avoidance of affect as avoidance of her. Again, usually such a girl is sensitive to parental feelings. What seems to be specific in this situation is that in the context of conflict (sometimes quite overt) between the parents, the child perceives the marital conflict as a situation in which the mother is unable to defend herself. This creates intense anxiety about the child's own self. Furthermore, the mothers of girls with gender identity disorder often feel acutely put down by their husbands, and the fathers tend to see females as less competent.

When a daughter tries out cross-gender behaviors in an initial effort to decrease anxiety (a pattern that may be consistent with her style of approaching and enjoying active play), her mother, who may consciously or unconsciously believe in the confidence and strength of males, in contrast to her own sense of inadequacy, fails to discourage the cross-gender behaviors. The father may in fact encourage the cross-gender behaviors. This permits the child the fantasy of being the mother's protector through identification with the aggressor. The continued need to use a fantasized other self to promote a sense of security is dependent on the family members' inability to resolve their conflicts and to promote a sense of strength and confidence in being female to counterbalance the cross-gender solution.

CHAPTER 9

Treatment

THERAPEUTIC INTERVENTION: RATIONALES AND ETHICAL ISSUES

The treatment of children with gender identity disorder has generated periodic controversies over the past three decades. In the 1970s, for example, behavior therapists, particularly Rekers and his colleagues, were criticized for their treatment of cross-gender-identified boys; this often consisted of extinguishing or punishing specific feminine behaviors, such as playing with female dolls (e.g., Barbie), and rewarding or encouraging specific masculine behaviors, such as playing with dart guns (e.g., Nordyke, Baer, Etzel, & LeBlanc, 1977; Winkler, 1977; Wolfe, 1979). It was argued against this approach that sex-stereotyped patterns of child rearing were thus reinforced, and that it was not inherently healthier for children to act in a manner typical of their own sex rather than the other sex. As a rule, critics arguing in this way doubted that childhood cross-gender identification was really associated with later gender dysphoria or homosexuality (e.g., Serbin, 1980). Most recently, Bem (1993, p. 108) has characterized the work of Rekers and colleagues as one of the "more coercive" approaches to therapeutic intervention with cross-gender-identified children.[1]

As the connection of gender identity disorder with later homosexuality became more apparent (see Chapters 3 and 10), new concerns arose regarding the implications of treating children, particularly boys, who might be "prehomosexual" (e.g., Morin & Schultz, 1978). According to Green (1987, p. 260), some of the critics who expressed these concerns objected to the treatment of cross-gender-identified boys

as "homosexual genocide." Although these objections have been responded to (e.g., Green, 1974, 1987; Rekers, 1977b), occasional critics
continue to question the ethics or the necessity of intervening in children's gender identity development (e.g., Coleman, 1986; Sedgwick,
1991; Woodhouse, 1989, pp. 136–137). Those clinicians (including
ourselves) who believe that the treatment of cross-gendered children
can be both therapeutic and ethical institute such treatment for a variety of reasons. These treatment rationales, which have been analyzed
by a number of other clinicians over the years (e.g., Bates, Skilbeck,
Smith, & Bentler, 1975; Curtis, 1985; Green, 1994b; Rekers, Bentler,
Rosen, & Lovaas, 1977; Rekers & Kilgus, 1995), are discussed below.

Reduction of Social Ostracism

As detailed in Chapters 3 and 5, clinical experience amply indicates
that cross-gender-identified children, particularly boys, are frequently
ostracized by their peers. In our experience, both boys and girls with
gender identity disorder are rejected by peers, but it appears to begin
earlier for the boys. Such ostracism, which can be very intense, often results in alienation, social isolation, and associated behavioral and emotional difficulties. Rekers, Bentler, et al. (1977) argued that "labeling
and peer rejection are perhaps the major sources of the [cross-gender-
identified boy's] extreme unhappiness and discontent" (p. 5). If this
thesis is correct, then these problems should become more prominent as
the child grows older—a claim that has some empirical support (see
Chapter 5). Thus, treatment interventions aimed at reversing a child's
cross-gender identification may not only alleviate short-term social distress by helping the child to mix more readily with same-sex peers, but
may also prevent the development of longer-term psychopathological
sequelae.

Treatment of Underlying Psychopathology

As discussed in Chapters 5 and 7, another perspective is that gender
identity disorder is secondary to more fundamental psychopathology in
the child and in his or her family. According to this model, childhood
cross-gender identification should receive clinical attention as part of a
larger problem in the child or family (e.g., Di Ceglie, 1995). As one example, if the separation anxiety hypothesis advanced by Coates and
colleagues is correct (see Chapter 5), then alleviation of the factors inducing and maintaining separation anxiety should have an indirect ef-

fect on the continuation of the defenses utilized to cope with it (i.e., the symptoms of cross-gender behavior). In fact, some therapists who subscribe to this perspective state that they do not focus their treatment on the cross-gender behavior or try to alter it in any direct way (e.g., Bleiberg, Jackson, & Ross, 1986; Gilpin, Raza, & Gilpin, 1979)—a technical issue to which we return later.

Prevention of Gender Identity Disorder (Transsexualism) in Adulthood

A third rationale for the treatment of cross-gender identification in children is that such treatment prevents transsexualism in adulthood. For many clinicians, there is little disagreement about this, given the emotional distress experienced by gender-dysphoric adults and the physically and often socially painful measures required to align an adult's phenotypic sex with his or her subjective gender identity (Blanchard & Steiner, 1990).

Prevention of Homosexuality in Adulthood

Among mental health professionals, the view that homosexuality per se is not a mental disorder is fairly well accepted by now (e.g., Friedman, 1988; Gonsiorek, 1991; Green, 1972; Spitzer, 1981; Stoller, 1980; see also Chapter 13) although dissenters can still be found (e.g., Berger, 1994; Nicolosi, 1991; Siegel, 1988; Socarides, 1978, 1988, 1990; Socarides & Volkan, 1991; Van den Aardweg, 1986). Given the relation between gender identity disorder in childhood and a later homosexual orientation, critics have questioned the therapeutic agenda of child clinicians. Regarding this matter, Green (1987) has mused:

> Should parents have the prerogative of choosing therapy for their gender-atypical son? Suppose that boys who play with dolls rather than trucks, who role-play as mother rather than as father, and who play only with girls tend disproportionately to evolve as homosexual men. Suppose that parents know this, or suspect this. The rights of parents to oversee the development of children is a long-established principle. Who is to dictate that parents may not try to raise their children in a manner that maximizes the possibility of a heterosexual outcome? If that prerogative is denied, should parents also be denied the right to raise their children as atheists? Or as priests? (p. 260)

Until it has been shown that any form of treatment affects a child's future sexual orientation, Green's point is moot. It is interesting to note that Rekers, who has been the primary researcher/clinician utilizing a behavior therapy approach in the treatment of cross-gender-identified children, has created some additional controversy by justifying clinical intervention on the religious ground that homosexuality is immoral (Rekers, 1982a, 1982b; for one critique, see Zucker, 1984). This treatment rationale is unlikely to appeal to more secular-minded child clinicians, who, if they set out to prevent homosexuality at all, probably do so because they believe that a homosexual lifestyle in a basically unaccepting culture simply creates unnecessary social difficulties. (Below, in our review of the behavior therapy literature, we consider the empirical efficacy of behavior therapy, and not the idiosyncratic ideological motivations of its individual practitioners.)

Pleak (1991) and Zucker (personal communication to R. A. Isay, September 16, 1991) have noted that clinicians of diverse theoretical persuasions have in fact justified the treatment of children with gender identity disorder for the same reason. For example, Zuger (1966), a child psychiatrist, described his therapeutic approach as follows:

> All parents were given guidance which it was thought would lead to a better masculine identification. . . . It appears that with guidance or treatment some of the younger boys could be induced to suppress their effeminate behavior. . . . What the eventual effect of such suppression may be on the potential for homosexuality cannot be predicted. . . . Feminine behavior beginning in early childhood would seem to constitute a clinical entity, possibly carrying with it serious consequences for future sexual identification. (pp. 1105–1106)

Newman (1976), also a child psychiatrist, wrote: "Because extreme boyhood femininity is often a precursor of adult transsexualism, transvestism, and homosexuality, the author recommends early intervention for boys who meet specific behavioral criteria of gender disturbance" (p. 683). Stoller (1978), a psychoanalyst, commented:

> The best treatment is prevention. . . . We are left with the ethical question whether one has the right to treat a child for an ego-syntonic condition others define as pathological. There are militant groups in society who demand that feminine boys not be treated because femininity in boys would be no problem, fundamentally no worse than masculinity, if a pathological society did not so define it. This is, I believe, an irresponsible position to take with children in our society as it presently functions, ignoring the painful consequences that accrue later in life. In contrast, for adults who already know full well

and accept these consequences, the choice to be left alone must be militantly protected. . . . Although it is not yet clear what boyhood behaviors indicate an adult homosexual outcome, femininity is one reliable marker. . . . Once an evaluation has revealed the femininity is intense, treatment should quickly begin. (pp. 555–557)

Money (1988), a medical psychologist, argued:

> The young son who becomes self-allocated to the role of daughter . . . reaches adulthood with a gender status that is homosexual or maybe, in a rare minority of cases, transexual or transvestophile. There is now new preliminary evidence, unpublished, that the gender-crosscoded course of events may be changed. (p. 83)

And Silverman (1990), a psychoanalyst with training in treating children, stated:

> The complexity, variability, and length of the path leading to adult male homosexuality . . . make it difficult to predict with certainty that any given child will ultimately develop such an orientation. We have learned, however, that the presence of certain factors in a significant combination signals so high a risk that vigorous intervention should be given serious consideration. (pp. 177–178)

Thus, the question of whether children with gender identity disorder should be treated with the explicit goal of averting a subsequent homosexual orientation does not seem to be merely an idiosyncratic concern of one or two clinicians. Given that most parents, not surprisingly, prefer that their children not develop a homosexual orientation, the contemporary clinician must carefully think through the ethics of instituting treatment for this reason and the empirical evidence that treatment can have this effect. We consider these issues in more detail below.

Summary

There are various rationales for offering treatment to children with gender identity disorder. Some of these rationales rest on firmer empirical or ethical grounds than others. At least three goals—elimination of peer ostracism in childhood, treatment of other psychopathology, and prevention of transsexualism in adulthood—are so obviously clinically valid and consistent with the ethics of our time that they constitute sufficient justification for therapeutic intervention.

The primary goal of avoiding adult homosexuality is considerably more problematic, especially if this is attempted for religious rather than pragmatic reasons. To anticipate information that we provide in more detail below and in Chapter 10, there are simply no formal empirical studies demonstrating that therapeutic intervention in childhood alters the developmental path toward either transsexualism or homosexuality. The hypothesis that treatment may alter the natural history of gender identity disorder so that it does not continue into adolescence or adulthood has some indirect support, but even this weaker evidence is lacking with regard to effects on later sexual orientation.

In Chapter 4, we have briefly discussed part of our therapeutic approach with parents regarding the question of later homosexuality. Here, we simply reiterate the position that treatment during childhood does not focus directly on eroticism; that it is unknown whether such treatment can affect later sexual orientation; and that other reasons make it legitimate to help children feel more secure about their gender identity as boys or as girls. In our clinical experience, we have found that many parents seem to feel comfortable with this perspective. At the same time, we recognize that for some parents the idea that their child has a disproportionate likelihood of developing a homosexual orientation triggers deep emotional reactions. The contemporary clinician, therefore, needs to consider these matters carefully and to develop a working relationship with families that is sensitive, empathic, and responsive to the complex reactions that issues pertaining to psychosexuality engender in most people.

TREATMENT OF THE CHILD

Behavior Therapy

There are 13 single-case reports of the use of a behavior therapy approach to the treatment of gender identity disorder; a majority of these are by Rekers and his associates (Dowrick, 1983; Dupont, 1968; Hay, Barlow, & Hay, 1981; Horton, 1980; Myrick, 1970; Rekers, 1979; Rekers & Lovaas, 1974; Rekers, Lovaas, & Low, 1974; Rekers & Mead, 1979; Rekers & Varni, 1977a, 1977b; Rekers, Willis, Yates, Rosen, & Low, 1977; Rekers, Yates, Willis, Rosen, & Taubman, 1976). Behavior therapy, like other forms of treatment for cross-gender-identified children, has been applied primarily to boys. (For a detailed outline of the subject and treatment characteristics of the case reports by Rekers and colleagues, see Zucker, 1985, Table 15.)

The classical behavioral approach assumes that children learn sex-typed behaviors much as they learn any other behaviors and that sex-typed behaviors can be shaped (at least initially) by encouraging some and discouraging others (cf. Mischel, 1966). Accordingly, behavior therapy for gender identity disorder systematically arranges to have rewards follow sex-appropriate behaviors and to have no rewards (or perhaps punishments) follow sex-inappropriate behaviors.

Targets and Techniques of Behavior Therapy

The behavioral targets of intervention have included a variety of cross-gender behaviors, including toy and dress-up play, role playing, exclusive affiliation with the opposite sex, and mannerisms. In addition, some treatments have focused on behavioral deficiencies, such as poor athletic ability. None of the case reports focused specifically on the child's verbal statements or fantasies about wanting to be of the opposite sex. Strictly speaking, therefore, the aim of the behavioral interventions has been to modify specific overt sex-typed behaviors rather than gender identity or gender dysphoria in general.

One type of intervention employed by Rekers and his associates has been termed *differential social attention* or *social reinforcement*. As stated by Rekers and Lovaas (1974), the therapeutic goal of such an intervention (for boys) was to "extinguish feminine behavior and to develop masculine behavior" (p. 179).[2] This type of intervention has been applied in clinic settings, particularly to sex-typed play behaviors. The therapist first establishes with baseline measures that the child (either when alone or in the presence of a noninteracting adult) prefers playing with cross-sex toys or dress-up apparel rather than same-sex toys or apparel. A parent or stranger is then introduced into the playroom and instructed to attend to the child's same-sex play (e.g., by looking, smiling, and verbal praise) and to ignore the child's cross-sex play (e.g., by looking away and pretending to read). Such adult response seems to elicit rather sharp changes in play behavior. Figure 9.1 provides an example of this procedure.

As noted by Rekers and colleagues, there have been two main limitations to the use of social attention or reinforcement in treating cross-gender behavior. First, at least some of the children studied reverted to cross-sex play patterns in the adults' absence or in other environments, such as the home—a phenomenon known as *stimulus specificity* (cf. Rekers, 1972, 1975). Second, there was little generalization to untreated cross-sex behaviors—a phenomenon known as *response specificity*. Rekers and Lovaas (1974) reported that the same limitations applied to the use of a token economy system in which a child was given points

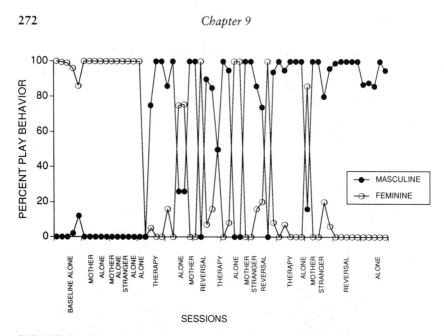

FIGURE 9.1. Percentage of feminine and masculine play behavior in a 5-year-old boy with gender identity disorder as a function of the mother's social reinforcement contingency in the clinic playroom. On the horizontal axis, "therapy" refers to the introduction of differential social attention by the mother; "reversal" refers to the withdrawal of this contingency. Adapted from Rekers and Lovaas (1974, p. 182). Copyright 1974 by the Society for the Experimental Analysis of Behavior. Adapted by permission.

for engaging in same-sex behaviors or penalized points for engaging in cross-sex behaviors.

The problems of stimulus and response specificity have led behavior therapists to seek more effective strategies of promoting generalization. One such strategy, *self-regulation,* has the child reinforce himself or herself when engaging in a sex-typical behavior. This eliminates the necessity of providing external reinforcement, which may not always be feasible. Blount and Stokes (1984) suggested that when the child is allowed to control his or her behavior, the "problems of generalization from one setting to another and from the presence to the absence of external behavior change agents may be avoided" (p. 196).

Rekers and Varni (1977a, 1977b) and Rekers and Mead (1979) reported on three cases in which self-regulation procedures were employed. In one of these reports (Rekers & Varni, 1977b), a 4-year-old boy was fitted with a wrist counter and told to press it only when playing with "boys' toys." This behavior was initially facilitated by "behavioral cuing," in which the boy wore a "bug-in-the-ear" device and was told when to press the counter. This self-monitoring procedure resulted in substantial decreases in cross-sex play, and there was also some evidence of generalization; however, as noted in detail elsewhere (Zucker, 1985, pp. 124–125), the reports of Rekers and his associates provide weak evidence for the claim that generalization is better promoted by self-regulation than by social attention.

Perhaps these difficulties can be understood in light of the work on children's gender schemas, discussed in Chapter 7. It is likely that the procedures used by behavior therapists do not fully alter internal gender schemas, and that as a result the children revert to their cross-gender behavioral preferences in the absence of external cues or incentives. For general discussions of how to induce changes in children's gender schemas, see Bem (1983); Flerx, Fidler, and Rogers (1976); Katz (1986); Katz and Walsh (1991); and Liben and Bigler (1987).

Evaluation of the Effectiveness of Behavior Therapy

An overall examination of the case reports cited above, particularly those by Rekers and his colleagues, suggests that behavior therapy techniques do have some immediate effect on the sex-typed behavior of children with gender identity disorder. For example, Rekers and his coworkers have provided short-term follow-ups of their cases (ranging from 5 weeks to 3.5 years after treatment), using a variety of formats: clinical interviews of the child and the family, home and school observations, and psychological tests. The general picture painted by Rekers and his colleagues is that all of their patients showed reductions in cross-sex behavior by the end of treatment, and that these reductions were being maintained at follow-up. Presumably, the children were also no longer wishing to change sex; this is not always specifically stated, but we believe that it can be safely inferred.

Although we believe that behavior therapy has had some success in treating children with gender identity disorder, a few critical comments are in order. First, it is obvious that behavioral improvements at follow-up cannot be unequivocally attributed to the treatment intervention without the use of a comparison group of untreated children to control for "spontaneous" remission or simple maturation effects. If the case reports by Rekers and his group are examined closely, as has been done elsewhere (Zucker, 1985), it becomes apparent that some of the changes noted at follow-up could not have been attributable solely to treatment, because these changes had not appeared by the time treatment was completed—unless one is willing to attribute the changes to "sleeper effects." Second, behavior therapists have not explained the apparent changes in gender identity (i.e., the child's desire to be of the opposite sex), which occurred even though this variable was not targeted for modification; this finding requires explanation, because the previously noted phenomenon of response specificity would lead one to expect the retention of untreated behaviors. Finally, it is unclear whether the cases reported can be generalized to all children with gender identity problems, since these cases may have been especially amenable to treatment because of particular characteristics (e.g., low levels of general psychopathology, highly motivated parents, and so on).

What do we know about the long-term outcome of children with gender identity disorder treated by behavior therapy techniques? Unfortunately, not very much. To date, Rekers and his group have provided only hints of what they have found over the long run. Rekers (1985, 687) reported that over 50 children had been "comprehensively treated" and that follow-up results suggested "permanent changes in gender identity." From this, one assumes that gender dysphoria was absent and there was no desire for sex reassignment surgery. Specific information, however, was not provided. More recently, Rekers, Kilgus, and Rosen (1990) provided group analysis of 29 boys treated by behavior therapy techniques. At a mean follow-up of 51 months after treatment, it was found that "completion" of treatment accounted for 20% of the variance in change scores, as defined by a reduction in ratings of cross-gender identification. Unfortunately, there have been no published reports on longer-term follow-ups that assess the adolescent gender identity and sexual orientation of the 29 boys. It is of interest, therefore, that Rekers (1986) has claimed, without formal substantiation, that from "the result[s] of my research studies, it now appears that a preventive treatment for transvestism, transsexualism, and some forms of homosexuality has indeed been isolated" (p. 28).

Psychotherapy

Numerous authors have reported on the treatment of cross-gender-identified children with psychoanalysis, psychoanalytic psychotherapy, or other forms of individual psychotherapy (Bleiberg et al., 1986; Bloch, 1976; Charatan & Galef, 1965; Chazan, 1995, Chap. 4; Eide-Midtsand, 1987; Fischhoff, 1964; Francis, 1965; Friend et al., 1954; Gilmore, 1995; Gilpin et al., 1979; Greenson, 1966; Haber, 1991a, 1991b; Herman, 1983; Holder, 1982; Hopkins, 1984; Karush, 1993; Lee, 1985; Loeb, 1992; Loeb & Shane, 1982; Lothstein, 1988; Lothstein & Levine, 1981; McDevitt, 1985; Meyer & Dupkin, 1985; Meyer & Sohmer, 1983; Pruett & Dahl, 1982; Sack, 1985; Sackin, 1985; Schrut, 1987; Schultz, 1979; Shane & Shane, 1995; Siegel, 1991; Silverman, 1990; Sperling, 1964; Stirtzinger & Mishna, 1994; Stone & Bernstein, 1980; Thacher, 1985; Volkan, 1979; Wallach, 1961; Wolfe, 1994; Zaphiriou, 1978). The psychoanalytic/psychotherapeutic treatment literature is more diverse than the behavior therapy literature, including varied theoretical approaches to understanding the putative etiology of gender identity disorder (e.g., classical psychoanalysis, object relations, and self psychology); nevertheless, a number of repeating themes can be gleaned from the published reports.

Psychoanalytic authors generally emphasize that cross-gender behavior emerges during the "preoedipal" years. Accordingly, they stress the importance of understanding how the gender identity disorder relates to other developmental phenomena that are salient during these years—for example, attachment (object) relations and the emergence of the self. Oedipal issues are also considered important, but these are understood within the context of prior developmental interferences and conflicts. Psychoanalytic clinicians also place great weight on the child's overall ego functioning, which they see as critical in determining the therapeutic approach to the specific referral problem (for further details, see Zucker, 1985, 1990c; Zucker & Green, 1989). In general, we have been impressed by the extent to which the putative risk factors for gender identity disorder that were reviewed in Chapter 7 can be detected in the individual case reports. Some of the more common themes are reviewed below.

Themes in Psychoanalytic Treatment

Mother–Child Relations. Some case reports of boys noted that an actual physical loss of the mother (or a mother surrogate) preceded the emergence of feminine behaviors (e.g., Gilpin et al., 1979; Wallach, 1961). This loss was understood to create a vulnerability in the child, which the child may have dealt with defensively, at least in part, by resorting to the use of behavioral enactments of gender representations (a "fetish" in the older analytic literature). In this view, the goal of therapy would be to help the child work through the loss of the attachment figure, which would presumably then alleviate the need to engage in cross-gender behavior.

In a chart review of our own cases, we found that 18 (10.6%) of 169 boys had experienced a long-term ($\geq$ 1 year) or permanent loss of their mothers after the age of 12 months (2 to death; 2 to separation/divorce; 13 to mothers' abandonment of their sons or inability to look after them, resulting in care by fathers or relatives, adoption, or foster placement; and 1 to abduction by the father). In a majority of these cases, however, an analysis of the history indicated that the feminine behavior had begun prior to maternal loss, so that at best the actual loss could be regarded only as a perpetuating factor. Given the circumstances of the remaining cases, it was very difficult (because of lack of a reliable informant) to discern whether the loss might have precipitated the onset of cross-gender behavior.

In some case reports, a psychological loss or withdrawal of the mother was deemed important (e.g., Pruett & Dahl, 1982; see also Chapter 5). Coates (1985) reported a high rate of adverse life events ("trauma") experienced by the mothers of boys with gender identity disorder during the putative sensitive period for gender identity formation. These events included physical and sexual assault, death of the boys' siblings, and husbands' extramarital affairs. Coates et al. (1991), Schultz (1979), and Thacher (1985), among others, have all provided detailed accounts of this perspective. The psychological sequelae (separation anxiety, feminine behavior, etc.) are then the same as those for boys who physically lose their mothers.

But other psychoanalytic psychotherapists have explained feminine behavior in boys in precisely the opposite way: Feminine identification is caused not by excessive distance from the mother, but by excessive closeness to her (e.g., Greenson, 1966; Loeb & Shane, 1982; Stoller, 1966, 1975, 1985b). In this view, the therapeutic task would be to help the boy individuate from his mother.

Father–Child Relations. The role of the father has received comment in many case reports. In a majority of these reports, the father was described as physically absent or psychologically peripheral (e.g., Haber, 1991a; Stoller, 1966), and hence as unavailable to counteract or buffer the distortions in the mother–son relationship. In other reports, the father was described as severely disturbed and unpredictably aggressive, and therefore as difficult for the son to identify with (e.g., Fischhoff, 1964).

If the father is truly remote or psychologically disturbed in his own right, part of the therapeutic task with the son who has gender identity disorder is to help the son develop a more diverse perception of men and maleness and thus to assimilate and work through the negative impact of the father's psychopathology and build on whatever strengths may exist in the father–son relationship. It is possible that when the therapist is a male, transference phenomena (e.g., idealization, identification) can be more readily used to facilitate a masculine identification.

Parental Encouragement of Cross-Gender Behavior. Stoller (1968b, 1975) stressed the effects of parental attitudes toward masculinity and femininity on the child's development. He argued that the mothers of extremely feminine boys had had gender identity conflicts as children (see Chapter 7), which led them to devalue men and masculinity. In Stoller's view, such devaluation is felt by a young boy, who somehow comes to believe that his mother will reject him if he is masculine but that he can preserve his relationship with her if he is feminine.

Other reports have also implicated mothers' (or grandmothers') encouragement of femininity and devaluation of men in the development of cross-gender identity in boys (e.g., Bleiberg et al., 1986; Loeb, 1992; Loeb & Shane, 1982; Lothstein, 1988). In fact, we were unable to identify in any case reports a clinician who felt that the parents unequivocally encouraged a masculine identity in their sons. But the motivations that were judged to underlie this aspect of parental behavior appeared to vary considerably. Nevertheless, it is of interest that the proximal variable of parental tolerance or encouragement of cross-gender behavior has been apparent in the intensive case reports offered by psychotherapists, which converge in this respect with the observations of those who hold other theoretical perspectives (see Chapter 7).

Eclectic Psychotherapy

Influenced by Stoller's (1968b) claim that extremely feminine boys did not experience internalized conflict and thus were not amenable to psychoanalysis, Green, Newman, and Stoller (1972) developed a more eclectic and multimodal approach to the psychotherapy of cross-gender-identified boys (see also Cohen, 1976; Green, 1974; Higham, 1976; Kosky, 1987; Lim & Bottomley, 1983; Metcalf & Williams, 1977; Money & Lehne, 1993; Newman, 1976; Stoller, 1970, 1978; Stoller & Newman, 1971; Wrate & Gulens, 1986; Zecca, Lertora, & Macchi, 1990). The therapeutic approach of Green, Newman, and Stoller (1972) had four stated objectives: (1) developing a relationship of "trust and affection" between the boy and a male therapist; (2) heightening parental concern regarding the boy's femininity; (3) increasing the father's involvement in the boy's life; and (4) sensitizing the parents to the dynamics of their own relationship, in order to alter the mother–son overcloseness and the father's peripheral role in the family. Green, Newman, and Stoller's (1972) therapy was intended to help feminine boys "understand" the motives for their cross-gender behavior and to indicate to such boys that being masculine is "good." Thus, approval was given for "any signs of masculinity" (p. 214) in either overt behavior or fantasy.

Sex of the Therapist

A technical question that is often asked in the psychotherapy of cross-gender-identified children is whether the therapist's sex should match that of the child. It has been argued that male therapists would be most therapeutic for feminine boys, because the close relationships of such children have usually been with women. Similarly, it has been argued that female therapists would be best for cross-gendered girls, whose normal feminine identification with their mothers has been impaired by the mothers' depression and devaluation of their own femininity (see Chapter 7).

These arguments seem plausible; on the other hand, one might argue that an opposite-sex therapist has the potential to "correct" distortions that have developed in a child's relationship with his or her opposite-sex parent. There have, in any event, been no systematic studies demonstrating that the sex of the therapist makes any difference. The most important qualification of the therapist is probably that he or she feel comfortable with the content issues arising in the treatment of cross-gender-identified children.

Evaluation of the Effectiveness of Psychotherapy

An overall examination of the available case reports suggests that psychotherapy, like behavior therapy, does have some beneficial influence on the sex-typed behavior of cross-gender-identified children. However, the effectiveness of psychoanalysis and other forms of psychotherapy, also like that of behavior therapy, has never been demonstrated in an outcome study comparing children randomly assigned to treated and untreated conditions. Moreover, many of the cases cited above did not consist solely of individual therapy with the child. The parents were often also in therapy, and in some of the cases the child was an inpatient and thus exposed to other interventions. It is impossible to disentangle these other potential therapeutic influences from the effect of the psychotherapy alone. (For a detailed outline of the subject and treatment characteristics of the majority of psychoanalytic case reports, see Zucker, 1985, Table 16.)

What do we know about the long-term outcome of gender-disordered children treated by psychotherapeutic techniques? Again, not very much. There have been no published long-term follow-up reports assessing gender identity or sexual orientation, and personal correspondence with several authors of psychotherapy case reports (Zucker, 1985) indicated that a majority (9 of 17) had no unpublished follow-up information either. Of the 8 cases for whom data were available, none were known to be transsexual, 6 were judged to be heterosexual, and 2 were judged to be homosexual.

Group Therapy

Another approach to the treatment of cross-gender-identified boys has involved group therapy. Green and Fuller (1973b) reported on the group treatment of seven boys (age range = 4–9 years). Each of these boys was reported to be aware, in varying degree, "of the reason for his inclusion in the group" (p. 55). Weekly sessions were held in a playground with a male therapist, who verbally reinforced the boys for nonfeminine, socially competent behaviors and verbally admonished them for feminine behaviors. At these sessions, the boys themselves often criticized one another for feminine behaviors. It was reported that both parental narratives and behavioral ratings of the boys indicated "change on a variety of parameters" (pp. 66–67) concerned with cross-gender identification. Detailed analyses were not available, however.

Bates et al. (1975) employed group therapy with gender problem boys who were mainly between the ages of 8 and 13. Their program emphasized the encouragement of masculine behavior and general social skills. In contrast to the approach of Green and Fuller (1973b), feminine behavior was not explicitly discouraged. Both modeling by the male therapists and more structured behavior modification techniques were used. Concurrent with the children's group, the parents also met in groups, with one of the main goals being to work on ways to improve father–son relationships. Although systematic data were not recorded, Bates et al. (1975) felt that the boys showed "recognizable improvement . . . both in terms of social skills development and in the development of masculine interests and abilities" (p. 154). Parental reports and the boys' self-reports indicated similar changes in the neighborhood and at school, including "less interest in cross-dressing, doll play, and imitating females" (p. 154).

Meyer-Bahlburg (1993c) has also emphasized the role of the peer group in facilitating behavioral change. The main strategy in Meyer-Bahlburg's treatment protocol was to have the parents of boys with gender identity disorder arrange consistent "play dates" for their sons with other boys. As noted in Chapter 2, many boys with gender identity disorder avoid boys as playmates and are often anxious about involvement in rough-and-tumble play. If the parents of such boys are able to find other boys whom their sons do not experience as too threatening, these boys may serve as role models for the development of more gender-typical play and activities. Meyer-Bahlburg indicated that this approach appeared effective in reducing cross-gender behavior after a short time, and that the boys successfully developed the friendships they formed in this way. Unfortunately, detailed information was lacking.

TREATMENT OF THE PARENTS

Two rationales have been offered for the involvement of parents in the treatment of their cross-gender-identified children. The first emphasizes the hypothesized role of parental dynamics in the genesis or maintenance of a child's disorder. From this perspective, individual therapy with the child will probably proceed more smoothly and quickly if the parents are able to gain some insight into their own contribution to their child's difficulties. Many clinicians, including ourselves, who have worked extensively with gender-disturbed children subscribe to this rationale (e.g., Coates, 1985; Green, Newman, Stoller, 1972; Newman, 1976; Stoller, 1978).

The second rationale is that parents need regular, formalized contact with the therapist to discuss day-to-day management issues that arise in carrying out the overall therapeutic plan. Our clinic, for example, suggests that parents not allow cross-dressing, discourage cross-gender role play and fantasy play, restrict play with cross-sex toys, tell the child that they value him as a boy or her as a girl, encourage same-sex peer relations, and help the child engage in more sex-appropriate or neutral activities. Some parents, especially the well-functioning and intellectually sophisticated ones, are able to carry out these recommendations relatively easily and without ambivalence. Many parents, however, require ongoing support in implementing the recommendations, perhaps because of their own ambivalence and reservations about gender identity issues (see, e.g., Newman, 1976). Some of these parents find it difficult to believe that their child has a gender identity problem; others are reluctant to restrict their child's favorite fantasies or activities. Regular involvement with such parents then benefits the child's treatment.

Although some case reports suggest that substantial therapeutic change can occur with minimal parental involvement (e.g., Sackin, 1985; cf. Karush, 1993), our experience is that parental involvement in therapy is required in the majority of cases. Although we concur with other clinicians in the importance of addressing familial and intrapersonal factors in therapy, we do not share the perspective of those clinicians whose therapeutic approach does not include the setting of limits on the cross-gender behavior. Our view is that limit-setting helps the child to become less confused about his or her gender identity (from the "outside in," as we explain to some parents), whereas the traditionally more open-ended approach within individual psychotherapy sessions helps the child to work through the various conflicts that have contributed to the consolidation of a cross-gender identity (from the "inside out"). In general, contact with the parents is important in gaining an understanding of, and helping the parents to understand, the day-to-day problems experienced by children with gender identity disorder (Pleak & Anderson, 1993).

Is there empirical evidence that working with the parents makes a difference? Again, systematic information on the question is scanty. The most relevant study (Zucker et al., 1985) found some evidence that parental involvement in therapy was significantly correlated with a greater degree of behavioral change in children at a 1-year follow-up, but this study did not assign families randomly to different treatment protocols.

IN THE BEST INTEREST OF THE CHILD: THERAPEUTIC OPTIMISM OR NIHILISM?

Most of the critics of therapy with children with gender identity disorder are not clinicians. Those critics who are clinicians appear to have had no experience in the area. Although we disagree with many of their objections, the fact that these critics are not "experts in the field" is not a sufficient reason for dismissing their concerns. Any clinician faced with the task of assessing, diagnosing, and considering options in the treatment of gender identity disorder must attempt to familiarize himself or herself with the disorder and then, with each child's family, decide what treatment plan (if any) should be followed. We hope that the information provided in this volume will be of use in that decision.

In this section, we offer some of our own views about the merits of offering therapeutic intervention. In our clinical experience, we have found no compelling reason not to offer treatment to a child with gender identity disorder. We have reviewed the evidence on the impact of marked cross-gender identification on the child's psychosocial functioning, documented the nature of the associated psychopathology, and summarized what is known about the familial psychopathology. We have found that many of the youngsters we have evaluated are very troubled, as are their families. In a small minority of cases, despite the presence of marked cross-gender identification, other aspects of the children's functioning are relatively intact. The range in parental functioning is also great. In regard to prognosis, it is necessary to take a guarded stance concerning the possibility of therapeutic change in very disturbed children and families, as is the case with any child psychiatric disorder. Thus, the severity of the disorder and the extent of familial risk factors must be considered. Another factor that must be considered is the age of the child. In general, we concur with those (e.g., Green, Newman, & Stoller, 1972; Newman, 1976; Stoller, 1978) who believe that the earlier treatment begins, the better. With children approaching puberty, it is often harder to effect therapeutic change; thus, one has to be especially cautious about what can be done with such children. Nevertheless, these generalizations can be made only with great care.

It has been our experience that a sizable number of children and their families achieve a great deal of change. In these cases, the gender identity disorder resolves fully, and nothing in the children's behavior or fantasy suggests that gender identity issues remain problematic. In a smaller number of cases, there is minimal or no evidence of change in the children's cross-gender identification and other behavioral difficulties. All things considered, however, we take the position that in such cases a clinician should be optimistic, not nihilistic, about the possibility of helping the children to become more secure in their gender identity. Research and clinical work pertaining to gender identity disorder is only a little over 30 years old, and only a small number of professionals have worked in the area. Much remains to be done.

NOTES

1. It is not clear whether Bem's objection pertains to behavior therapy per se, to the particular brand of behavior therapy practiced by Rekers and his colleagues, to the putative goals of that brand of behavior therapy, or to a more general ethical/ideological concern regarding the treatment of children with gender identity disorder.

2. Perhaps because of the criticisms directed at Rekers's work, Rekers and his colleagues made what seems to be a post hoc revision of their therapeutic aim: "[Our] intent and . . . practice [have been] . . . to enhance supporting masculine behaviors, *while maintaining the coexisting feminine behaviors*" (Rosen, Rekers, & Brigham, 1982, p. 372, italics added). This revision is inconsistent with their actual accounts of treatment, and we are not persuaded that it makes clinical sense. Consider, for example, a preschool boy who, among other things, cross-dresses both at home and at nursery school. What would the rationale be for allowing the cross-dressing to continue? It is unlikely that this would allay social ostracism—one of the rationales that Rekers and colleagues offer for intervention.

CHAPTER 10

Follow-Up

Several follow-up studies of cross-gender-identified children (almost all of boys) have provided information on postpubertal gender identity and sexual orientation. Green's (1987) prospective study, the most comprehensive of these studies and the only one that included a comparison group, can be used as a frame of reference for the other studies (Bakwin, 1968; Davenport, 1986; Kosky, 1987; Lebovitz, 1972; Money & Russo, 1979; Zuger, 1978, 1984). The available follow-up data on case reports published prior to 1985 have been summarized elsewhere (Zucker, 1985, pp. 143–153).

GREEN'S (1987) STUDY AND OTHER STUDIES

Green's (1987) study began with a sample of 66 feminine and 56 control boys, assessed initially at a mean age of 7 years (range = 4–12 years). About two-thirds of the boys from each group were available for follow-up at a mean age of 19 years (range = 14–24 years). At the follow-up, a semistructured interview protocol was used to assess sexual orientation. Sexual orientation was assessed separately for fantasy and behavior; in each of these domains, it was rated on a 7-point scale ranging from exclusive heterosexuality (0) to exclusive homosexuality (6) (Kinsey et al., 1948).

Table 10.1 shows the sexual orientation of the two groups. Of the 44 feminine boys seen for follow-up, 33 (75%) were classified as bisexual or homosexual in fantasy (Kinsey ratings of 2–6), and 11 (25%) were classified as predominantly or exclusively heterosexual in fantasy (Kinsey ratings of 0–1). All 35 control boys seen for follow-up were classified as heterosexual in fantasy. Of the 30 feminine boys who had

TABLE 10.1. Sexual Orientation in Fantasy and Behavior at Follow-Up in Green's (1987) Study

Kinsey rating	Feminine boys ($n = 44$)	Control boys ($n = 35$)
Fantasy		
0	9 (20.5%)	33 (94.3%)
1	2 (4.5%)	2 (5.7%)
2	6 (13.6%)	0 (0.0%)
3	0 (0.0%)	0 (0.0%)
4	9 (20.5%)	0 (0.0%)
5	10 (22.7%)	0 (0.0%)
6	8 (18.2%)	0 (0.0%)
Behavior		
0	5 (16.7%)	24 (96.0%)
1	1 (3.3%)	0 (0.0%)
2	3 (10.0%)	1 (4.0%)
3	1 (3.3%)	0 (0.0%)
4	7 (23.3%)	0 (0.0%)
5	5 (16.7%)	0 (0.0%)
6	8 (26.7%)	0 (0.0%)

Note. Data from Green (1987, pp. 102–103). Not all subjects had experienced overt, interpersonal sexual behaviors, so the *n* is smaller for this rating. 0, exclusively heterosexual; 6, exclusively homosexual.

had overt sexual experiences, 24 (80%) were classified as bisexual or homosexual, and 6 (20%) were classified as heterosexual. All but one of the 25 control boys who had had overt sexual experiences were classified as heterosexual. (The one control boy with bisexual behavior was an identical twin of a proband; see Green, 1987, Chap. 8, and Green & Stoller, 1971.) Thus, Green's (1987) study produced quite strong evidence that feminine boys have a greatly increased probability of ending up homosexual in adulthood. This finding converged closely with the findings of the retrospective literature on the relation between childhood sex-typed behavior and sexual orientation (see Bailey & Zucker, 1995).

A word is in order here regarding the combining of Green's bisexual and homosexual cases—a procedure whose validity is sometimes contested (e.g., Paul, 1993). It is common for homosexual men to recall bisexual behavior during adolescence; thus, it is likely that adolescent subjects who describe themselves as bisexual will move toward a more exclusively homosexual orientation. This prediction is based in part on extensive clinical experience, in the course of which it has been found that most bisexual men are more strongly aroused by homosexual stimuli than by heterosexual stimuli (e.g., Langevin, 1983), although they may not label themselves as "homosexuals" (see, e.g., Ross, 1983). Moreover, it is known that the age at which many people "come out" as gay or homosexual extends into the early 20s, if not later.

Green (1987) also assessed the gender identity of his participants at follow-up, although the precise procedures used in making this assessment were not reported. Only 1 (2%) of the 44 feminine boys was seriously entertaining the notion of sex reassignment surgery. This boy was 18 years old at the time of follow-up (see Green, 1987, pp. 115–132).

How do Green's data compare with the data from the other six published follow-up studies of boys with gender identity disorder? The data from these six studies are presented in Table 10.2. A total of 55 boys were seen in follow-up, usually in late adolescence or young adulthood (range = 13–36 years). At follow-up, 5 of these boys were classified as transsexual (with a homosexual sexual orientation), 21 were classified as homosexual, 1 was classified as a (heterosexual) transvestite, 15 were classified as heterosexual, and 13 could not be rated with regard to sexual orientation. If one excludes the 13 "uncertain" cases in these six studies, then 27 (64.2%) of the remaining 42 cases had "atypical" (i.e., homosexual, transsexual, or transvestitic) outcomes.

TABLE 10.2. Sexual Orientation in Six Other Follow-Up Studies of Boys with Gender Identity Disorder

Study	Homosexual	Heterosexual	Uncertain	Lost to follow-up
Bakwin (1968)	2	2	3	4
Lebovitz (1972)	3	3	4	19
Zuger (1978)	9	2	1	—
Money & Russo (1979)	9	0	0	2
Davenport (1986)	3	6	1	0
Kosky (1987)	0	2	4	1
Total	26	15	13	26

Note. Only subjects who were first assessed during childhood, not adolescence, are listed. An additional subject in Lebovitz's report was described as a "heterosexual transvestite." Number of subjects lost to follow-up in Lebovitz's study may include some who were first assessed during adolescence (the age of these subjects when first assessed was not provided). Zuger (1984) reported a subsequent follow-up, indicating that 35 subjects were homosexual, 3 were heterosexual, 7 were uncertain, and 7 were lost to follow-up. Unfortunately, 16 of these subjects were first assessed during adolescence, and follow-up of these subjects was not reported separately from those who were first assessed during childhood.

These outcomes are obviously quite comparable to Green's (1987) finding.

A full appreciation of these follow-up data requires one to consider certain general methodological issues in the prospective study of feminine boys. First, it should be understood that the percentage of atypical outcomes is likely to be underestimated in such studies, given the sensitive material involved. This underestimation may be especially great if the reporting authors have little rapport with their subjects, perhaps because their involvement with the subjects has been minimal over the years. Second, some of the published follow-up studies were rather vague about how they assessed and classified psychosexual status (e.g., Kosky, 1987). Third, some of the classifications in these studies were based solely on maternal report (e.g., Bakwin, 1968). Fourth, the age of subjects at follow-up may affect the proportion of atypical outcomes observed, with longer follow-ups revealing larger percentages of homosexual or transsexual outcomes. As noted elsewhere (Zucker, 1988), data from Green's (1987) study indicate that older adolescents or young adults were more likely than younger adolescents to acknowledge a homosexual orientation (Table 10.3). This finding is reinforced by the fact that Money and Russo's (1979) and Zuger's (1978, 1984) relatively thorough studies, which examined most of their subjects in young adulthood, found a somewhat higher proportion of atypical outcomes than that found by the other studies: 90% of Money and Russo's and Zuger's combined cases were homosexual or transsexual. It would be of interest, therefore, to have further follow-up on the heterosexual

TABLE 10.3. Relation between Age and Sexual Orientation in Green's (1987) Study

	Age (in years)	
Sexual orientation	*M*	*SD*
Fantasy[a]		
Homosexual/bisexual (*n* = 33)	19.7	2.0
Heterosexual (*n* = 11)	16.8	2.1
Behavior[b]		
Homosexual/bisexual (*n* = 24)	20.3	1.6
Heterosexual (*n* = 6)	17.2	1.2
No behavior (*n* = 14)	17.6	2.7

Note. Data from Green (1987, p. 102). The correlation between age and sexual orientation (continuous rating) in fantasy was .51 (*n* = 44, *p* < .001), and in behavior was .43 (*n* = 30, *p* < .01).
[a]$t(42) = 4.07, p < .001$.
[b]$F(2, 41) = 10.5, p < .001$.

minority in Green's (1987) study once they are within the age range of the bisexual/homosexual majority.

EVIDENCE REGARDING THE LONG-TERM EFFECTS OF THERAPY

The behavior therapy and psychotherapy case report literatures (see Chapter 9) have not provided a satisfactory database for evaluating the long-term effects of treatment on gender identity or sexual orientation. A few of the prospective studies of feminine boys included children who underwent various forms of treatment. These studies, therefore, are an alternative source of information on the outcome of therapy for cross-gender-identified children.

Green (1987) reported that 12 of the 44 feminine boys on whom follow-up data were available "entered a formal treatment program," such as behavior therapy, group therapy, individual therapy, or therapy with the parents. Green further noted that "most parents . . . elected not to seek therapy for their child's cross-gender behaviors, but rather to try gently to discourage the behaviors as they occurred" (p. 260).

The one boy in Green's study who was transsexual at follow-up had not received treatment. The feminine boys who later developed a bisexual or homosexual orientation did not differ from those with a heterosexual orientation as a function of involvement in therapy. Green felt that these data indicated the "apparent powerlessness of treatment to interrupt the progression from 'feminine' boy to homosexual or bisexual man" (p. 318). He did find, however, that at follow-up the feminine boys who received treatment had self-concept scores somewhat higher than those of the feminine boys who did not receive treatment, and that the boys themselves "look[ed] back favorably" on the treatment experience.

In our view, Green's (1987) conclusions must be regarded cautiously. First, it should be recognized that the primary aims of Green's study were descriptive and etiological, not therapeutic. Cases were not randomly selected to receive or not to receive treatment. Second, one must question what constituted treatment. Green did not provide basic information about the therapies, such as their length, the experience of the therapists, the short-term effects on the children, and so on.

Zuger (1966) also provided some information on the treatment experiences of his patients. He noted that "all parents were given guidance which it was thought would lead to a better masculine identification. They were advised to discourage effeminate activities and to reinforce masculine ones" (p. 1105). The treatment of Zuger's one eventual transsexual consisted of "consultations and several inter-views." One of Zuger's two eventual heterosexuals was seen in therapy over a 3-year period, as were his parents, but the other received no treatment except for advice given to his parents at the time of the assessment. The patients who were later classified as homosexual received varying amounts of treatment during childhood, but generally not for very long. Because the great majority of Zuger's feminine boys later proved to be homosexual, one can conclude that, whatever the treatment interventions may have been, they clearly did not produce heterosexuality. Zuger's research, like Green's, was not designed to evaluate the effects of therapy; and in Zuger's study, as in Green's, what actually constituted treatment is unclear.

As noted in Chapter 9, Rekers, Kilgus, and Rosen (1990) reported short-term data on therapy outcome. To our knowledge, however, Rekers and his colleagues have not published results concerning postpubertal sexual orientation and gender identity. Thus, Rekers's (1986) claim to have isolated "a preventive treatment for . . . transsexualism, and some forms of homosexuality" (p. 28) is puzzling.

It appears, then, that the (largely unspecified) treatments administered to feminine boys in the two major prospective studies had little or no impact on adult sexual orientation (see also Money & Russo, 1979). There is suggestive evidence that therapy might have had a beneficial effect on adult gender identity, in that none of the patients who ended up transsexual had received treatment during childhood.

At this point, formal outcome studies of cross-gender-identified children are needed to determine whether some types of treatment are better than others, and whether any type of treatment is significantly better than no treatment. Process studies are also needed to learn why, with or without intensive treatment, the vast majority of cross-gender-identified children eventually relinquish the desire to change sex. Finally, research is needed to determine the best age for clinical intervention. Our own clinical experience suggests that treatment is most effective prior to puberty and that in adolescence it becomes much more difficult to affect the desire to change sex, as is discussed in Chapter 11.

CORRELATES OF SEXUAL ORIENTATION
AND TRANSSEXUALISM

It has been well established by studies of children at risk for major mental disorders, such as schizophrenia or major depression, that the outcome is variable: Some of these children remain well, whereas others develop the full-blown syndrome. It is possible, therefore, to examine predictors of outcome within a group of children at risk (cf. McNeil & Kaij, 1979).

As noted in Chapter 3, adult transsexuals, particularly those with a homosexual orientation, invariably recall a childhood cross-gender history. The follow-up studies of cross-gender-identified children (again, mainly of boys) found that only a very small percentage persisted in their wish to change sex after puberty, although that percentage does appear to be considerably higher than the percentage one would expect on the basis of general population rates for transsexualism. Why is this? There are several possibilities. One possibility is that because of the low base rate of transsexualism, even within the population of cross-gender-identified children, identifying the few transsexual cases requires a large sample size (Weinrich, 1985). Another possibility—a stronger one, in our view—is that the severity of the condition varies, even among children with gender identity disorder who meet the complete diagnostic criteria. Apart from other influences, such as perpetuating factors, it is conceivable that many of the children with gender identity disorder are simply not disturbed enough to be at bona fide risk for subsequent transsexualism. A third possibility is that the assessment process and (when it occurs) therapeutic intervention alter the natural history of cross-gender identification, thus reducing the risk of later transsexualism. Unfortunately, we do not have good predictive data that explain why a small minority of children followed prospectively eventually seek sex reassignment surgery.

Clinically, it has been our impression that children who do not move away from extreme cross-gender identification as they enter adolescence may be at greater risk for later transsexualism. In our experience, the persistence of gender dysphoria, including the desire to change sex, is considerably higher among patients who are first assessed during adolescence and followed up later than among patients who are first assessed during childhood and followed up later. This suggests that the clinical situation at or near the transition from childhood to adolescence may be crucial in differentiating a transsexual outcome from other outcomes.

Green (1987; Green, Roberts, Williams, Goodman, & Mixon, 1987) compared on a number of childhood variables the feminine boys who were subsequently classified as bisexual or homosexual with the feminine boys who were subsequently classified as heterosexual. Although some feminine behaviors distinguished the two subgroups, a composite childhood femininity score only approached conventional levels of significance, and only for the rating of sexual orientation in fantasy (not behavior). The lack of a stronger correlation is somewhat surprising, since one might have expected an association between the degree of cross-gender identification and long-term outcome; however, Green did find that the continuation of certain feminine behaviors throughout childhood was associated with later homosexuality. Thus, it may be that the persistence of these feminine behaviors is more important than their extent during the early childhood years. Less father–son shared time in the first 2 years of life was also found to be associated with later homosexuality, but the amount of mother–son shared time was not.

THE TORONTO FOLLOW-UP STUDY: PRELIMINARY RESULTS

To date, we have followed 45 children into adolescence or young adulthood. Our follow-up strategy has been to conduct an initial assessment in midadolescence, in which we obtain information on gender identity, sexual orientation, and general socioemotional functioning. In this section, we provide a glimpse of the preliminary results pertaining to gender identity and sexual orientation.

Gender identity and sexual orientation were assessed by means of a structured interview (which was audiotaped) and paper-and-pencil self-report questionnaires. The interview always preceded the self-report questionnaires, which provided an immediate cross-check of the interview and served additional quantitative purposes. Discrepancies between the interview and the self-report questionnaires were resolved by further discussion with the youngster. (As it turned out, such discrepancies were very rare, so they are not considered further here.) In the assessment of gender identity, questions pertaining to gender dysphoria were asked, including questions on the subject's desire to change sex and on the subject's feelings about his or her gender status as a male or female. In addition, the participants completed a paper-and-pencil questionnaire pertaining to gender dysphoria.

The assessment of sexual orientation used Green's (1987) procedure. Regarding fantasy, the participants were asked about crushes, visual arousal, dream imagery, and masturbation imagery. Regarding behavior, the participants were asked about dating, holding hands, kissing, genital touching, and engaging in intercourse. Kinsey et al. (1948) ratings were assigned to each item, and global ratings were then made for fantasy and behavior, respectively. Only ratings for the 12-month period prior to the interview are reported here. A number of the sexual orientation interviews were scored by a second rater, who was unaware of the primary interviewer's ratings; there were no major discrepancies in these ratings.

Rapport with the subjects appeared to be good in most cases—at least in the sense that most of the participants were well known to us, inasmuch as we had conducted the original assessment, had followed many of the participants and their families over time, and in a few cases had conducted the treatment (when it occurred) with the subject and/or the family. This rapport might also be reflected in our refusal rate. To date, only two youngsters have declined to participate in the follow-up study; interestingly, in both cases their mothers did not want them to be interviewed. At the time of follow-up, none of the participants were in treatment with either of us, although a few were in therapy with other practitioners. Table 10.4 provides demographic information on the sample.

TABLE 10.4. Demographic Characteristics of the Toronto Follow-Up Sample

Variables	Data
Age at assessment (in years)	
M	8.3
SD	2.7
Range	3.1–14.3
Age at follow-up (in years)	
M	16.7
SD	2.3
Range	13.1–23.5
Interval (in years)	
M	8.4
SD	2.6
Range	2.8–14.9
IQ	
M	105.8
SD	18.5
Range	53–144
Social class[a]	
M	35.8
SD	15.6
Range	8–66
Marital status	
Two parents (n)	26
Mother only/reconstituted (n)	19

[a]Hollingshead's (1975) Four-Factor Index of Social Status.

Gender Identity

Table 10.5 provides information on gender identity. Participants were classified as gender-dysphoric if they indicated during the clinical interview that they desired sex reassignment surgery, wished that they had been born as a member of the opposite sex, and/or wondered whether they would be happier as a member of the opposite sex. On this basis, 9 (20%) of the participants were classified as gender-dysphoric at follow-up. Of these 9 youngsters, 6 desired sex reassignment surgery, 7 wished that they had been born as a member of the opposite sex, and 9 wondered whether they would be happier as a member of the opposite sex. In part because of their age, only two of these youngsters have thus far been referred for further evaluation to the Clarke Institute's Adult Gender Identity Clinic. It is, of course, unclear whether their gender dysphoria will persist and lead to eventual sex reassignment surgery. The following vignettes illustrate the clinical status of these youngsters.

CASE EXAMPLE 10.1

José was initially assessed at age 10 (IQ = 104). Although he did not meet the full DSM-III criteria for gender identity disorder, he was markedly cross-gender-identified. He had been referred by school authorities because of his effeminacy and the attendant social ostracism that he experienced. His parents, who did not speak English, denied that he had any problems and refused to receive feedback. José was referred again by school authorities at age 13 because of similar concerns. At this time, both José and his parents were more receptive to receiving help, but they did not follow through. When José was seen for an initial follow-up at age 15, he reported no gender dysphoria and an exclusively heterosexual orientation. He claimed that he had just been elected class president and that he had received A's in his schoolwork; however, he could provide no documentation of these claims. A year later, José requested an interview. At that time, he was cross-dressing and passing socially as a female. He had dropped out of school and run away from home, and he was abusing recreational drugs and engaging in prostitution. He reported an exclusively homosexual orientation and urgently requested sex reassignment surgery. He stated that in the initial follow-up he had "lied" about his feelings because he had been "embarrassed."

CASE EXAMPLE 10.2

Chris was initially assessed at age 12 (IQ = 144). Chris was referred by school authorities, after it was learned that this youngster, who had registered in a new school as a male was in fact a female. Her name and appearance did not provide phenotypic cues to her actual sex. Chris's mother was quite distraught about her gender development, but her father was unconcerned. Her parents did not pursue the recommendation of therapy. When seen for follow-up in midadolescence, Chris reported that she felt very unhappy about being a girl but did not know what to do about it. She reported that she had had no sexual experiences in either fantasy or behavior, describing herself as "sexually dead." She also reported intense suicidal ideation. Nevertheless, Chris rejected efforts to engage her in therapy. A teacher to whom she felt close was able to provide her with some support and structure.

CASE EXAMPLE 10.3

Jethro was initially assessed at age 8 (IQ = 78). He had been in either foster care or day treatment since the age of 2. His family life was extremely chaotic, and his single mother was unable to provide him with appropriate care. His general functioning was very poor. Subsequent to the initial assessment, Jethro never returned to his mother, remaining in various foster care arrangements or group home settings. At the time of follow-up at age 15, he was extremely preoccupied with sexuality and constantly looking for older male sexual partners. He wanted to cross-dress publicly and strongly requested sex reassignment surgery.

CASE EXAMPLE 10.4

Greg was assessed initially at age 5 (IQ = 100). The referral was somewhat unusual, in that he had been seen in another child psychiatric setting, to which his teacher had referred him because of aggressive behaviors directed at girls. During this assessment, the interviewers noted that Greg was extremely preoccupied with femaleness and femininity. This behavior was denied by his mother but not by his father. When the issue was explored with his parents, his mother fled the assessment room in tears. Greg and his parents were seen for several years in psychotherapy. Although his gender dysphoria diminished during this period and his functioning at school improved, he retained many elements of cross-gender identification. In early adolescence, Greg initiated further therapeutic involvement. He talked strongly about wanting sex-reassignment surgery. In therapy, he became able to talk about his sexual attraction to males, but he felt unable to share this information with his family. He used therapy as a forum for the discussion of his sexual orientation and his feelings about being a male.

TABLE 10.5. Gender Identity and Sexual Orientation in the Toronto Follow-Up Study

ID	Sex	Age at assessment (in years)	Age at follow-up (in years)	Kinsey ratings		Gender identity	DSM
				Fantasy	Behavior		
01.	M	6.4	18.2	6	6	Dysphoric	+
02.	M	5.7	15.1	0	—	WNL	+
03.	M	8.2	17.7	0	0	WNL	−
04.	M	6.4	18.3	0	0	WNL	+
05.	M	5.1	15.1	0	—	WNL	+
06.	F	5.4	16.3	—	—	WNL	+
07.	M	8.9	19.6	(6)^a	(6)^a	WNL	−
08.	M	9.5	17.7	0	—	WNL	+
09.	M	5.9	15.1	0	—	WNL	+
10.	F	5.9	17.4	0	0	WNL	−
11.	M	8.0	16.1	0	0	WNL	+
12.	F	14.3^b	23.0	0	—	Dysphoric	−
13.	M	12.9	20.1	5	6	WNL	+
14.	M	5.3	20.2	5	—	WNL	+
15.	M	8.8	19.0	2	—	Dysphoric	+
16.	M	6.2	14.2	—	—	WNL	−
17.	M	4.7	14.3	0	—	WNL	−
18.	M	10.4	17.3	0	—	WNL	+
19.	M	7.0	14.2	0	0	Dysphoric	+
20.	M	7.2	14.7	0	—	WNL	−
21.	M	12.4	18.8	0	0	WNL	−
22.	M	10.7	19.4	6	6	Dysphoric	+
23.	M	6.5	14.3	0	0	WNL	+
24.	F	3.2	14.8	0	—	WNL	+

25.	M	5.9	16.6	3	0	Dysphoric	+
26.	M	5.1	15.8	0	—	WNL	+
27.	M	11.1	23.5	6	6	WNL	−
28.	M	10.5	19.1	6	6	Dysphoric	+
29.	M	5.3	16.8	0	0	WNL	+
30.	M	8.6	15.3	3	—	WNL	+
31.	M	11.1	16.7	0	4	WNL	+
32.	M	8.5	14.8	0	—	WNL	+
33.	M	5.6	15.0	0	—	WNL	−
34.	M	9.1	16.5	0	—	WNL	+
35.	M	3.8	13.1	2	—	WNL	+
36.	M	9.3	14.1	3	—	WNL	−
37.	M	12.3	15.1	0	—	WNL	−
38.	M	7.2	14.5	0	—	WNL	−
39.	M	11.0	18.0	0	—	WNL	+
40.	M	8.6	15.0	0	0	WNL	−
41.	M	10.7	14.6	5	—	WNL	−
42.	F	12.7	17.1	—	—	Dysphoric	−
43.	M	9.0	15.5	5	6	Dysphoric	+
44.	M	12.0	14.8	—	—	WNL	−
45.	M	9.7	16.0	0	0	WNL	−

Note. M, male; F, female. For Kinsey ratings, 0, exclusively heterosexual; 6, exclusively homosexual. A dash indicates that the subject reported no sexual fantasies or behaviors. For gender identity, WNL, within normal limits (i.e., the patient did not report any distress about being a male or a female). For DSM, a plus sign means that the patient met the complete DSM-III or DSM-III-R criteria for gender identity disorder of childhood at initial assessment.

[a]In the clinical interview, this subject reported an exclusively heterosexual orientation in fantasy and in behavior; however, there was compelling evidence that she was in fact involved in an enduring lesbian relationship, so for conservative reasons she has been classified as homosexual.

[b]This subject was severely retarded (IQ = 53), so we have elected to include her in the follow-up although she was seen initially in early adolescence.

Sexual Orientation

Ratings of Fantasy and Behavior

The sexual orientation ratings, which are given for each participant in Table 10.5, were classified as no experience, heterosexual (Kinsey ratings of 0–1), and bisexual/homosexual (Kinsey ratings of 2–6). Regarding sexual orientation in fantasy, 4 (8.9%) participants reported no sexual fantasies. Of the remaining 41 participants, 27 (60.0%) were classified as heterosexual, and 14 (31.1%) were classified as bisexual or homosexual. Regarding sexual orientation in behavior, 26 (57.8%) participants reported no interpersonal sexual experiences. Of the remaining 19 participants, 11 (24.4%) were classified as heterosexual, and 8 (17.8%) were classified as bisexual or homosexual.

Compared to Green's control sample, a significantly larger percentage of the participants in our study was bisexual or homosexual in fantasy (χ^2 [2] = 18.1, p < .001); however, compared to Green's probands, a significantly smaller percentage was bisexual or homosexual in fantasy (χ^2 [2] = 18.4, p < .001). Similar results were found for behavior (χ^2 [2] = 16.4 and 13.1, p's < .001 and .01, respectively).

At the time of the current follow-up, our participants were an average of 2.3 years younger than Green's (1987) probands—a significant difference, t (87) = 4.7, p < .001. The relation between age and sexual orientation ratings showed effects comparable to those shown in Green's (1987) study. Regarding fantasy, a one-way analysis of variance showed that the participants with a bisexual or homosexual orientation were significantly older than those with a heterosexual orientation (p <

TABLE 10.6. Relation between Age and Sexual Orientation in the Toronto Follow-Up Study

	Age (in years)	
Sexual orientation	M	SD
Fantasy		
Homosexual/bisexual (n = 14)	18.0	2.7
Heterosexual (n = 27)	16.1	2.0
No fantasy (n = 4)	15.6	1.3
Behavior		
Homosexual/bisexual (n = 8)	19.0	2.4
Heterosexual (n = 11)	16.5	1.5
No behavior (n = 26)	16.0	2.2

.10) and those who did not report sexual fantasies ($p < .05$), F (2, 42) = 3.9, $p < .03$. The latter two groups did not differ from each other. Regarding behavior, the age effects were similar, F (2, 42) = 6.5, $p < .01$ (see Table 10.6).

It is apparent from these preliminary results that the rate of an eventual bisexual or homosexual outcome is going to be greater than the rate that one would observe in the general population; this buttresses the findings of the previously conducted follow-up studies. Because our group at follow-up was still relatively young, it remains unclear whether the rate of a heterosexual outcome will ultimately prove different from that of Green's (1987) follow-up study, as well as those of some of the other follow-up studies. Because we are still following our participants, it will ultimately be possible to answer this question.

Clinical Impressions

As noted earlier, social desirability is a key validity issue in the assessment of sexual orientation during the adolescent years. Thus, one would expect youngsters to underreport an atypical sexual orientation. Among the youngsters who reported a bisexual or homosexual orientation, the majority appeared to be comfortable about their emerging sexuality. Many of these youngsters had already "come out" to friends or family. A minority, however, were closeted, and the interviewer (Zucker) was the first person with whom they had spoken about their sexuality. All of these youngsters seemed to find this experience supportive and were receptive to the suggestion that they develop links with other adolescents of a similar orientation.

Among the youngsters who reported a heterosexual orientation or who reported no sexual experiences, some seemed to be very constricted and inhibited with regard to sexuality. Others, however, seemed to feel more confident about their emerging heterosexuality and were able to describe their experiences in detail, as in the following cases.

CASE EXAMPLE 10.5

Trevor was initially assessed at age 5 (IQ = 129). At that time, he met the DSM-III criteria for gender identity disorder. Other aspects of his psychosocial functioning have been described briefly in Chapter 5 (see Case Example 5.3). Trevor was seen for several years in individual therapy by a resident in child psychiatry, and his mother was also seen in therapy for her own psychiatric difficulties. During his childhood and early adolescence, Trevor's functioning was

compromised, and he experienced difficulties in his academic functioning and
social relationships.

Trevor's most recent follow-up was at the age of 16.3 years. He reported
no gender dysphoria. When asked about his sexual development, Trevor commented that there was "not a whole hell of a lot" to talk about. "I'm afraid I'm
not into it . . . it's basically nonexistent." He reported no sexual fantasies or interpersonal sexual experiences, although he acknowledged nocturnal emis-
sions. He seemed "apathetic" and affectively removed when talking about sexuality. He stated that he had always thought that sex was "kind of bizarre."
When asked to imagine his later sexuality, Trevor commented that he was pretty sure that he would develop interests, but stated, "I don't think I'll be one of
the bone people." (The term *bone* is used by some adolescents and young
adults to describe intense sexual interactions.) Trevor commented that he
thought that he would be attracted to girls, that "sex toward guys repulses
me."

CASE EXAMPLE 10.6

Abe was initially assessed at age 8 (IQ = 123). At that time, he was not
markedly cross-gender-identified. He preferred to play with girls and showed a
marked avoidance of rough-and-tumble play and competitive athletics, but
gave no other signs of cross-gender behavior. In addition to these behaviors,
Abe was also an anxious youngster, and his anxiety affected his peer relationships. Abe was seen in weekly individual therapy by a child psychiatry resident for a year, with the primary focus on social skills, anxiety reduction, and
the encouragement of friendships with same-sex peers. Abe's family then
moved to another Canadian province, and he was not seen again until the age
of 17.

Abe was eager to participate in the follow-up study. He was doing well in
school and had both male and female friends. He reported, however, that
same-sex peer relationships had remained problematic through his early adolescent years, and that he had experienced a lot of teasing. He felt, however,
that he had become more assertive in the past several years. He attributed this
to an event that had happened when he was 15. He was working in a store and
a "beautiful girl" came in. He was extremely anxious about serving her, but
said to himself, "I either do it or I'm fired." To his surprise, this girl showed an
interest in him, and this boosted his self-esteem. Since then, he reported that he
felt much more confident in his heterosocial interactions.

In fantasy, Abe's sexual orientation was exclusively heterosexual. He re-
ported that he had engaged in heterosexual dating, holding hands, and kissing.
He was, however, clearly anxious about more intimate sexual involvements.
For example, Abe commented that genital touching was "sleazy." His main

masturbatory fantasy involved "potential girlfriends." He described orgasm as "okay, I guess, it's not unpleasant; it's nothing fantastic, though." Abe denied fantasizing about sexual intercourse while masturbating, commenting, "I'm probably thinking about just being on a date, being at her house, sitting on a sofa . . . messing a bit . . . kissing above the waistline . . . and that's basically the ideal fantasy." He then expressed concerns about contracting a sexually transmitted disease or impregnating a girl.

Abe's childhood gender development seemed more consistent with Friedman's (1988) concept of *juvenile unmasculinity* than with gender identity disorder. He had apparently struggled with his sense of masculinity until the event with the girl described earlier. During the follow-up interview, he presented in a much more gregarious and extraverted fashion than he had in childhood. It was the impression of the interviewer, however, that his confidence about sexual relationships was still uneven and affected by anxiety.

CASE EXAMPLE 10.7

Calvin was initially assessed at age 6 (IQ = 113). At that time, he met the DSM-III criteria for gender identity disorder. He was also an anxious youngster who had trouble concentrating at school. After the assessment, the parents chose not to bring Calvin to the child psychiatrist who had referred him. According to the father, this was because the psychiatrist "yawned a lot" and seemed uninterested. At a 1-year follow-up, Calvin's gender identity confusion and general psychosocial difficulties had persisted. A referral to a social worker proved more successful; by late childhood, Calvin had relinquished many of his cross-gender behaviors and was no longer gender-dysphoric.

Calvin was seen for follow-up at the age of 14.5 years. He seemed to enjoy the testing and interviewing thoroughly. He presented as a much more outgoing youngster who had developed stable friendships with boys. Calvin felt that he was popular and that he fit in with his peer group. He noted, however, that he enjoyed sports less than his male peers, but stated that this was not a problem and he was not ostracized for his relative lack of interest. He particularly enjoyed going to a dance club for teenagers. He expressed concern about notable gynecomastia, and a referral was made to a pediatric endocrinologist. The examination revealed no underlying endocrine abnormality, and Calvin was assured that the gynecomastia would lessen as he matured.

Calvin reported no gender dysphoria. In fantasy, his sexual orientation was exclusively heterosexual, including crushes, arousal to visual stimuli, sexual dream imagery, and masturbation imagery (which involved females whom he "didn't know"). Although Calvin had dated a few girls, he had had no interpersonal sexual experiences. He felt confident that these would occur as he got older.

CASE EXAMPLE 10.8

Leonore was initially assessed at age 3 (IQ = 144). At that time, she met the DSM-III criteria for gender identity disorder. After the assessment, the parents resisted the recommendation for therapeutic intervention. Leonore continued to show severe gender dysphoria at a 1-year follow-up; the parents were now more receptive to therapeutic intervention, and Leonore was seen for several years by a child psychiatrist who was also in training as a psychoanalyst. Follow-ups in late childhood indicated a complete resolution of the gender dysphoria and marked cross-gender identification.

Leonore was seen most recently for follow-up at the age of 14.8 years. She reported no gender dysphoria. In fantasy, Leonore's sexual orientation was exclusively heterosexual, including crushes and arousal to visual stimuli. Leonore described the experience of having a crush on someone as "when you like someone, you like being around them, [you] like seeing them . . . you feel kind of nervous around them." She described several such crushes on boys. Leonore reported that several "guys" had had crushes on her, which she experienced as "flattering." When asked what it would be like if a girl had a crush on her, Leonore commented, "I'd be flattered, but it would feel kind of weird." Regarding visual attraction, Leonore commented, "I just feel attracted to them [boys] . . . and sometimes I'm lucky enough to get to know them." Leonore could not recall any instances of sexual dream imagery. She stated that she had masturbated on only a few occasions, but could not describe sexual content. Although the interviewer had the impression that her masturbation fantasies were about boys, her descriptions were too vague to be classified as heterosexual, bisexual, or homosexual, and she was not pressured to do so; however, on the self-report questionnaire concerning sexual fantasy, Leonore indicated that she had not masturbated during the past 6 months. Although Leonore had dated (primarily in the context of "group dating," a common social ritual among contemporary young middle-class adolescents), held hands with, and kissed boys, she had not done so in the 12-month period prior to the follow-up.

Information obtained at the follow-up interview also indicated that Leonore was struggling academically and was in full-scale "rebellion" against her parents concerning issues such as alcohol use and curfew. It was the interviewer's impression that the parents continued to have the same kinds of disagreements about child rearing that they had had when Leonore was a preschooler. Thus, Leonore and her parents were referred back to the child psychiatrist who had treated her during childhood.

As noted earlier, the validity of our sexual orientation assessments, particularly for the younger adolescents classified as heterosexual, must be viewed cautiously. Follow-up of these youngsters into late adolescence or early adulthood will be required in order to assess the stability of the classification. Ideally, cross-validation with psychophysiological techniques would be desirable. In addition, it will be important to understand our adolescents' emerging sexuality within the context of their more general functioning, including their capacity for intimate relationships and psychosocial adaptation.

CHAPTER 11

Gender Identity Disorder in Adolescence

Adolescents with gender identity disorder experience a profound sense of discomfort about their status as members of their biological sex, and strongly identify themselves psychologically as members of the opposite sex. For some individuals this cross-gender identification appears fixed, whereas for others it may intensify or weaken with time and life events.

There is a very small literature, entirely descriptive, on the clinical presentation and treatment of adolescents with gender identity disorder (Barlow, Reynolds, & Agras, 1973; Bradley, 1980, 1990; Cohen-Kettenis & Everaerd, 1986; Davenport & Harrison, 1977; Dulcan & Lee, 1984; Kronberg, Tyano, Apter, & Wijsenbeek, 1981; Lothstein, 1980; Newman, 1970; Philippopoulos, 1964; Westhead, Olson, & Meyer, 1990). There have been no epidemiological studies on gender identity disorder during the adolescent years, so there are no data on its prevalence or incidence. It is likely, however, that the prevalence of the disorder among adolescents is reasonably comparable to its prevalence among adults (see Chapter 3).

Although disturbances in gender identity have been recognized for many years, the advent of sex reassignment surgery, with its accompanying public and professional debate, has given gender identity disorder a greater prominence than might seem justified by the number of people affected. Some would argue that this prominence may have even shifted the natural history of the disorder. Most individuals with gender identity disorder are aware of the highly publicized stories of such persons as Christine Jorgensen (see Hamburger, 1953) and others. The widespread awareness of a surgical solution to the psychological distress accompanying the disorder has led to the somewhat artificial distinction between individuals seeking sex reassignment ("transsexuals") and individuals with gender dysphoria who less clearly meet the diagnostic criteria for reassignment generally accepted in specialized gender identity clinics, such as gender identity disorder of adolescence or adulthood, nontranssexual type, and gender identity disorder not otherwise specified (American Psychiatric Association, 1987). That distinction was apparent in the DSM-III-R, but it has been modified in the DSM-IV (American Psychiatric Association, 1994) to reflect the notion that we are dealing with a broad spectrum of disturbance in gender identity, regardless of the solution sought or the treatments available (see Tables 11.1–11.3).

There have been several good recent overviews on the clinical presentation and management of adults with gender dysphoria (e.g., Blanchard & Steiner, 1990; Levine & Lothstein, 1981; Lothstein, 1983; Steiner, 1985b; Tully, 1992; Walters & Ross, 1986). Males outnumber females presenting to adult gender identity clinics. This may reflect the fact that the male population consists of two subgroups, *early-presenting* and *later-presenting* (Blanchard, 1990b, 1994). Early-presenting males typically have a history of childhood cross-gender identification and sexual attraction toward males; in contrast, later-presenting males typically have a history of transvestic fetishism and sexual attraction toward females. Early-presenting males usually request sex reassignment surgery in their 20s, whereas later-presenting males are usually first seen in their 30s and 40s. Adult females with gender dysphoria do not include a subgroup that corresponds to later-presenting males, and gender-dysphoric females almost invariably experience same-sex attraction (Blanchard, 1990a; see also Chapter 3, note 1).

The course of the disorder is generally chronic, although spontaneous remission and a few "cures," mainly in adolescents, have been

---

TABLE 11.1. DSM-III-R Diagnostic Criteria for Transsexualism

A. Persistent discomfort and sense of inappropriateness about one's assigned sex.

B. Persistent preoccupation for at least two years with getting rid of one's primary and secondary sex characteristics and acquiring the sex characteristics of the other sex.

C. The person has reached puberty.

Specify history of sexual orientation: **asexual, homosexual, heterosexual,** or **unspecified.**

Note. Reprinted with permission from the *Diagnostic and Statistical Manual of Mental Disorders,* Third Edition, Revised (p. 76). Copyright 1987 by the American Psychiatric Association.

TABLE 11.2. DSM-III-R Diagnostic Criteria for Gender Identity Disorder of Adolescence or Adulthood, Nontranssexual Type

---

A. Persistent or recurrent discomfort and sense of inappropriateness about one's assigned sex.

B. Persistent or recurrent cross-dressing in the role of the other sex, either in fantasy or actuality, but not for the purpose of sexual excitement (as in Transvestic Fetishism).

C. No persistent preoccupation (for at least two years) with getting rid of one's primary and secondary sex characteristics and acquiring the sex characteristics of the other sex (as in Transsexualism).

D. The person has reached puberty.

Specify history of sexual orientation: **asexual, homosexual, heterosexual,** or **unspecified.**

Note. Reprinted with permission from the *Diagnostic and Statistical Manual of Mental Disorders,* Third Edition, Revised (p. 77). Copyright 1987 by the American Psychiatric Association.

reported (e.g., Barlow, Abel, & Blanchard, 1977; Barlow et al., 1973; Davenport & Harrison, 1977; Kronberg et al., 1981). Individuals with gender dysphoria appear to be at high risk for psychiatric impairment, including character pathology, substance abuse, depression, suicide, and difficulties with the law (Dickey, 1990). Females appear to be somewhat less at risk for such impairment than males (Levine & Lothstein, 1981).

To reduce the chances of a poor outcome, most authors recommend careful evaluation of candidates prior to sex reassignment, with the expectation of a lengthy period (usually 2 years) of living as the other sex (Clemmensen, 1990; Levine & Lothstein, 1981; McCauley & Ehrhardt, 1984). Most gender identity clinics follow the Harry Benjamin International Gender Dysphoria Association Standards of Care ("Standards of Care," 1985) criteria for sex reassignment surgery (Peterson & Dickey, 1995). These include careful evaluation and monitoring, cross-gender living for a lengthy period, and evidence of stability in work or school and social functioning. Not all of the individuals who present with a firm belief that sex reassignment surgery is the solution to their difficulty persist in that belief (Lothstein, 1980; McCauley & Ehrhardt, 1984). Some of them continue to endure a chronic gender dysphoria, but will not actively pursue sex reassignment. Others accept a homosexual adaptation, and a very few, usually after extensive psychological treatment, apparently become free of their cross-gender wishes and pursue a heterosexual orientation (Barlow et al., 1973; Davenport & Harrison, 1977; Kronberg et al., 1981). Psychotherapeu-

TABLE 11.3. DSM-IV Diagnostic Criteria for Gender Identity Disorder (Adolescent and Adult Criteria)

A. A strong and persistent cross-gender identification (not merely a desire for any perceived cultural advantages of being the other sex).

   In adolescents and adults, the disturbance is manifested by symptoms such as a stated desire to be the other sex, frequent passing as the other sex, desire to live or be treated as the other sex, or the conviction that he or she has the typical feelings and reactions of the other sex.

B. Persistent discomfort with his or her sex or sense of inappropriateness in the gender role of that sex.

   In adolescents and adults, the disturbance is manifested by symptoms such as preoccupation with getting rid of primary and secondary sex characteristics (e.g., request for hormones, surgery, or other procedures to physically alter sexual characteristics to simulate the other sex) or belief that he or she was born the wrong sex.

C. The disturbance is not concurrent with a physical intersex condition.

D. The disturbance causes clinically significant distress or impairment in social, occupational, or other important areas of functioning.

Specify if (for sexually mature individuals):
   Sexually Attracted to Males
   Sexually Attracted to Females
   Sexually Attracted to Both
   Sexually Attracted to Neither

Note. Reprinted with permission from the *Diagnostic and Statistical Manual of Mental Disorders*, Fourth Edition (pp. 537–538). Copyright 1994 by the American Psychiatric Association.

tic support is generally recommended even for individuals who are considered good candidates for surgery (Levine & Lothstein, 1981; McCauley & Ehrhardt, 1984).

Patient satisfaction is usually said to result from sex reassignment surgery, although objective indices have not always confirmed this judgment (Abramowitz, 1986; Blanchard, 1985b; Blanchard & Sheridan, 1990; Levine & Lothstein, 1981). Female-to-male transsexuals appear to have more stable relationships (Dixen, Maddever, Van Maasdam, & Edwards, 1984; Köckott & Fahrner, 1988) and a slightly better economic outcome (postsurgery) than that of male-to-female transsexuals (Blanchard, 1985b).

Levine and Lothstein (1981) have addressed the clinical and ethical dilemmas faced by therapists who work with gender-dysphoric individuals (see also Lothstein, 1982). These problems include establishing a therapeutic alliance; dealing with the countertransference feelings engendered by difficult patients; deciding whether or not to accept a "surgical solution" (i.e., the patients' solution) to a complex psychological disorder; and carrying on despite lack of adequate knowledge about the etiology of the disorder and the most appropriate treatment for it. Caution and careful monitoring are urged for all who choose to treat such individuals.

CLINICAL PRESENTATION

Table 11.4 shows the demographic characteristics of our sample of 44 gender-dysphoric adolescents (26 males, 18 females). It can be seen that the youngsters were generally in their midadolescence, of average intelligence, and from lower-middle-class to middle-class backgrounds. The majority of the males were from broken homes, whereas a slight majority of the females were from two-parent families. There were no significant sex differences on any of these demographic variables.

Younger adolescents, and adolescents who are ambivalent about their disorder or uncomfortable about acknowledging their cross-gender feelings, may be harder to assess. Older adolescents tend to resemble adults with gender identity disorder and present their gender dysphoria and cross-gender identification more clearly.

Younger adolescents are frequently brought for assessment because of behaviors that signify their cross-gender identification. They may attempt to pass as members of the opposite sex at school or in other social situations. Such passing may result in clinical referral when school officials or other adults bring it to the attention of the adolescents' parents. Older adolescents who are more comfortable about acknowledging their cross-gender wishes, or those adolescents whose parents have been supportive of their cross-gender interests, may present with a request for sex reassignment. In examining 27 clinically referred adolescents, Lothstein (1980) reported that the wish for sex reassignment intensified with experiences of loss or reaction to pubertal changes.

In our experience, most adolescents with gender identity disorder have had a history of gender identity disorder during childhood (Bradley & Zucker, 1984); in some cases, however, they may not have had a full-blown history of gender identity disorder at that time, or such a history may not be recalled clearly by either the parents or the adolescent. Some adolescents recall a desire hidden from parents to be of the opposite sex and a history of cross-gender behaviors carried out in secret. It is sometimes difficult to assess the extent to which these

TABLE 11.4. Demographic Characteristics of Gender-Dysphoric Adolescents

Variables	Males ($n = 26$)	Females ($n = 18$)
Age (in years)		
M	15.8	15.7
SD	1.2	1.0
Range	14.1–19.0	14.1–17.4
Verbal IQ		
M	95.4[a]	90.7[b]
SD	15.9	17.2
Range	65–124	64–139
Performance IQ		
M	101.0[a]	104.4[c]
SD	15.9	13.3
Range	62–128	83–123
Social class[d] (n and %)		
I	3 (11.5%)	1 (5.6%)
II	2 (7.7%)	4 (22.2%)
III	11 (42.3%)	5 (27.8%)
IV	7 (26.9%)	4 (22.2%)
V	3 (11.5%)	4 (22.2%)
Family status (n and %)		
Mother and father	10 (38.4%)	10 (55.5%)
Mother only[e]	7 (26.9%)	3 (16.6%)
Mother and stepfather	6 (23.0%)	0 (0.0%)
Father only[e]	0 (0.0%)	2 (11.1%)
Father and stepmother	0 (0.0%)	0 (0.0%)
Foster care[f]	3 (11.5%)	3 (16.6%)

[a]$n = 22.$ [b]$n = 15.$ [c]$n = 16.$

[d]For social class, Hollingshead's (1975) five-category system was used, where I indicates major business executives and professionals, and V indicates unskilled laborers and menial service workers.

[e]Single, divorced, separated, or widowed.

[f]Adopted after infancy, foster care, group home.

adolescents are reporting their own stories and the extent to which they are reporting the account they believe is expected from a person seeking sex reassignment surgery. Parents have typically ignored or tolerated earlier cross-gender behaviors. Seldom have the adolescents been seen clinically during childhood with respect to their cross-gender behavior.

Clinical assessment of the young adolescent with gender identity disorder is often difficult. Despite such behaviors as passing, some adolescents, when confronted about the meaning of the behaviors or about wishes to be of the opposite sex, deny the significance of cross-gender identification or gender dysphoria. This denial may reflect the adolescents' ambivalence with regard to these wishes or the adolescents' perception that others will find them unacceptable.

Adolescents with gender identity disorder are often lonely, feeling uncomfortable about relating to same-sex peers toward whom they may experience erotic attraction. They report being more comfortable in the company of opposite-sex peers with whom they share interests. Generally, they have not divulged their sexual feelings or their wishes to be of the opposite sex to these peers, and so they tend to feel distanced even in these relationships.

As these adolescents mature, they generally become more prepared to acknowledge their gender dysphoria and their cross-gender identification. Often they experience crushes and erotic feelings toward same-sex individuals. Some of them may engage in dating, but they often feel very inhibited in intimate situations in which it is difficult to conceal their sexual anatomy. Typically, they regard a homosexual adaptation as unacceptable, if not repugnant, and do not define themselves as gay or lesbian (for further discussion on this point, see Sullivan, Bradley, & Zucker, 1995).

Some adolescents with gender identity disorder have an almost delusional sense that they are really the opposite sex or can really be the opposite sex. For example, one female patient called in a perplexed state when her girlfriend, who knew that the patient was biologically female despite passing as a male, insisted that she was pregnant by "him." The patient appeared unable to confront the reality that this was not possible. Another female adolescent had created a penis with various materials, and kept it in place by running wire through her underwear. As a relationship with a female partner became more intimate, she believed that it would be possible to experience fellatio "with the lights on" if only she could find better material for her penis. It is common for gender-dysphoric adolescents to believe that they are in some sense "hermaphroditic," and that physical examination will reveal that they are actually of the opposite sex.

Adolescents who have decided that sex reassignment is the solution to their dilemma often become very impatient with the time requirements for cross-gender living before surgery. They may become depressed because of what appear to be impossible delays in their pursuit of reassignment. Males in particular may find their growth in stature, facial hair, and musculature very distressing. Females experience frustration in concealing breast development, particularly in the summer, when light tops and swimsuits are fashionable.

ASSOCIATED FEATURES

Like their adult counterparts, adolescents with gender identity disorder have been described as having a borderline personality organization (Bradley, 1990; Lothstein, 1980). Although such labeling is at times useful, what is clinically most relevant is that individuals with gender identity disorder have poor anxiety tolerance. This may manifest itself in character pathology, frank anxiety, substance abuse, and depression. Dynamically oriented investigators have consistently regarded the act of cross-dressing as a form of anxiety relief (Bradley, 1990; Coates et al., 1991; Kirkpatrick & Friedman, 1976; Person & Ovesey, 1974a, 1974b, 1983; Oppenheimer, 1991). Thus, when adolescents with gender identity disorder are significantly stressed and the process of achieving sex reassignment surgery (the intrapsychic solution) is delayed, their anxiety increases; this may lead to a variety of acting-out behaviors.

Suicidal ideation occurs in many of these adolescents and requires monitoring, especially at times of isolation from peers or family. Depression is a common response to the failure of these adolescents in sociosexual relationships and to the many hurdles that they must surmount at most gender identity clinics. Character pathology may interfere with their ability to comply with the requirement of stability in work, school, and social functioning over the 2 years prior to recommendation for surgery. Many of these adolescents drop out of school or experience academic failure.

Maternal or surrogate mother CBCL ratings were available for about half of our sample (the majority of adolescents for whom data were missing had been assessed prior to the publication of the CBCL; most of the remaining youngsters had attended our clinic without their parents' knowledge, and in a few other cases parents did not speak or read English). It can be seen in Table 11.5 and Figure 11.1 that for both sexes behavioral difficulties were common. On the CBCL, there were, on average, four narrow-band elevations; the CBCL sum score was well within the clinical range, as were the Internalizing and Externalizing T scores. Thus, on average, our sample of gender-dysphoric adolescents showed very severe levels of behavioral disturbance that cut across the internalizing and externalizing domains of psychopathology.

Correlations between CBCL ratings and demographic variables showed no relation with age and parents' marital status (two parents vs. all other combinations). Social class was highly correlated with CBCL psychopathology (r's ranged from $-.54$ to $-.64$, all p's $< .001$), indicating that youngsters from lower social class backgrounds were more disturbed. Verbal IQ was also significantly correlated with three of the five CBCL indices of psychopathology (significant r's ranged

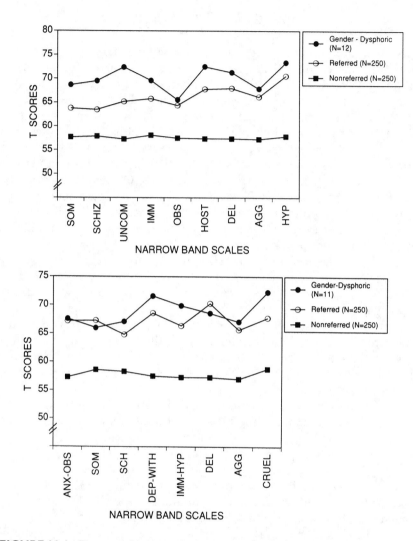

FIGURE 11.1. Top panel: Narrow-band factors on the CBCL, 12- to 16-year-old boys. SOM, Somatic Complaints; SCHIZ, Schizoid; UNCOM, Uncommunicative; IMM, Immature; OBS, Obsessive–Compulsive; HOST, Hostile Withdrawal; DEL, Delinquent; AGG, Aggressive; HYP, Hyperactive. Bottom panel: Narrow-band factors on the CBCL, 12- to 16-year-old girls. ANX-OBS, Anxious–Obsessive; SOM, Somatic Complaints; SCH, Schizoid; DEP-WITH, Depressed Withdrawal; IMM-HYP, Immature–Hyperactive; DEL, Delinquent; AGG, Aggressive; CRUEL, Cruel. Nonreferred and referred group data are from the standardization study (Achenbach & Edelbrock, 1983, Appendix D).

TABLE 11.5. Mothers' or Surrogate Mothers' Ratings of Behavioral Disturbance on the CBCL in Gender-Dysphoric Adolescents

	Males					
	Gender-dysphoric ($n = 12$)		Nonreferred ($n = 250$)		Referred ($n = 250$)	
Measures	M	SD	M	SD	M	SD
No. elevated narrow-band scales	5.0	3.4	—	—	—	—
Number of items	50.0	22.5	—	—	—	—
Sum of items	69.5	34.4	21.7	15.0	58.9	24.0
Internalizing *T*	70.4	10.2	51.2	9.1	65.6	8.9
Externalizing *T*	66.8	11.2	51.0	9.3	68.1	8.7

	Females					
	Gender-dysphoric ($n = 11$)		Nonreferred ($n = 250$)		Referred ($n = 250$)	
Measures	M	SD	M	SD	M	SD
No. elevated narrow-band scales	3.4	2.5	—	—	—	—
Number of items	47.2	23.0	—	—	—	—
Sum of items	66.0	34.7	16.6	14.1	55.8	26.3
Internalizing *T*	64.7	8.5	49.8	8.0	64.3	8.4
Externalizing *T*	65.9	10.6	49.4	7.5	64.0	8.6

Note. Nonreferred and referred samples consist of boys or girls aged 12–16, from Achenbach and Edelbrock (1983, Appendix D). For the probands, all CBCL items pertaining to gender identity disorder scored 1 or 2 were set to 0 to avoid artificial inflation of general psychopathology.

from $-.40$ to $-.50$, all p's $< .05$), which was probably mediated by the relation between social class and Verbal IQ ($r = -.62$, $p < .001$).

COURSE

It is not clear what proportion of adolescents with gender identity disorder proceed to sex reassignment. To date, 19 (43.2%) of our 44 adolescents have been referred for assessment to the adult clinic at the Clarke Institute. Of these cases, three patients have received both hormonal and surgical sex reassignment; a number of the others have been placed on cross-sex hormonal treatment, but as yet have not been approved for surgery. Many adolescents continue with chronic gender dysphoria, being unable or unwilling to comply with the requirements for reassignment. A few fluctuate between self-definition as homosexual and intermittent wishes for reassignment, typically at stressful times in their lives.

The following cases illustrate some aspects of the course of gender identity disorder in adolescence.

CASE EXAMPLE 11.1

Helen, a 17-year-old female who was born and raised in an Eastern European country, was brought for assessment by her aunt, to whom she had indicated her wish to change sex. Her mother was excluded from the assessment for fear that news of her daughter's feelings would be too much for her. The parents had been separated for a number of years, following a stormy marriage during which Helen's alcoholic father had physically abused her mother.

Helen had had a difficult birth, with some anoxia and a subsequent toxic period that delayed her discharge from the hospital. She had progressed through school at a normal pace until Grade 6, when she became uninterested and her grades declined. She recalled being a tomboy while growing up, but was unaware of wishing to be a boy while young. She was concerned about her parents' conflict and felt a need to look after her mother, who was frequently depressed. At about age 12, she began to feel that she was different from other girls, as she did not share their romantic interest in boys. These feelings of being different became much more intense at age 15, when she became involved in a lesbian relationship. She felt very uncomfortable about being in love with a girl and so experimented with a heterosexual relationship for a while; she found this physically unsatisfying and returned to her relationship with her female lover. The relationship continued until Helen was forced to leave her native country, as she and her mother were emigrating to Canada. Subsequent to the loss of this relationship, she experienced intensification of her fantasies of being male. She continued at the time of assessment to imagine that she would be able to reunite with her female lover as a male.

On revealing her feelings to her aunt, the aunt had tried to encourage Helen's feminine identification by supporting her wearing of makeup and dresses. Helen had gone along with this effort and acknowledged that she enjoyed it. It was felt that Helen had some gender identity confusion, but had been able to deal with that until the loss of her lover. Removal from the abusive relationship with her father, and her aunt's encouragement to work on a feminine identification, were felt to be factors that might support her being able to use psychotherapy either to accept her lesbian orientation or (conceivably) to attempt a heterosexual adaptation.

On the basis that the cross-gender wishes were of recent onset, in the context of loss of a love relationship, and because of the presence of some acknowledged heterosexual interest and Helen's willingness to work on her feminine identification, a trial of insight-oriented psychotherapy was recommended. Helen agreed to be involved in psychotherapy, although the process was complicated by the need to find a therapist who could speak her language and who was acceptable to the family in this small ethnic community. After several months, Helen refused to continue in psychotherapy.

Follow-up after 18 months was occasioned following a suicide attempt, after a breakup with a girlfriend who had discovered that Helen was not male. She was referred to the adult gender identity clinic, as she insisted that the solution was sex reassignment surgery.

CASE EXAMPLE 11.2

Stella, a 16-year-old female, was referred by her youth group therapist when she revealed that she felt she was a boy and was interested in sex reassignment surgery. She had begun treatment with the referring therapist following several minor suicide attempts.

Background history revealed moderate cross-gender interests, a preference for boys as playmates, and a role as protector when socializing with girls. Intense interest in sex change surgery began to emerge at about age 13, after Stella watched a TV show about this. She began to feel that surgery would make her feel "complete the way I am and feel" and would make her physically acceptable. At about this same time, Stella changed her appearance to look very punk and began to ask that she be called "Spike." Subsequently, she referred to herself as "Sid" after Sid Vicious, a punk rock musician. She became involved in the drug culture and was sexually involved with a girl, to whom she introduced herself as a male with a congenitally absent penis. She liked to be identified as male and would get upset when her maleness was challenged.

Reaction to puberty had been very negative, with Stella refusing to wear a bra. She had also been concealing her breasts and using feminine napkins to simulate male genitals. At the time of assessment, she maintained that she still had not begun her periods—a concern that was only later revealed to have been a deception. She refused to use the girls' washroom, maintaining that she didn't urinate at school.

Stella's parents were disapproving of both her sexual orientation and thoughts about sex change surgery, although her father felt he could accept her as a lesbian. Stella was very negative about her mother, whom she perceived as "wimpish." She had more positive feelings about her father, with whom she shared an interest in repairing cars.

It was felt that Stella's gender dysphoria had remained relatively mild in childhood, but that for reasons that were not entirely clear during the assessment (aside from her hearing about sex reassignment surgery on TV), it had intensified amid the psychosexual demands of early adolescence. She was followed in supportive psychotherapy; she gradually clarified a more appropriate (less antisocial) male identity and went on to sex reassignment. At follow-up, she was functioning well and was attending university. The parents appeared gradually to have accepted Stella as male.

CASE EXAMPLE 11.3

Harvey, an 18-year-old male, requested an assessment for sex reassignment. He was seen with his mother who had remarried a year prior to the assessment.

Harvey had been conceived in a stressful marital relationship, and his mother had been sick throughout the pregnancy. Following his birth, the mother had a depressive episode, which resulted in a 6-week hospitalization when he was 3 months of age. She felt that the early years of her son's development were stressful because of her husband's lack of involvement in the family and his infidelity. She was also burdened with the finding of a breast lump (which required surgery) and with her difficulty in managing her son's behavior. Following his parents' separation at age 3, Harvey and his mother entered a further stormy period related to his marked noncompliance, demanding behavior, and angry outbursts, and to the mother's inconsistency. This pattern continued until early adolescence, when he became more compliant.

Although Harvey's mother had had little concern during her son's childhood about his gender identity, he displayed avoidance of rough-and-tumble activities, an interest in dolls, some preference for female peers, and occasional dress-up and female role play. These behaviors diminished somewhat in early adolescence with involvement in a male peer group, although Harvey reported an ongoing fantasy of being female. This fantasy became even more active at about age 12, when he began a sexual relationship with a slightly younger male cousin. In this relationship, which involved frequent sexual activity, Harvey fantasized himself as female. Although the relationship was kept relatively secret, both boys were active members in a fantasy group game (akin to *Dungeons and Dragons*) in which Harvey always played the female role. Shortly before the assessment, the cousin, who had begun to establish a heterosexual relationship, indicated his desire to end their relationship. Harvey was actively suicidal following this breakup, but was eventually able to console himself with the belief that his cousin would return to the relationship.

At the time of assessment, Harvey acknowledged homosexual feelings but also described himself as transsexual. He did not appear particularly homophobic (nor did his mother), but he did express the desire to be able to have a "normal" sexual relationship with a male. The mother was supportive of her son but dismayed at the idea of his changing sex. She was feeling particularly overwhelmed in her present marital situation with a noncompliant stepdaughter and an uninvolved husband—a pattern that seemed a repetition of her first marriage. Her relationship with her own father had been negative, related in part to his alcoholism and abuse of her mother.

It was considered likely that Harvey would proceed toward sex reassignment, given the long-standing nature of his fantasy of himself as a female; however, as he had had little opportunity to explore the gay world and appeared open to this as an option, it was recommended that he spend some time exploring options other than reassignment. Follow-up contact with his therapist after 2 years indicated that he was gradually pursuing a cross-gender identity.

TREATMENT

Treatment is largely supportive, the intent being to help the adolescent clarify his or her gender identity and, when appropriate, to provide support in surmounting the many hurdles on the path toward sex reassignment.

Although there have been several reports of treatment resulting in resolution of cross-gender wishes and assumption of a heterosexual orientation (e.g., Barlow et al., 1973; Davenport & Harrison, 1977; Kronberg et al., 1981; Philippopoulos, 1964), most authors have not found psychotherapy efficacious in achieving such a resolution; however, several authors have reported the achievement of gains in helping adolescents with gender identity disorder to accept a homosexual orientation and to relinquish the wish for sex reassignment (Barlow, Abel, & Blanchard, 1979; Kirkpatrick & Friedman, 1976; Levine & Lothstein, 1981; Lothstein, 1980; McCauley & Ehrhardt, 1984). The frequency with which such gains have been achieved with severely gender-disordered adolescents is unclear.

Several factors interfere with attempts at treatment. As indicated earlier, adolescents with gender identity disorder have poor anxiety tolerance. Seeking sex reassignment surgery is a defensive solution and a mechanism for control of anxiety. The thought of not having a "solution" for their distress increases their anxiety, thus making it very difficult to achieve a therapeutic alliance. Despite an understanding (at least at a superficial level) of why they have cross-gender wishes, these adolescents are often unable to relinquish their defense, as they feel too overwhelmed to face their anxiety without it. This leads to demanding behavior and impatience with the therapist as he or she tries to help them explore feelings and behaviors. Many adolescents who seek sex reassignment withdraw from therapy because of their inability to tolerate the anxiety connected with exploration of their wish for surgery.

In those cases in which a complete reversal of cross-gender behaviors and fantasies has apparently occurred, that reversal has been achieved by means of intensive (usually residential) long-term treatment employing behavior modification and insight-oriented psychotherapy (e.g., Davenport & Harrison, 1977; Kronberg et al., 1981). Such treatment is probably critical to providing adolescents with gender identity disorder the "holding" they need to explore new behaviors and wishes. It also removes them from a family environment that has probably been reinforcing their need for a defensive solution to their anxiety. However, given changes in sensibility regarding treatment choice, adolescents with gender identity disorder who are competent enough to make these decisions are unlikely to accept residential treatment for their condition. In fact, there have been no reports of such treatment over the last 10 years.

In our experience, attempts at psychotherapy with these adolescents have not yielded dramatic changes in gender identification. We do, however, have one case of a young man who presented at age 16 requesting sex reassignment and at follow-up 2 years later, with no treatment, reported that he had relinquished his desire to change sex, was comfortable as a male, and wished to forget about his contact with the clinic. His father (who had also undergone some gender identity confusion) felt that his son's involvement in a church group, together with an improvement in their relationship, had been instrumental in effecting his son's change of mind.

Some young adolescents who present with an earlier gender identity disorder and residual effeminate mannerisms may respond to behavioral treatment focused on reduction of these mannerisms; however, efforts to encourage such adolescents to explore same-gender roles have generally proved very difficult.

Families need support in accepting their adolescents' cross-gender difficulties and possible sex reassignment. Some families are unable to accept their adolescents' change of gender role and identity; other families come to accept these changes because of the improved adjustment and increased independence that appear to result from them.

For the adolescent who is going to pursue sex reassignment, support will be needed in such concrete but necessary details as name changes on documents and registration at school or job. Occasionally, contact with a reassigned individual can be helpful in discussing personal experiences, the importance of the period of cross-gender living, family reactions, and sociosexual relationships (for a more thorough discussion, see Clemmensen, 1990).

Certain countertransference reactions are commonly elicited by adolescents with gender identity disorder. Some therapists experience such adolescents' wish for sex reassignment as an unacceptable solution to an intrapsychic dilemma, and cannot work supportively with the adolescents to achieve a reasonable resolution of the problem. For many of the therapists who choose to work with adolescents pursuing sex reassignment, there is a gradual shift from viewing the individuals as members of one sex to an acceptance of them as members of the other sex. This may involve self-monitoring of references to the patient (e.g., choice of male or female pronouns). Therapists who believe that sex reassignment is unnecessary should probably avoid treating individuals with extreme gender identity disorder, as countertransference feelings may make it difficult for these therapists to support such individuals adequately if they pursue reassignment.

Finally, as individuals with gender identity disorder may also have comorbid personality and other disorders (Lothstein, 1980), it is important to clarify the nature of these other disorders, since their existence may significantly affect the course of treatment.

FOLLOW-UP

Adolescents who pursue sex reassignment surgery will experience the same range of complications as that experienced by adults (e.g., vaginal strictures and breast scarring). Those adolescents who remain gender-dysphoric after surgery may require long-term follow-up, as their lives may be unstable in many dimensions. After reassignment, some individuals want long-term support in their relationships with spouses and children. Many of these individuals do not feel well equipped for such roles as husband and father or wife and mother, and so may seek help intermittently if stressed by the new demands. On the other hand, there are individuals who do not wish further therapeutic contact after reassignment, as they wish to "wipe the old slate clean and begin anew."

DIFFERENTIAL DIAGNOSIS

Clinically, there are two situations that require differentiation in approaching an adolescent with gender dysphoria. These are (1) homosexuality, in which the gender dysphoria may be transient (as an initial manifestation of difficulties in accepting a homosexual identity) or fluctuating (as in some effeminate homosexuals); and (2) transvestic behavior, in which the intermittent cross-gender behavior does not reflect a sustained cross-gender identification.

Some homosexual adolescents experience a period of intense cross-gender identification that may reflect unresolved earlier cross-gender feelings. For some male adolescents, these feelings may be manifested in involvement in "drag queen" activities or other forms of female impersonation. Such behaviors undoubtedly reflect unresolved cross-gender identification, but they are seldom accompanied by prolonged gender dysphoria or a psychological identification as female. Although some of the adolescents who engage in these behaviors use hormones to enhance aspects of their appearance, they appear accepting of their homosexual identification and value their genitals (in contrast to the adolescent with gender identity disorder, who finds them repugnant). Occasionally, an adolescent who becomes aware of homoerotic feelings but views such feelings as unacceptable will experience a desire for sex reassignment. If the source of concern can be identified and the adolescent can be integrated into an accepting gay or lesbian community, such cross-gender wishes may become less salient. Conversely, in both of the situations described above, the cross-gender wishes may become more clearly established and the individual may request sex reassignment.

The male adolescent with transvestic fetishism typically denies cross-gender wishes, although he may acknowledge feeling like a woman when he puts on female clothing (see Chapter 12). He seldom has a childhood history of gender identity disorder, although he may have begun wearing such items as pantyhose in early childhood. Sexual orientation is typically reported as heterosexual. Occasionally, a transvestic adolescent also manifests gender dysphoria. Such an adolescent may be assigned both diagnoses or may receive a DSM-IV diagnosis of transvestic fetishism with gender dysphoria (American Psychiatric Association, 1994).

Lastly, a floridly psychotic adolescent may present with the statement that he or she is of the opposite sex. Such statements are typically part of the delusional system and generally cease with treatment of the psychosis (see, e.g., Commander & Dean, 1990; Connolly & Gittleson, 1971; Gittleson & Dawson-Butterworth, 1967; Gittleson & Levine, 1966).

CHAPTER 12

Transvestic Fetishism in Adolescence

Transvestic fetishism is defined in the DSM-IV (American Psychiatric Association, 1994) as a disorder occurring in heterosexual males in which the individual acts upon, or is distressed by, recurrent, intense sexual urges and sexually arousing fantasies involving cross-dressing (Table 12.1). As such, it is designated as a paraphilia; in the DSM-IV, the paraphilias are described as involving sexual behaviors, fantasies, or objects that "lead to clinically significant distress or impairment (e.g., are obligatory, result in sexual dysfunction, require participation of nonconsenting individuals, lead to legal complications, interfere with social relationships)" (p. 525).

In this chapter, we discuss transvestic fetishism in male adolescents. We draw heavily on our clinical experience with 79 adolescents referred because of transvestic behaviors. Table 12.2 shows the demographic characteristics of this sample. It can be seen that the youngsters were, on average, in their early adolescence, from lower-middle-class to middle-class backgrounds, and more often than not from broken homes.

Most of the adolescents met Criterion A for transvestic fetishism. The minority who did not reported that they did not experience sexual arousal when cross-dressed. Our clinical impression was that this was true for some of these adolescents, particularly those around the age of 13 years; however, in the remaining cases it most likely reflected denial. Regarding Criterion B, the majority of our adolescents met this criterion because they had cross-dressed, not because they were distressed by it. Only a small minority of the adolescents reported being distressed by their cross-dressing. Lack of sexual arousal (as inferred from masturba-

319

TABLE 12.1. DSM-IV Diagnostic Criteria for Transvestic Fetishism

A. Over a period of at least 6 months, in a heterosexual male, recurrent, intense sexually arousing fantasies, sexual urges, or behaviors involving cross-dressing.

B. The fantasies, sexual urges, or behaviors cause clinically significant distress or impairment in social, occupational, or other important areas of functioning.

Specify if:
With Gender Dysphoria: if the person has persistent discomfort with gender role or identity

Note. Reprinted with permission from the *Diagnostic and Statistical Manual of Mental Disorders,* Fourth Edition (p. 531). Copyright 1994 by the American Psychiatric Association.

tion when cross-dressed) during adolescence has also been noted in interview studies of adults with transvestic fetishism (e.g., Croughan, Saghir, Cohen, & Robins, 1981).

Because no epidemiological studies have established how common transvestic behaviors are in a nonclinical population, and because we

TABLE 12.2. Demographic Characteristics of Male Adolescents (*n* = 79) with Transvestic Fetishism

Variables	Data
Age (in years)	
M	14.8
SD	1.3
Range	11.5–17.6
Social class[a] (*n* and %)	
I	8 (10.1%)
II	14 (17.7%)
III	24 (30.4%)
IV	19 (24.1%)
V	14 (17.7%)
Family status (*n* and %)	
Mother and father	29 (36.7%)
Mother only[b]	10 (12.7%)
Mother and stepfather	4 (5.0%)
Father only[b]	1 (1.2%)
Father and stepmother	14 (17.7%)
Foster care[c]	21 (26.6%)

[a]For social class, Hollingshead's (1975) five-category system was used, where I indicates major business executives and professionals, and V indicates unskilled laborers and menial service workers.
[b]Single, divorced, separated, or widowed.
[c]Adopted after infancy, foster care, group home.

do not know how many adolescents continue transvestic behaviors into adulthood, whether adolescents referred for such behaviors display the early manifestations of transvestic fetishism remains an open question. Studies of adults typically suggest a childhood or adolescent onset (Croughan et al., 1981; Prince & Bentler, 1972). In our experience, many of the adolescents referred for transvestic behaviors eventually become more extensively involved in cross-dressing if no attempt is made to control this activity. Thus, it is likely that these behaviors are the developmental precursors of the adult disorder, so we will treat them as such and refer to the largely adult literature where appropriate.

PHENOMENOLOGY OF TRANSVESTIC FETISHISM IN ADULTS

Adult men with transvestic fetishism often report an onset of cross-dressing before the age of 10. For the remainder of such men, cross-dressing usually begins at about the time of puberty (Croughan et al., 1981; Prince & Bentler, 1972). Cross-dressing is usually accompanied by masturbation in adolescence and by sexual intercourse in early and middle adulthood, with an eventual decline in sexual arousal over time (Croughan et al., 1981). The cross-dressing behavior is reported to provide a sense of relaxation and comfort or relief from what are experienced as "masculine demands" (Buhrich, 1978). The course of the disorder is chronic, with many individuals making sporadic attempts to stop or control the behavior (Croughan et al., 1981). However, most of these individuals return to cross-dressing fairly quickly and have little motivation to stop what they regard as a pleasurable activity. In addition, many individuals fantasize about expanding the extent of what they experience as feminine role behaviors (Prince & Bentler, 1972). Generally, transvestites appear to have elevated levels of anxiety, depression, and alcoholism (Buhrich, 1981; Croughan et al., 1981; Fagan, Wise, Derogatis, & Schmidt, 1988; Levine, 1993). These men usually define themselves as heterosexual. Although some of them may engage in sexual activity with men, they tend to regard themselves as heterosexual, and often see themselves as female in such encounters. Many transvestites marry, and their wives' reactions may range from encouragement of their cross-dressing to hostility (Prince & Bentler, 1972; Woodhouse, 1989).

Buhrich and McConaghy (1979) categorized transvestites as *nuclear, marginal,* or *transsexual.* The nuclear group displays little or no feminine identification and is largely heterosexual; the transsexual group displays more extensive cross-dressing, sexual interest in men, and a feminine gender identity; and the marginal group is intermediate between the nuclear and transsexual groups. Although Buhrich and McConaghy argued that these categories are discrete, the evidence for this is scanty, and other authors have held that transvestites exist at an intermediate point between heterosexuals and transsexuals on a continuum of gender dysphoria (Fagan et al., 1988).

The natural history of transvestism indicates that some individuals continue a pattern of cross-dressing with little change in their gender identity, whereas others develop an increasing cross-gender identification that may ultimately result in the desire for surgical sex reassignment (Blanchard, 1990b; Blanchard & Clemmensen, 1988). Whether this pattern is the result of extensive cross-dressing with fantasized elaboration of the self as the opposite sex, or whether the cross-gender identification is present from childhood and simply becomes more manifest with time and/or cross-dressing, is not clear. We do know that these individuals do not manifest the pattern of cross-gender identification seen in boys with gender identity disorder or in transsexual men with a homosexual orientation (Bradley & Zucker, 1984). In the DSM-IV, the presence of cross-gender identification is noted through the use of a subtype "with gender dysphoria."

REVIEW OF THE LITERATURE ON TRANSVESTIC FETISHISM IN ADOLESCENTS

The literature on adolescent transvestism is entirely descriptive (Adams, Klinge, Vaziri, Maczulski, & Pasternak, 1976; Krueger, 1978; Liakos, 1967; Spensley & Barter, 1971). Unfortunately, this literature has been confusing because precise definitions of transvestic fetishism were lacking, and in some instances it appeared to use the term *transvestism* to describe gender identity disorder or transsexualism. Adams et al. (1976), for example, reported on six adolescent patients. Four of these youngsters appeared actually to have gender identity disorder and were involved in homosexual activity. Of the two youngsters who did appear to have transvestic fetishism, one was also exhibitionistic and the other one was involved in pedophilic behavior.

Spensley and Barter (1971) described the family patterns of 18 adolescents to whom they referred as "transvestites." They defined a "core" group of 12 youngsters whom they considered to be "homogeneous" adolescent transvestites. In contrast, the other six youngsters—including one who was transsexual, one who was homosexual, and two who exhibited other paraphilias—were considered to be "partial" cross-dressers. Because Spensley and Barter did not provide adequate information about the actual behaviors of their 12 core subjects, it is difficult to assess whether these subjects would meet the DSM-IV criteria for transvestic fetishism. Spensley and Barter noted that masturbation was not a prominent feature, but was "intermittently associated with excitement stimulated by wearing female clothing in about half the cases" (p. 350). They described the mother–son relationship as of the "symbiotic hostile type" (p. 350), characterizing the mothers as "masculine [and] dominant" (p. 350) and the fathers as "passive and dependent" (p. 351).

CLINICAL FEATURES

Adolescents who engage in transvestic behaviors seldom present to the clinician of their own volition. Most typically, parents become concerned upon discovering that missing items of women's clothing have been hidden in their son's room. Occasionally, they discover their son wearing pantyhose or women's underwear while in bed. Occasionally, they will report that when younger, their son wore pantyhose under his clothing. The parents' reactions to such behavior usually include anger, confusion, and concern about gender identity and sexual orientation. Some parents, however, view the behavior as adolescent experimentation and do not give a clear message that it is of any particular concern. Clinical referral is likely to result if the behavior is prolonged or leads to the stealing of a neighbor's underwear or items from stores. As the adolescent and his family may feel very embarrassed by the behavior, it is often kept secret from relatives. Assessment of transvestic behaviors is sometimes made more difficult by the reluctance of the adolescent or other family members to talk about them.

Most of the youngsters seen in our clinic were referred in their early to middle adolescence with a history of use of female undergarments that began near puberty; some of the youngsters recalled sporadic use of their mothers' or sisters' pantyhose or undergarments from a much earlier age. Often such behaviors begin at a time when an adolescent's mother is absent, unavailable, or in conflict with the teenager. Initially, the garments are used for anxiety relief. A sexual connotation appears to develop when the joint use of the garments and masturbation becomes an anxiety-relieving mechanism. If allowed to pursue this strategy with little interference, the adolescent tends to increase the extent of cross-dressing to include shoes, outer garments, wigs, and makeup. These behaviors may occur sporadically, especially in response to stressful interactions with maternal or other important female figures; however, they may also become the preferred method of sexual arousal and they may be practiced several times a week with masturbation.

Obviously, the situation is affected by the extent of the individual's privacy, as these behaviors are seldom practiced when others are around. Some adolescents soil (masturbate, defecate, or urinate on) and mutilate the transvestic garments. Some contain the behaviors because they fear parental reaction, court involvement, or the impact of the behaviors on their sexuality in later life. Some try to stop their transvestic activities, but experience significant stress as a result and therefore sporadically return to them. Others make no effort to curb these activities, as they are not convinced that there is any particular reason to do so.

In the interview situation, an adolescent who engages in transvestic behaviors usually appears inhibited and has difficulties in expressing himself verbally. Most typically, he will state that he has a heterosexual orientation and no history of cross-gender behavior apart from the transvestic cross-dressing, which may have begun in childhood. Such adolescents do not manifest childhood cross-gender interests and activities, which are commonly found in the developmental histories of adolescents with gender identity disorder and adolescents presenting with homosexual concerns (Figure 12.1). Although gender identity confusion is acknowledged by some adolescents who engage in transvestic behaviors, most of them are quite clear about their identity as males. Such adolescents frequently experience discomfort in heterosocial situations, and they may also be somewhat distanced from their male peers.

Most of these adolescents find it difficult to discuss feelings, but the more insightful are able to describe their use of transvestic garments following stressful interactions with their mothers. Typically, following an argument with his mother, an adolescent retreats to his room feeling overwhelmed by his anger. Using female garments provides him with a sense of inner calm. As the adolescent also uses masturbation for self-soothing, the sexual connotation of the garments appears to arise out of the combination of these two anxiety-relieving mechanisms. With more prolonged use of female garments, the adolescent will report facilitation of sexual arousal through fantasies of himself cross-dressed or through cross-dressing itself. Although otherwise denying a wish for sex reassignment, some adolescents who engage in transvestic behaviors state that cross-dressing makes them feel like women. This feeling may be reinforced by self-observation in a mirror while cross-dressed.

A common characteristic of adolescents who engage in transvestic behaviors is that they perceive their mothers as impossibly dominating (Krueger, 1978; Liakos, 1967). In some families, this perception is shared by the boys' fathers and is corroborated in the interview. In oth-

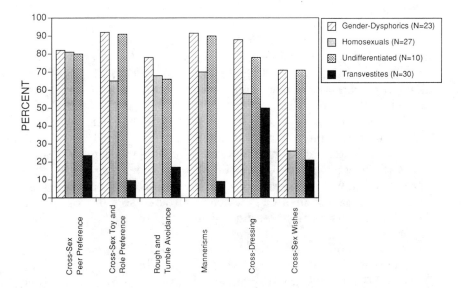

FIGURE 12.1. Percentage of subjects by diagnostic group with a childhood history of cross-sex-typed behaviors as derived from clinical interview data. The group labeled "Undifferentiated" consisted of adolescents who were referred for current cross-gender behavior, but who did not report concurrent gender dysphoria or a homosexual sexual orientation.

ers, however, sensitive, unassertive adolescents appear to be overwhelmed by their mothers' anger, which may have resulted from the sons' own behavioral difficulties. In many situations of this kind, the fathers have been unable to understand the sons or to help the sons in working out the conflict with the mothers (Krueger, 1978).

Adolescents with transvestic behaviors commonly have a history of behavioral and academic difficulties. Many of the referrals to our clinic were living in foster care families or in group homes. In part, this was a result of the adolescents' behavioral difficulties, but many also came from very disturbed families in which the parents were unable to look after their children (Table 12.2). In an alternate care situation, such an adolescent's frustration with his biological mother may continue or may develop in interaction with caregivers at the group home.

At some point prior to the onset of the transvestic fetishism, the number of our adolescents who had experienced either a long-term or a permanent separation from their mothers was high. Table 12.2 shows that 36 of the 79 adolescents were not living with their biological mothers at the time of assessment; another 4 adolescents had experienced a separation from their mothers, but were living with them again at the time of the assessment. Thus, the rate of maternal separation was 50.6%, which was considerably higher than the rates of maternal separation among our samples of gender-dysphoric and homosexual adolescents (Bradley & Zucker, 1984; see also Table 11.4). Many of these adolescents were aware of resenting their mothers, who they felt had rejected or abandoned them.

The connection of transvestic behaviors with other paraphilias (e.g., autoerotic asphyxia) and suicide has been reported (Shankel & Carr, 1956). The presence of transvestic behaviors in a sample of adult rapists (Langevin, Paitich, & Russon, 1985), in case reports of adult murderers (Snow & Bluestone, 1969), and in one unreported case of transvestic behavior in an adolescent murderer seen by one of us (Bradley) suggests the need for inquiry about aggressive fantasy and behavior.

As noted above, behavioral difficulties were common. Table 12.3 and Figure 12.2 show mothers' or surrogate mothers' CBCL ratings. On the CBCL, there were, on average, almost five narrow-band elevations; the CBCL sum score was well within the clinical range, as were the Internalizing and Externalizing *T* scores, which did not differ signif-

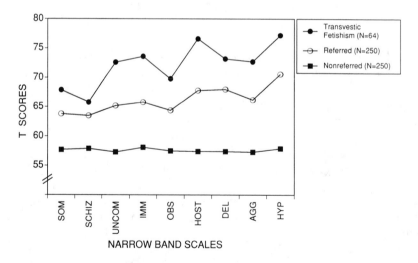

FIGURE 12.2. Narrow-band factors on the CBCL, 12- to 16-year-old boys. SOM, Somatic Complaints; SCHIZ, Schizoid; UNCOM, Uncommunicative; IMM, Immature; OBS, Obsessive–Compulsive; HOST, Hostile Withdrawal; DEL, Delinquent; AGG, Aggressive; HYP, Hyperactive. Nonreferred and referred group data are from the standardization study (Achenbach & Edelbrock, 1983, Appendix D).

TABLE 12.3. Mothers' or Surrogate Mothers' Ratings of behavioral Disturbance on the CBCL in Male Adolescents with Transvestic Fetishism

Measures	Transvestic fetishism (*n* = 64)		Nonreferred (*n* = 250)		Referred (*n* = 250)	
	M	*SD*	*M*	*SD*	*M*	*SD*
No. elevated narrow-band scales	4.9	2.8	—	—	—	—
Number of items	54.3	14.6	—	—	—	—
Sum of items	78.3	29.4	21.7	15.0	58.9	24.0
Internalizing *T*	71.1	6.8	51.2	9.1	65.6	8.9
Externalizing *T*	72.0	8.4	51.0	9.3	68.1	8.7

Note. Nonreferred and referred samples consist of boys aged 12–16, from Achenbach and Edelbrock (1983, Appendix D). For the probands, all CBCL items pertaining to transvestic fetishism (e.g., item 73, "Sexual problems") scored 1 or 2 were set to 0 to avoid artificial inflation of general psychopathology.

icantly from each other. On the narrow-band scales, peak scores were found for Hyperactivity and Hostile Withdrawal. The majority of the narrow-band scales were considerably higher than those for the referred sample in the standardization study (Achenbach & Edelbrock, 1983). Thus, on average, our sample of adolescents with transvestic fetishism showed very severe levels of behavioral disturbance that cut across the internalizing and externalizing domains of psychopathology. The most common other DSM-III-R diagnoses were conduct disorder, oppositional defiant disorder, attention-deficit hyperactivity disorder, and overanxious disorder. Formal learning disabilities (particularly language disorders) and failing a grade at school were also quite common.

Table 12.4 shows the correlations between CBCL ratings and de-

TABLE 12.4. Correlations between CBCL Ratings and Demographic Variables

Measures	Age	Full Scale IQ	Social class	Marital status[a]
No. elevated narrow-band scales	−.04	−.08	−.28*	.25*
Number of items	−.08	.03	−.18	.10
Sum of items	−.09	.03	−.14	.12
Internalizing *T*	.04	.02	−.09	.21
Externalizing *T*	−.07	.11	−.13	.08

[a]1 = mother and father; 2 = all other combinations (see Table 12.2).
*$p < .05$.

Chapter 12

mographic variables. Only 2 of 20 correlations were significant. Since the sample was somewhat biased demographically (lower IQ, lower social class, high rate of broken families), it was of interest that the demographics were virtually unrelated to the extent of behavioral psychopathology.

Intellectual testing confirmed the clinical impression of relative deficits in verbal expression (Table 12.5). It can be seen that Verbal IQ was significantly lower than Performance IQ. On Cohen's factor scores (Cohen, 1957), Verbal Comprehension and Freedom from Distractibility were both significantly lower than Perceptual Organization, but they did not differ from each other. This pattern of intellectual functioning was consistent with that found in two previous studies of adult men with transvestic fetishism (Bowler & Collacott, 1993; Steiner, Sanders, & Langevin, 1985). Although Verbal IQ and Performance IQ were each significantly correlated with social class (r's = $-.45$ and $-.39$, respectively, both p's $< .001$), the difference score was not correlated with social class ($r = .03$) or any of the other demographic variables; thus, the discrepancy between Verbal and Performance IQ appeared to be representative of the sample as a whole.

Referral for neurological assessment to rule out a temporal lobe focus (see below) has revealed only one significant abnormality by history and electroencephalographic (EEG) testing. However, three other adolescents had a documented history of epilepsy or EEG abnormality prior to the onset of the transvestic fetishism, and a fourth had Tourette's syndrome. In one of the adolescents with an established seizure disorder, the frequency of transvestic behaviors escalated, and a diaper fetish (cf. Malitz, 1966; Tuchman & Lachman, 1964) also began as seizure control diminished. Several other youngsters had had severe head injuries as toddlers, and several had been exposed to very severe

TABLE 12.5. IQ and Factor Scores of Male Adolescents with Transvestic Fetishism

	M	SD	Range	n
Verbal IQ[a]	92.1	17.1	47–131	66
Performance IQ[a]	98.5	10.6	45–138	66
Full Scale IQ	94.7	19.3	41–138	66
Verbal Comprehension[b]	8.9	3.0	1.75–15.75	64
Perceptual Organization[b]	10.3	3.4	1.25–16.25	64
Freedom from Distractibility[b]	7.7	2.8	1.00–13.33	64

Note. The IQ test used was the WISC, WISC-R, or WISC-III.
[a]$t (65) = 4.10, p < .001.$
[b]$F (2, 126) = 35.4, p < .001.$

environmental deprivation; both of these factors are suggestive of cerebral insult.

The following cases illustrate some aspects of the clinical presentation of adolescents with transvestic fetishism.

CASE EXAMPLE 12.1

Joe, a 15-year-old Native American, was referred to our clinic because he had been taking underclothes belonging to an older foster sister. He often would defecate on them. At the time of presentation, he was living in a group home following a physically aggressive outburst against his foster father. This outburst had been preceded by a period of very frustrating interaction between Joe and his foster parents over control of his cross-dressing, which had been revealed to the foster family some months previously.

Joe's cross-dressing behaviors had begun at about age 6, while he was living in an abusive adoptive family. Shortly after the onset of these behaviors, he had come to live with his foster family. Joe had significant developmental difficulties—nighttime fecal soiling, extreme slobbering owing to difficulty in swallowing his saliva, and an expressive language problem that often made it hard for others to understand him. Nevertheless, both the foster family and Joe felt that they were getting along all right and that Joe was gradually overcoming his difficulties. They acknowledged, however, that Joe's difficulty in dealing with angry feelings had continued, and his foster father was concerned about the possibility that he could become violent. This concern stemmed in part from the fact that Joe's natural mother had murdered two members of her family.

There was no evidence of gender identity disorder. Joe had always been withdrawn and quiet. He was not well coordinated, but was able to become competent at baseball and hockey. He also enjoyed hunting with his foster father. The foster family indicated that Joe had never been very able to express his feelings, especially angry ones. He reached a point at which he was able to cry, and the family felt that some progress was being made.

Despite Joe's difficulties, the family saw him as having a good sense of humor and as having been a very talkative youngster. Joe became quite anxious when his natural mother showed up unexpectedly. He began having nightmares at that time, and he expressed the fear that she might take him away. Aside from the difficulties reported above, he showed no evidence of conduct problems until shortly before the disclosure of his cross-dressing to his foster family. He had also been doing reasonably well at school.

When Joe decided, in collaboration with his child welfare worker, to reveal what he had been doing, the family supported his efforts in trying to find treatment. The process of finding a therapist dragged on, and during this period Joe's cross-dressing escalated. The welfare worker reported that he ejaculated and urinated on the clothing, poured salad oil on it, and burned it. The family became very upset with his behavior and tried to control it by locking doors to prevent his access to others' clothing. The situation climaxed in the fight with his father that led to his move to a group home. In the group home, he was seen as alternating between depression and hyperactivity. He ran away several times, was truant from school, shoplifted, and broke into his foster family's home.

In the individual interview, Joe acknowledged his cross-dressing, his masturbatory fantasies of himself dressed as a woman, and his occasional thoughts about feeling like a girl when he put on the female underwear. He also acknowledged that he was concerned about his temper and that he sometimes had vengeful fantasies. He was somewhat worried that he might act on these fantasies and even murder someone. He denied concerns about homosexuality. Apart from the fantasies of himself dressed as a woman, he could not report other masturbatory sexual fantasies. He agreed that he had always found it difficult to express himself, because he frequently had trouble finding words. He saw himself as being sensitive and as feeling things deeply. He had had suicidal feelings at one time, and he had tried to hang himself after a fight with his best friend. There was no evidence of other abnormalities of thought content or process.

In discussing his relationship with his foster family, Joe said that life had been much better for him in that family than in his adoptive family. He did, however, report that he experienced anxiety about fights or arguments with his foster mother. He did not want to get mad at her, as he was afraid that if he lost his temper, he might end up hitting her. He was also worried about his foster mother being angry with him. In contrast, he found it much easier to get angry with his foster father and did not seem uncomfortable about occasionally getting into a fight with him. He felt that both he and his foster father had a sense of winning if they fought and that both of them would end up forgetting about it.

Following the assessment, Joe was referred back to his individual therapist with recommendations for working on his angry feelings. Efforts were made to support an ongoing positive relationship between Joe and his foster family.

Our formulation of Joe's situation was that the cross-dressing had developed as a form of self-soothing in his initial adoptive family, in which this very sensitive boy at times felt overwhelmed by feelings that he was unable to express. We felt that the continuation of the cross-dressing was a reflection of Joe's marked vulnerability in dealing with his affects, his failure to resolve feelings related to earlier traumas, and his concern about the impact of expressing anger toward his foster mother. Despite occasional fantasies of himself as female while he was masturbating or cross-dressed, Joe was not significantly cross-gender-identified. Thus, we felt that the most important therapeutic intervention was to assist this adolescent in finding alternative ways to deal with his feelings, especially his anger.

CASE EXAMPLE 12.2

John was a 13-year-old Grade 7 student who was referred after a 1-year history of taking panties, bras, and pantyhose belonging to his mother and sister. These objects were found intermittently in his bedroom. His mother was suspicious that he was using these articles for masturbatory purposes, as she had also found "girlie" pictures in his room over the same period. His parents were concerned that he might be "gay."

John was the result of a planned pregnancy but a toxemic birth. There were no concerns about his development, although his mother felt that he was "oversexed." This comment originated from the observation that he seemed to jump up and down on his bed a lot and to squirm around frequently on his stomach. He had had two transitional objects—a blanket and a teddy bear—until about age 6, when his mother discarded them. He was always somewhat shy with other children. He had been put in day care at about age 2, when his mother returned to work. John's father perceived this as indicating his mother's lack of affection for him, and believed that John's present problems resulted from his mother's difficulty in relating to her son. There was no history of a gender identity disorder. John's interests were largely in animals and the outdoors. He had a good same-sex friend with whom he shared his interests. He belonged to a bowling team and expressed a special interest in a girl on the team.

In the joint interview, the parents, who had recently separated, demonstrated difficulty in looking at each other or talking freely. Separately, father and son expressed their frustration at John's mother, whom they saw as non-nurturing, overbearing, and aggressive. Both John and his father tended to see themselves as lesser members of the family, able to get along only by giving in to the desires of the women in the family (including John's mother's mother) rather than by speaking out. John's mother perceived her husband as gradually becoming more lethargic, as uninterested in a sexual relationship with her, and as passive in his relationship with John. She also acknowledged having a history of depression, severe enough to require taking time off work.

During the joint interview, John mumbled when under stress, but he was more articulate when seen individually. He acknowledged his anger at his mother, whom he perceived as restricting and rejecting him. He described feelings of low self-esteem and inadequacy, and expressed a desire to be more manly. His favorite animal was the ichthyosaurus, which he described as having various protuberant parts (fins, tails, flippers, and a long beak). He also expressed the desire to be a "dominant" fish like a shark and to "rule everything." He denied homosexual feelings, describing masturbatory fantasies about and crushes on girls or women. He was reluctant to talk about his use of female undergarments. He indicated that he did not know why he took them, and he was sure that he wouldn't "fool around" with them any more. He appeared aware that his oppositional behavior at home was related to his anger at his mother.

This family was seen in supportive therapy. The parents were able to make modest changes, with the father becoming more involved with and supportive of his son. The mother was able to back off somewhat and to be more positive toward John. John responded by controlling his transvestic urges and trying to be more compliant at home. His parents saw him as calmer and more at ease with himself. They decided to try living together again after discussing ways in which they both needed to be more accommodating. John refused individual psychotherapy, indicating that he felt he was in control of his problem.

ETIOLOGY

There have been three main theoretical approaches to understanding the development of transvestic behavior: psychoanalytic, learning, and biological. Each of these approaches is reviewed below. Because we believe that no one theory adequately addresses the complexity of transvestic fetishism and that all three approaches have some merit, an integration of these approaches follows this review.

Psychoanalytic Theory

Transvestism, defined as a form of fetishism, was seen in the classic psychoanalytic literature as an individual's response to learning about genital differences (Fenichel, 1945). The fetish (in this case, the cross-dressing) was thought to represent a disavowal of the "penis-less" mother; thus cross-dressing was seen as enabling a boy or a man to protect himself against castration anxiety. This theory failed to adequately explain the differences that led to homosexual object choice as opposed to transvestism (both resulting from castration anxiety), except to posit early fixations in transvestism (Fenichel, 1945). Later analysts questioned the overriding importance of oedipal conflict for the development of transvestic behaviors. With an increased emphasis on the role of family interaction and self psychology, the idea of preoedipal traumas emerged as a way of explaining both the early onset of transvestism and the presence of gender identity confusion in it (Bak, 1953; Berman, 1953; Glasser, 1979; Greenacre, 1955). Conceptualizing the fetish as an extreme form of a transitional object, these etiological theories focused on separation anxiety. Although many analytic writers continue to view transvestic behavior as a solely oedipal solution, most analytic writers also acknowledge the contribution of preoedipal factors to the boy's extreme castration concerns. Greenacre (1968) described the development of perversions (among which she included transvestism) as follows:

> Due to early disturbances in the mother–infant relationship there is a severe impairment of object relationships which combines with a specifically determined weakness of the body and self images, especially involving the genitals. This becomes more significant during the phallic and oedipal periods when castration anxiety is extraordinarily acute, due to the quality of the aggression aroused at these times. The maturing sexual drives are distorted in the interest of bolstering the body image. There is then a vicious circle of recurring castration panic for which the fetish or the ritualized behavior serve almost literally as a stopgap permitting the semblance of a more nearly adequate sexual performance or relationship. This may have more narcissistic than object related value. (p. 57)

Thus, preoccupation with viewing oneself in a mirror (a commonly observed behavior in transvestism) would be seen to act as a stabilizer of body image—perhaps illustrative of a supposed defect of "parental mirroring" in early childhood.

Person and Ovesey (1978) conceptualized transvestism as part of a spectrum between transsexualism and effeminate homosexuality. They viewed the cross-dressing in each of these disorders as an attempt to deal with separation anxiety at three different levels, the transsexual's solution being the most primitive and the effeminate homosexual's the most advanced. Stoller (1985a, 1985b) presented a particularly vivid account of the treatment of a mother whose 2½-year-old son was displaying transvestic interests. Although cautious in extrapolating from this case history to all cases of transvestism, he believed several factors to be important in the development of transvestic behavior:

> Early boyhood fetishism is the consequence of a constellation of events, not a single event. It is, therefore, very rare since few boys are exposed to the whole constellation. To explain any case, much less all cases, as a splitting of the ego in the effort to substitute the fetish for mother's absent penis leaves out too much. (p. 135)

Other factors that Stoller (1985b) deemed important were "a mother–infant symbiosis in disarray, primeval separation anxiety, and intense physical trauma, especially when augmented by a terrified mother" (p. 135).

Cooper (1991), in an effort to provide an integrated perspective on analytic views of fetishism, concluded that "the perversion dynamic is present whenever an action or fantasy is dominated by the denial of unconscious passivity through the triple fantasies of dehumanizing the object, dehumanizing the self, and securing masochistic pleasure" (p. 34).

Because the analytic literature consists almost entirely of case reports, it is hard to know how much weight should be assigned to such theories. What does seem to emerge, however, is a general agreement that transvestic boys have suffered difficulties in their early relationships with their mothers (Friedemann, 1966; Hora, 1953; Lihn, 1970; Stoller, 1985a, 1985b). This may involve intense frustration, parental neglect or abandonment, exposure to traumatizing situations, and/or early seductions. Although case reports demonstrate significant anger toward the mother or toward mother surrogates, most of the focus has been on understanding the transvestism as a defense against castration or separation anxiety. Anxiety about anger per se has been relatively neglected, although there is some consensus with regard to the view that transvestic behavior serves both an anxiety-relieving and a reparative function by creating a closeness to the mother or by recreating the mother as unharmed (i.e., noncastrated).

Learning Theory

Fetishistic responses can be conditioned (Junginger, 1988). Rachman (1966), for example, showed that sexual arousal could be conditioned to a boot. Others have replicated such conditioned arousal to different stimuli (e.g., geometric figures), but with smaller effects, suggesting that conditioning of this kind is unlikely to play a major role in the development of fetishistic behaviors (Langevin & Martin, 1975; McConaghy, 1967; see also O'Donohue & Plaud, 1994). Theoretically, therefore, transvestic behaviors could be viewed as a conditioned response, although there is no empirical literature demonstrating that a complex behavior such as transvestic fetishism can be conditioned. Learning may be operative when sexual arousal (response) is connected with female clothing (stimulus), in that orgasm is rewarding and thus may make the behavior difficult to extinguish (cf. Laws & Marshall, 1991).

Biological Theory

Although "brain mechanisms" responsible for sexual arousal have not been definitively identified, there is a general consensus that limbic and temporal lobe structures are important for both sexual interest or arousal and for inhibition of sexual behaviors (Blumer & Walker, 1975). Generally, temporal lobe epilepsy (TLE) produces a state of hyposexuality. However, case reports of hypersexuality, and of fetishistic and transvestic behaviors associated with TLE, led Epstein (1960, 1961, 1969, 1973) to hypothesize that some forms of transvestism or fetishism arise as a result of inhibition or release of limbic regions with seizure activity (see also Kolarsky, Freund, Machek, & Polak, 1967). Other reports have linked transvestic fetishism and other types of fetishism with head injury (e.g., Miller, Cummings, McIntyre, Ebers, & Grode, 1986; Pandita-Gunawardena, 1990). This theory is supported by the fact that in several cited cases transvestic and fetishistic impulses have been reduced or eliminated through either surgical removal of the irritating focus or medication to control the seizures (e.g., Davies & Morgenstern, 1960; Hunter, Logue, & McMenemy, 1963; Mitchell, Falconer, & Hill, 1954; Walinder, 1965). The idea that abnormalities in limbic structures may facilitate transvestic behavior is illustrated by a case report in which such behavior, previously extinguished by behavioral treatment, returned with the development of a seizure-provoking mass and then diminished with treatment of the seizures (Ball, 1968). Nevertheless, as noted earlier, neurological examination of transvestic adolescent males referred to our clinic has revealed only one case of previously undiagnosed TLE. However, high levels of anxiety (Fedoroff, 1988) and learning and behavioral difficulties among such males have raised issues regarding neurological intactness at a higher or integrative level in transvestic individuals (Bradley & Zucker, 1984).

Elevated testosterone levels, which at one time were suspected of being etiologically relevant in sexual deviations, generally do not appear to play a significant role. Buhrich and Theile (1979) found testosterone levels in 26 volunteers from a transvestic club to be within the normal range.

Although the exhibition of transvestic behavior by more than one family member has been reported (Buhrich, 1977; Liakos, 1967), Croughan et al. (1981) did not find a higher than expected number of family members with transvestism in a study of 70 transvestites.

An Integrative Formulation

We believe that adolescents who display transvestic behavior are vulnerable to difficulties with anxiety regulation. These adolescents are described as having been sensitive children who were never comfortable when talking about feelings. Frequently, they also have language or learning disorders that have resulted in academic failure and/or behavioral difficulties. Low self-esteem may result from intrafamilial conflict, behavioral or academic problems, and peer difficulties.

Although there is seldom a history of other cross-gender activities and interests, some of these adolescents do report having used such items as pantyhose for anxiety relief in childhood. Withdrawal and avoidance are other strategies commonly used to cope with stressful situations.

We do not believe that separation anxiety or oedipal factors alone provide an adequate explanation for the onset of transvestic behaviors. We do believe that many of the adolescents who engage in such behaviors have experienced early (preoedipal) difficulties, as well as self-esteem difficulties during the latency period, and that these have interfered with the development of effective anxiety regulation. In early adolescence, conflict with a maternal figure produces intense frustration for which such a poorly regulated, relatively nonverbal adolescent has few coping strategies. Resort to self-soothing through silky garments may provide him with a sense of connectedness to his mother, which he may find necessary to assure himself that he has not harmed her by his anger. Masturbation has a similar self-soothing function. The proximity of the two hypothalamic centers that control sexual and affective arousal (MacLean, 1962, 1965; MacLean & Ploog, 1962), combined with the possibility of a spreading arousal via a kindling-type mechanism (Adamec & Stark-Adamec, 1986; Post, Weiss, Uhde, Clark, & Rosen, 1993), may be a factor in the choice of masturbation for self-soothing.

If the individual persists in the use of cross-dressing accompanied by masturbation as his preferred strategy for dealing with states of inner tension, he may elaborate a gradually increasing sexual fantasy of himself as a female. This may become the preferred way of achieving arousal. Learning theory suggests that this pattern may be very hard to unlearn, especially if the stresses continue and anxiety relief is needed.

Although our formulation appears to be an adequate description of the adolescents we have seen, it is important to acknowledge the likely bias in our clinical population. The fact that the adolescents referred to us have both behavioral and academic difficulties may indicate that we are seeing a more disturbed subgroup of individuals with transvestic behavior. This issue can be only addressed through epidemiological studies of larger populations.

TREATMENT

The treatment of transvestic fetishism in adults, aside from psychoanalysis, has focused largely on behavioral interventions such as aversive conditioning, satiation, and shaming. Langevin (1983) provided a thorough review of these interventions; he cautioned that although their success rates were above 50%, follow-up had been limited, samples had not been well defined, and motivation of subjects in many studies had been questionable (see also Gelder, 1979; Gelder & Marks, 1969). Anecdotal reports of analytically oriented approaches (Stoller, 1985b) and of antianxiety medication (Fedoroff, 1988, 1992) suggest that some change can be achieved with such interventions as well.

Our formulation points to the need to focus on stress reduction within the family—specifically, to help the adolescent and his parents resolve conflict with less tension. This should include helping parents understand the difficulties their son is having with self-assertion in his relationship with his mother. Frequently, the adolescent's mother has felt frustrated by her son's behavioral difficulties, has reacted angrily, and has imposed unreasonable limits out of distrust. The adolescent needs help in negotiating control over his life. In addition, both the parents and the adolescent need to understand that transvestic behavior does not imply a homosexual orientation, as worry over this possibility frequently creates even further distance in the parent–child relationship.

The adolescent requires a conceptual framework to understand that the anxiety-relieving function of his transvestic behavior has been necessary because of his difficulties in dealing with his angry feelings. He needs to understand that continued use of such anxiety-relieving mechanisms—especially if the cross-dressing becomes more extensive and is used in behavior or fantasy for sexual arousal—will make him very vulnerable to full-blown transvestism in adulthood. Individual work focusing on alternative ways of dealing with anger and the associated anxiety should be pursued.

This approach has enabled some adolescents to relinquish their transvestic behaviors. Unfortunately, many of the adolescents and their families are reluctant to engage in treatment. Given the poor response of the paraphilias (including fetishism and transvestism) to psychological treatment, interest lately has focused on psychopharmacological approaches. For example, there are several case reports describing the benefits of fluoxetine for different types of paraphilias, including transvestic fetishism (e.g., Kerbeshian & Burd, 1991; Masand, 1993; Perilstein, Lipper, & Friedman, 1991). In a double-blind crossover comparison of the effects of clomipramine and desipramine in paraphilic subjects, Kruesi, Fine, Valladares, Phillips, and Rapoport (1992) found that both medications reduced the severity of paraphilic symptoms in those who completed the study (see also Clayton, 1993). Epstein's (1973) theory of a relationship between temporal lobe seizures and fetishism suggests that such medications as carbamazepine might also be effective. To date, there have been only anecdotal reports as indicated in the section on etiology. Theoretically, antianxiety agents should be useful, and the successful use of buspirone has been reported in an uncontrolled trial in one adult with transvestic fetishism (Fedoroff, 1988) and in another adult with an atypical paraphilia (Fedoroff, 1992).

CHAPTER 13

Homosexuality in Adolescence

Some will question why we have included a chapter on homosexuality in adolescence, given that it is no longer considered a psychiatric disorder. As noted by Meyer-Bahlburg (1990–1991, 1993b), the reason is that clinicians are frequently consulted about, or by, gay or lesbian youth. Thus, they should be knowledgeable about homosexual development and the issues faced by gay youth in order to provide proper care for these individuals. Despite the progress made toward greater acceptance of homosexuality during the early stages of the gay liberation movement, there is little doubt that the AIDS epidemic has led to a significant setback in the acceptance of homosexuality in the broader community. The clinical community has a responsibility not to worsen the stigma through inadequate understanding or belief in outdated theories.

Although our clinical experience has been derived from our work in a gender identity clinic for children and adolescents, we are regularly consulted by parents or group home workers who are concerned about adolescents' homosexual behavior. More occasionally, we are contacted by adolescents themselves who are concerned about their homosexual feelings or behaviors.

CLINICAL PRESENTATION

Adolescents may divulge their concerns about homosexual feelings or behavior to professionals, but more frequently do so to friends. Most typically, professionals are consulted by parents or other family members to whom an adolescent has "come out" or who have discovered the adolescent's homosexual behavior or interests. Occasionally, the discovery of involvement with a younger child, the finding of gay pornography in the adolescent's bedroom, or conflict over friends or curfews leads to clinical referral. Female adolescents are brought less regularly than males by family members for consultation, perhaps in part because they begin their sexual involvement later than gay males, but also because they may be better able to disguise the nature of their same-sex relationships. Some adolescents may be referred because of involvement in prostitution. Although many such males are homosexual, not all would acknowledge a homoerotic preference (Coleman, 1989). Some adolescents will be seen by professionals through contact for treatment of sexually transmitted diseases, substance abuse, or suicide attempts (Owen, 1985; Remafedi, 1987a, 1987b; Remafedi, Farrow, & Deisher, 1991; Rigg, 1982). Homosexual youth appear more at risk than nonhomosexual youth in several psychosocial domains, as evidenced by high frequencies of running away, drug and alcohol abuse, suicide attempts, and contact with the law (e.g., Erwin, 1993; Kourany, 1987; Prenzlauer, Drescher, & Winchel, 1992; Remafedi, 1987a; Remafedi et al., 1991; Rich, Fowler, Young, & Blankush, 1986; Roesler & Deisher, 1972; Rotheram-Borus, Hunter, & Rosario, 1992; Saunders & Valente, 1987; Schneider, Farberow, & Kruks, 1989). There is also some evidence that homosexual men, but not homosexual women, with a childhood history of cross-gender behavior are at greater risk for parasuicide (i.e., attempts or suicidal feelings) (Harry, 1983).

Adolescents presenting with the above-noted psychosocial problems may not easily acknowledge their sexual orientation and it is important for clinicians to inquire sensitively about sexual issues. For some adolescents, depression or a suicide attempt may be the first indication to others that the individual is struggling with homosexual feelings. Males typically have their first homosexual experience in middle adolescence, in contrast to females whose involvement tends to begin in late adolescence or early adulthood (Bell et al., 1981; Saghir & Robins, 1973).

The following case vignettes provide some sense of the issues with which these adolescents present.

CASE EXAMPLE 13.1

Sunny, an 18-year-old female, came to the clinic on the advice of her group home worker because of her concerns about the "rightness" of being lesbian. She also indicated that she was worried about how to deal with her parents' negative reaction to her disclosure. When she announced that she was lesbian to her parents, they had reacted angrily, insisting that she couldn't be. Their response made Sunny depressed, and she began to question whether they might in fact be right and whether she should try to be heterosexual.

Sunny had grown up in a family with an abusive alcoholic stepfather, who (in her view) had treated her differently from either her older brother or younger sister. Her stepfather, a karate instructor, had hit her on several occasions, having told her to remain still while purportedly demonstrating moves to her. Furthermore, he had touched her on the breasts and genitals and indicated that he would take her to a motel room, take off her clothes, and show her the vulnerable spots to hit someone. She had since avoided him.

In contrast, Sunny viewed her mother positively and seemed to excuse her mother's inability to prevent the stepfather's abuse. She was convinced that she was the cause of her parents' fighting—a view that was reinforced when, after she left home, she was told that her stepfather had stopped drinking and his blood pressure had come down. Sunny's relationships with her siblings were generally positive.

In the individual interview, Sunny acknowledged long-standing difficulties with anxiety and an inner tenseness which frequently resulted in self-mutilatory behavior. She was aware of feeling very distressed by her angry feelings, having grown up in a family in which she couldn't get angry at her stepfather, for fear of his reaction, or at her mother for fear it might hurt her. When very angry, she worried about losing control. Sunny acknowledged feeling depressed with some suicidal feelings, but was prevented from acting on these out of concern for her parents.

Since the age of 16, Sunny had been involved in several lesbian relationships. These tended to be romantic relationships lasting several months. She experienced no sexual attraction to men, although she had several male friends.

Her developmental history was that of a very tomboyish girl, with avoidance of girls' clothing, preference for play with boys, and concerns about breast development and menarche, but no overt wish to change sex. Sunny experienced difficulties at school, partly because of a learning disability but also because of social isolation. In midadolescence she became withdrawn to such an extent that her parents sought psychiatric help. While in the hospital, she developed "seizures," which were eventually considered reactive to the stresses she was experiencing. She was then referred to a group home and given medication for depression. In addition, she had some difficulties with use of street drugs and one shoplifting charge.

Sunny agreed to be seen in individual psychotherapy, the focus of which was to help her achieve a more positive lesbian identity and to explore more adaptive ways of dealing with her anger. Over a 2-year period, she succeeded in moving out of the group home; joined an Outward Bound experience; found regular work; and, as she became more comfortable in dealing with her feelings, reduced her involvement with drugs. She continued a relatively positive relationship with her mother and siblings, but she continued to avoid her stepfather. She became actively involved in a gay and lesbian movement to provide support and counseling for gay and lesbian students. At termination, she was continuing to have difficulty with relationships but chose to try to manage without therapy.

CASE EXAMPLE 13.2

Leslie, a 16-year-old female, presented following an admission to an inpatient unit for depression. In addition to concerns about her family and friends, she indicated that she was very distressed by homosexual feelings and believed she must be a lesbian.

Leslie had grown up in a family marred by parental discord. She viewed her mother as weak because of her inability to deal with her husband's unfaithfulness and chronic work difficulties. Leslie felt particularly conflicted about loyalties to her parents in early adolescence and felt she had to make a choice between them. Her relationship with her sister had been one of chronic put-downs, which had significantly undermined her self-esteem.

Developmentally, there was little of note. In particular, there was no early history of cross-gender behavior, and Leslie reported that she did not consider herself tomboyish. Difficulties in sustaining friendships, related to problems with assertiveness and a tendency to be sarcastic, left her feeling socially isolated and inadequate.

At age 15, Leslie became aware of strong feelings of attraction to a friend of her sister—a girl whom her sister also admired. Being an obsessive worrier, she began to brood about these feelings. When she was depressed about other things, her preoccupation with these feelings would become particularly intense and would make her feel even more despondent. Over the 1-year period prior to being seen in therapy, she became aware of attractions to other women. She had not, however, had any sexual involvement with a female, nor had she discussed her feelings with anyone. Although she also had experienced crushes on boys, she had little dating experience, tending to feel awkward and unlikable despite the fact that she was physically very attractive. She was particularly anxious in social situations and felt that she had nothing to say or would say the wrong thing. Despite attempts to confront her social difficulties, her natural avoidance reaction when anxious made her feel that she would never learn to cope socially, and thus furthered her sense of failure.

Because Leslie did not wish to pursue a homosexual orientation and because the clinician (Bradley) did not see her homosexual feelings as indicating a fixed sexual orientation, an agreement was reached to begin a trial of therapy. Despite significant discomfort with discussing negative feelings in general, Leslie was able to recognize that her concern about homosexual feelings became more intense when she was feeling inadequate or depressed. When she was coping reasonably well and feeling better about herself, she became less bothered by these concerns and began to pursue heterosexual relationships. Her initial relationships were frustrating, as she tended to involve herself with men who had their own personality problems. The relationships became obsessively focused on sexual functioning and inevitably became frustrating, because they were not balanced by other qualities such as mutual interests. Over time, however, she became more certain that she could become aroused in heterosexual situations and was much less concerned about her occasional homosexual feelings.

After a struggle as to whether she was prepared to commit herself to more intensive psychotherapy to deal with recurrent bouts of depression, Leslie was transferred to an adult therapist and has continued to work productively on her depression.

CASE EXAMPLE 13.3

Billy, a 14-year-old adolescent male, was brought by his parents for treatment after he revealed to them that he had been sexually involved with a boy.

Billy grew up in a family in which the parents, who came from very different backgrounds, were openly antagonistic to each other. The father, an Eastern European refugee, had lost his own father during the war. Despite limited education, he had become reasonably successful in a small business in North America. Billy's mother, who was the unwanted last child in her family, had lost her father when she was 9 months old. She felt that she was a chronic burden to her often bitter mother. The couple married, despite the realization that they did not love each other, because it was "time" for each to marry. The early years of the marriage were difficult. The father worked long hours in his business, in which the mother was also involved. Billy spent a lot of time with his older sister, who took on a nurturing role.

Developmentally, Billy was described as sensitive and anxious, frequently worrying, and having difficulty asserting himself with male peers. He preferred playing with girls, enjoyed girls' activities and toys (e.g., Barbie dolls), and was quite avoidant of competitive or rough-and-tumble play. As he grew older, the more overt cross-gender interests declined, but he continued to be teased by male peers and was unable to defend himself against their attacks.

Billy presented as a somewhat obese, talkative youngster. He acknowledged his homosexual involvement and was uncomfortable that he had found it so arousing. He had no heterosexual interests, but he indicated that he did not want to be gay. He had limited erotic fantasy, most of which was homosexual.

Although it was felt that Billy was most likely homosexual, he was offered a trial of therapy because of his motivation to try to develop heterosexual interests and the family's marked difficulty in accepting the idea of his homosexuality. It was explained to him that he would have to work on developing heterosocial interests, as well as skills in self-assertion to enhance his very low self-esteem. He had difficulty making a commitment to work on these areas; he alternated between being convinced he was gay and could do nothing about it and feeling he must be able to change. Over a period of several years of somewhat irregular contact, he chose to work on his increasing self-assertion and improving his academic and social situation. During this period, he recalled an experience from late childhood in which he had been beaten up by a girl in his neighborhood. This memory, coupled with an exceedingly high level of social anxiety, prevented him from pursuing social contact with women.

Efforts to help the family be more supportive were quite frustrating. The father was unable to accept his son as homosexual and continued to be highly critical of almost everything he did. Billy fought back in a passive–aggressive fashion, which further fueled his father's rage. The mother tried to act as an intermediary; however, she often found herself torn among affection for her son, sympathy for her husband's viewpoint (which she shared to some extent), and worry that her son was going nowhere (which was reinforced by his prolonged difficulty in sorting out academic and career goals).

Over many years, Billy gradually moved away from the family and was able to consolidate a more comfortable identity as a gay person. He continued a supportive relationship with his sister. An anxious orientation to the world persisted, however, manifested particularly in his concern about finding the right partner.

"COMING OUT"

"Coming out" as a gay or lesbian person is a complex process in a predominantly heteroerotic society (Herdt, 1989; Martin, 1982; Zera, 1992). Such individuals usually identify themselves as different in late childhood or early adolescence. For some, this sense of being different is defined fairly quickly with respect to sexual preference. For others, the process may take several years and may include heterosexual experimentation.

Troiden (1979, 1988, 1989) has conceptualized the "coming-out" process as consisting of four phases. The initial phase is one of *sensitization* regarding the nature of one's attractions and feelings, the significant aspect of which is the meaning one attaches to such feelings. The second phase involves a sense of *identity confusion,* which Troiden (1989) feels is affected by altered perceptions of oneself, the experience of heterosexual and homosexual arousal and behavior, the stigma surrounding homosexuality, and inaccurate knowledge about homosexuals and homosexuality. The third stage, which Troiden labels *identity assumption,* involves the designation and acceptance of oneself as homosexual and contact with other homosexual individuals in social and sexual relationships. *Commitment* is the final stage and is marked internally by "the fusion of sexuality and emotionality into a significant whole" (Troiden, 1989, p. 63), as well as by same-sex love relationships and some degree of self-disclosure to nonhomosexual individuals. Troiden (1989) has described various patterns of adaptation to these stages, such as avoidance during identity confusion, as well as group alignment and passing during identity assumption. Awareness of how youth may present when using these various strategies will aid clinicians working with young gay and lesbian individuals.

Lesbians and gay males differ somewhat in the typical context of early sexual experiences. Girls are more inclined to become sexually involved in the context of a romantic relationship, whereas for boys initial homosexual contact more often involves brief sexual encounters (Bell et al., 1981; Saghir & Robins, 1973). (However, Troiden, 1989, has noted that this difference may already have begun to shift with changing patterns of male sexual behavior as a result of the AIDS epidemic.) Such a difference, if it is real, may reflect male–female differences as described by Gilligan (1982), who has theorized a female orientation toward relationships and ties as opposed to a male orientation toward separation and autonomy. It may also be influenced by the slightly later age at which females define themselves as homosexual. Lastly, because of the need to hide their sexual feelings, both gay and lesbian individuals may be generally later in exploring developmental issues of middle to late adolescence, such as identity and intimacy (Schneider, 1988).

Disruption in relationships with parents and siblings often follows an individual's announcement of same-sex erotic preference (Anderson, 1987, 1990; Malyon, 1981; Newman & Muzzonigro, 1993; Savin-Williams, 1989, 1990). Some parents are able to come to an acceptance of a child's homosexual orientation, while others are not. Parents' lack of acceptance may result in long-term tension or may be manifested in acute rejection and ejection of the youngster from the home. This issue may be particularly problematic for ethnically diverse youth, although Tremble, Schneider, and Appathurai (1989) have described ways in which some ethnically diverse families have arrived at acceptance of their sons' or daughters' sexuality. Some adolescents react to parental conflict by moving out, running away, engaging in prostitution, or using drugs or alcohol. Those adolescents who are able to maintain reasonably positive relationships with parents appear to be best able to maintain positive self-esteem (Savin-Williams, 1989). Parents generally go through various stages of mourning their "lost heterosexual child" before coming to a new acceptance of their child as homosexual (Robinson, Walters, & Skeen, 1989).

SOME THEORETICAL APPROACHES TO UNDERSTANDING HOMOSEXUAL DEVELOPMENT

As with other aspects of development, there are many ways of attempting to understand the phenomenon of homoerotic preference. In contrast to other areas of human development, however, discussions of possible factors contributing to the formation of same-sex attraction are invariably more heated. Some of the conflicts arise because of concern as to how etiological theories of homosexuality will be used. Some groups feel that study in this area inevitably implies blaming of parents. Others, who view homosexuality as a variant of normal sexual functioning, are critical of study in this area because they see it as implying abnormality. Some prefer to take the position that, whatever has caused the development of a same-sex preference, this preference is established very early in life and is therefore irreversible. None of these positions is intellectually very satisfying. Although we know relatively little as well about the establishment of heterosexual object choice, to choose not to study or theorize about the development of sexuality and its many forms is academically irresponsible. What is done with such information or theories is another issue—one that requires much consideration and discussion.

In Chapter 6, studies of biological influences on sexual orientation have been reviewed. These efforts span a variety of areas: molecular genetics, behavior genetics, prenatal sex hormones, neuroanatomy, neuropsychology, and familial demographic variables. Although each of these approaches has yielded positive findings (but also negative findings), our review, as well as those of others (e.g., Byne & Parsons, 1993; Friedman & Downey, 1993a; Meyer-Bahlburg, 1984), suggests that no single factor can as yet explain sexual orientation development. It may well be the case that there are multiple biological influences (which may or may not be interrelated), and a cautious conclusion is that they are likely to be contributory but not determining. Below, a brief review is provided of psychoanalytic and social learning accounts of sexual orientation development, in order to give the clinician working with homosexual adolescents an appreciation of the diverse views on this topic.

Psychoanalytic Theories

Despite the fact that the psychoanalytic approach to homosexuality has recently received serious critical scrutiny, especially in regard to the equation of homosexuality with psychopathology (see Lewes, 1988), an understanding of sexual development cannot ignore its important theoretical contributions.

Freud (1905/1953) regarded homosexual erotic preference as an "inversion"—that is, a deflection of sexual aim away from a biologically "appropriate" object. Although later analysts interpreted homosexual object choice as a pathological form of development, Freud described it as a variant of sexual object choice. Although he did not regard such a choice as necessarily pathological, he did see it as very resistant to change.

Freud (1905/1953) regarded sexual object choice as dependent on oedipal resolution, and heterosexual development as abandonment of same-sex strivings through identification with the parent of the same sex. He postulated that homosexuality could develop as a negative oedipal resolution resulting from castration anxiety. In males, this anxiety was thought to produce a symbolic flight from "penis-less" women and a search instead for objects with penises, or identification with the mother and desire for the father as a sexual object. In females, the pre-homosexual girl was presumed to react to her discovery of genital differences through a regression to her original love object (her mother) and a concomitant identification with her father. Fenichel (1945) has provided a summary of Freud's views, extracted from a variety of sources.

As investigators began to provide evidence that gender identity is normally established by age 3 (i.e., prior to oedipal resolution) (Money & Ehrhardt, 1972; Stoller, 1968c), doubts arose about the overriding importance of oedipal factors (i.e., identification with the mother or father) in gender development and thus in sexual orientation. Moreover, with the emergence of object relations theories, interest in earlier phases of the individual's intrapsychic life began to develop. For example, attachment and separation–individuation phases were seen as critical in the development of a sense of self. This approach also placed a greater emphasis on familial, as opposed to constitutional, factors.

Although Freud (1905/1953) considered parental factors as contributory, later analysts espoused a particular family pattern as etiological in the development of male homosexuality. Specifically, Bieber et al. (1962) argued that homosexuality in males occurs in the context of a close-binding, overprotective relationship with the mother and a distant, rejecting relationship with the father. Although this work has been criticized because the subjects were in psychoanalysis, and the specificity of this particular family dynamic has not held up, more general findings of difficulties in relationships with parents have been replicated in many different groups of homosexual men (Bell et al., 1981; Saghir & Robins, 1973; for a review, see Friedman, 1988) and homosexual women (Siegel, 1988; Siegelman, 1974, 1981). However, parental difficulties are not reported uniformly in all samples of homosexual men and women. Male homosexuals who score lower on femininity and neuroticism report fewer differences in parental relationships than do homosexuals who score higher on these factors (Siegelman, 1974). These findings may be taken to underscore the lack of a single, simple familial etiology in the development of homosexuality, but they may also result from the fact that homosexuals who establish a better level of adjustment report fewer earlier difficulties.

Freud (1905/1953) emphasized the presence of a constitutional predisposition as necessary for the development of homosexuality. Although he was unable to define this predisposition specifically, he presumed a certain sensitivity that may contribute to the creativity seen in many homosexual men (see Lewes, 1988, p. 54). Although some authors would argue that this constitutional predisposition is the biological basis for homosexuality (e.g., Diamond, 1976; Dörner, 1976), others believe that such a predisposition does not absolutely determine that an individual will develop homosexuality (Bradley, 1990; Friedman, 1988). More recently, retrospective studies have identified a factor that appears consistently across most categories of homosexual men—avoidance of competitive, rough-and-tumble, or aggressive activities during childhood. Although cross-gender interests and activities are also more common in homosexual than in heterosexual men, this factor is not as universally present in the boyhood histories of gay men as is avoidance of aggressive activities (Bell et al., 1981; cf. Bailey & Zucker, 1995).

Friedman (1988) has developed a theory, articulated similarly by Van den Aardweg (1986), that boys who avoid masculine, aggressive activities experience a lowering of their sense of masculinity, and therefore of their sense of themselves as adequate. This avoidance may be influenced or intensified by an earlier history of cross-gender interests or identification. Such behavior alienates a boy from peers and leads to a sense of being different in the period of late childhood or early adolescence. In contrast to earlier analysts, who viewed the development of erotic preference as being largely determined by oedipal factors, these authors see homoerotic preference as developing in late childhood and early adolescence, partly out of a yearning for same-sex affiliation to counteract a sense of inadequacy. Although neither Friedman (1988) nor Van den Aardweg (1986) explains why such yearnings become sexual preferences, their theory underscores the fact that homosexuality in itself does not necessarily imply psychiatric pathology. Friedman (1988) asserts that a sense of masculine adequacy may proceed despite a homosexual orientation, and that it is more dependent on one's life experiences, relationships, and achievements. He acknowledges, however, the difficulties all gay individuals must experience in establishing comfortable self-esteem in an essentially homophobic society.

Social Learning Theory

Those who believe in the overriding importance of learning propose that homosexuality can develop from homosexual experience (Churchill, 1967; West, 1967), which is conditioned through masturbatory erotic arousal (McGuire, Carlisle, & Young, 1965). These authors do acknowledge the importance of this learning's occurring in individuals who are already predisposed to the development of homosexuality. Similarly, unsatisfying heterosexual experience is seen as contributory in other cases (Bradley, 1985). Gagnon and Simon (1973) have expanded this notion within the idea of *sexual scripts,* which become internalized programs reinforced through experience. Although there have been few controlled studies in this area, clinical and anecdotal evidence supports the importance of experience and learning in the development of other domains of sexual functioning, so that one cannot dismiss the possible contribution of learning in the development of same-sex attraction.

Questions are often raised about the impact of homosexual parents on the gender identity or sexual orientation of their offspring. A recent review of studies in this area provides clear confirmation of the lack of differences between children raised by homosexual parents and controls (Patterson, 1992). In this vein, it is important to point out that most homosexuals grow up in families with heterosexual parents.

Comment

It is reasonably clear that the development of sexual object choice can hardly be explained by a single factor. Friedman's (1988) theory allows for the incorporation of constitutional and familial factors and acknowledges the importance of later periods of development (e.g., adolescence). Although the role of biological factors such as those proposed by Dörner (1988) awaits clarification, it is highly unlikely that a

single factor could be more than contributory, given the overlap between heterosexual and homosexual subjects in most studies and the
importance of other factors as identified by Friedman.

In our own work with children, we have become convinced that
difficulties with gender identity emerge in the interaction between temperamental or constitutional factors and factors within the family environment. The boys referred to our clinic typically have poor anxiety
tolerance, which contributes to their avoidance of rough-and-tumble
play and to their sensitivity to intrafamilial factors such as parental discord. They generally feel inadequate as males and have difficulty inter-
acting with same-sex peers. This pattern appears to be consistent with
Friedman's theory of masculine inadequacy, which can also develop for
other reasons. These feelings of gender inadequacy predispose such individuals to seek same-sex affiliations. What is missing in Friedman's
theory is the link between yearning for same-sex affiliation and actual
homoerotic preference. We believe that it is the meaning attached to
such yearnings that defines the feelings as sexual (see Troiden, 1989).
Idealization of others produces attraction and emulation, and in current North American society such intense feelings may be equated with
sexual desire. The homosexual youth may be more conditioned to
make this connection for constitutional or intrapsychic reasons, but
this remains an area requiring further clarification. We also support the
idea that, beginning in early adolescence, learning and experience interact with these other factors to promote the further development of homosexual patterns.

Although there is a comparative lack of recent theorizing in the
area of female homosexual development, our clinical experience suggests that a similar framework can be applied to the understanding of
female sexual orientation. Others have suggested that whereas females
may choose a homosexual orientation, most males do not experience
their orientation as chosen.

CLINICAL MANAGEMENT

The clinician faces different issues, depending on whether an adolescent
is referred for homosexual behavior or conflict, or a self-defined gay or
lesbian adolescent presents with other medical or psychosocial concerns. In the first instance, the clinician is being asked to clarify
whether or not the adolescent is or is likely to become homosexual. It is
important to help both the family and the adolescent define clearly
what their questions or concerns are. Some adolescents may be comfortable with the fact that they are gay or lesbian, while their parents

may want to know whether their children's orientation can or will change. In addition, lack of information, misinformation, myths, and stereotypes about homosexuality need to be explored and (where possible) clarified. Issues for the self-defined gay or lesbian adolescent may include health-related concerns such as sexually transmitted diseases, "coming-out" issues, contact with other gay or lesbian adolescents in socially acceptable situations, and relationships with family members (Myers, 1982; Schneider, 1988).

Assessment of homosexual orientation requires more than an examination of behavior. Kinsey et al.'s (1948) original study and subsequent studies (e.g., McConaghy, Armstrong, Birrell, & Buhrich, 1979) indicate that a substantial proportion of males (roughly 30%) experience some degree of homoerotic arousal or behavioral experience. But, as noted in Chapter 3, the percentage of adult males who would define themselves as preferentially homosexual is considerably lower. It is necessary, therefore, to understand the current context of homosexual behavior (e.g., adolescent sexual experimentation, individual romantic relationships, involvement with a younger child) and the developmental history that may have contributed to the individual's difficulty with a sense of masculine or feminine adequacy. Earlier cross-gender identification and interests, as well as present and past erotic fantasy (including dream imagery, fantasies during masturbation, and sexual attractions), need to be explored.

Adolescents who present with a childhood history of gender identity disorder or masculine inadequacy (Friedman, 1988), who have experienced little or no heteroerotic arousal, and who are reasonably comfortable with either their homoerotic fantasy or experience present little difficulty for the clinician. Treatment should focus on development of a positive gay identity; support with respect to acculturating into the gay community; and help for parents, who may be quite distressed at the loss of their dreams for their children and the hazards they believe the adolescents will confront as gay or lesbian persons.

Adolescents who consult a professional on their own initiative are typically less clear about their sexual identity. They may have had a somewhat distant or unsatisfying relationship with a parent, may have felt different from other children by late childhood or early adolescence, and may not have experienced significant sexual arousal toward either males or females. In middle to late adolescence, they find themselves experiencing some heterosexual and some homoerotic arousal but have had little sexual experience. The issue in such a case becomes one of helping the individual clarify a sexual orientation. It is important in this situation that the clinician maintain a neutral stance, working with the adolescent to define what is most comfortable for him or her. The initial effort may involve having the adolescent attempt further heterosocial and heterosexual experience, to clarify whether issues emerge that can be addressed in psychotherapy. Some adolescents will become profoundly distressed about their competence when they try to engage in heterosocial behaviors. This anxiety may be related to the assumption that any heterosocial encounter implies that they must feel aroused and be able to respond sexually. Behavior modification approaches to alleviate this anxiety can be helpful. Some adolescents, with the support of a neutral therapist and opportunities to explore their sexual feelings, will become more accepting of their homosexual feelings and more convinced that they are gay, and will choose to act on that. The therapist should, however, look for premature closure on this decision, exploring an adolescent's need to idealize same-sex individuals and other motivations that may be promoting same-sex attractions. Frequently, despite the therapist's feeling that dynamic factors are contributing to such attractions, the adolescent may be unable or unwilling to address these issues, and over a period of time both the adolescent and therapist will see a homosexual orientation as most comfortable for the individual.

When an adolescent experiences undesired homoerotic attractions and wishes to function as a heterosexual, the clinician may work with the individual using the approach outlined by Masters and Johnson (1979) or Nicolosi (1991). Although there is currently considerable pessimism view regarding the ability of individuals to shift from a homosexual to a heterosexual orientation, it is clear that some individuals who do not want or cannot accept a gay or lesbian identity can make such changes (see Nicolosi, 1991). Mitchell (1981) has provided a well-articulated analysis of the hazards of some of the earlier analytic approaches to treatment. However, if an individual experiences little heterosexual arousal, and his or her discomfort about homoerotic feelings is related largely to fear about societal reaction, an effort to help the individual adopt a more comfortable view of the gay or lesbian community may be more useful. Involvement with gay and lesbian youth groups can be particularly supportive to those individuals who appear to be essentially homosexual but who are struggling with self-acceptance.

For the young adolescent male presenting with a history of involvement with a younger boy, questions about his sexual orientation frequently arise. Quite regularly, such adolescents have been sexually abused or have come from families with minimal constraints or boundaries on sexual behavior. Seldom will these adolescents acknowledge homoerotic attractions, and they often have difficulty talking about their behavior. The issue here is to clarify family expectations, history of sexual abuse, the adolescent's knowledge of appropriate and inappropriate behavior, the consequences of sexually inappropriate behavior in the past, and the adolescent's ability to empathize with the younger child's feelings about such involvement. Typically, the sexual orientation of these individuals will remain in question until they move further into adolescence. Peer relationship difficulties, which may interfere with appropriate social and sexual contacts, should be addressed.

The female adolescent presenting with homosexual concerns is more typically involved in an intense romantic attachment to an older and admired female. There may or may not be homosexual behavior. Such adolescents often have felt less competent than female peers in feminine activities or have experienced conflict with parents, either of which may have caused self-esteem difficulties. They are particularly vulnerable to developing idealizing relationships with older females, whose respect and admiration in return bolster their self-esteem. For some, these relationships develop out of shared athletic, political, or cultural interests. Self-definition as lesbian may develop when there is little heteroerotic attraction and such homosexual involvement provides a sense of self-validation. For others, who may also experience heterosexual arousal, such romantic involvements may be seen as transitory. These individuals may label themselves as bisexual or predominantly heterosexual. As with the homosexual male adolescent, the clinician's role is to support a positive lesbian identity where that is clearly in the best interests of the individual, but to take a more neutral stance when the adolescent is less clear.

Parents of gay adolescents often need social support (Kaufman, 1991). Recently, parent support groups have emerged in major urban areas, and these can be very helpful for those parents who are able to become involved. Parents need information about gay lifestyles and AIDS, access to more positive images of gay men and women, and help with their own feelings of loss. When parents can mourn the loss of their son or daughter as heterosexual, they may be able to create a new and positive relationship with their homosexual child. Siblings may also have conflicted feelings that will need to be addressed.

Finally, the gay or lesbian teenager who presents with depression, a suicide attempt, or other psychiatric difficulties will require the same attention as would a heterosexual individual with such difficulties. However, sensitivity to the issues that such teenagers face in grappling with their identity may make the difference between a therapeutic and a nontherapeutic contact (Remafedi et al., 1991).

References

Abelove, H. (1986). Freud, male homosexuality, and the Americans. *Dissent, 33,* 59–69.

Abelove, H., Barale, M. A., & Halperin, D. M. (Eds.). (1993). *The lesbian and gay studies reader.* New York: Routledge.

Abraham, F. (1931). Genitalumwandlung an zwei maenlichen Transvestiten. *Zeitschrift für Sexualwissenschaft, 18,* 223–226.

Abramovitch, R. (1977). Children's recognition of situational aspects of facial expression. *Child Development, 48,* 459–463.

Abramovitch, R., Corter, C., Pepler, D. J., & Stanhope, L. (1986). Sibling and peer interaction: A final follow-up and a comparison. *Child Development, 57,* 217–229.

Abramowitz, S. I. (1986). Psychosocial outcomes of sex reassignment surgery. *Journal of Consulting and Clinical Psychology, 54,* 183–189.

Absi-Semaan, N., Crombie, G., & Freeman, C. (1993). Masculinity and femininity in middle childhood: Developmental and factor analysis. *Sex Roles, 28,* 187–206.

Achenbach, T. M. (1978). The Child Behavior Profile: I. Boys aged 6–11. *Journal of Consulting and Clinical Psychology, 46,* 478–488.

Achenbach, T. M. (1979). The Child Behavior Profile: An empirically based system for assessing children's behavioral problems and competencies. *International Journal of Mental Health, 7,* 24–42.

Achenbach, T. M. (1980). DSM-III in light of empirical research on the classification of child psychopathology. *Journal of the American Academy of Child Psychiatry, 19,* 395–412.

Achenbach, T. M., & Edelbrock, C. S. (1979). The Child Behavior Profile: II. Boys aged 12–16 and girls aged 6–11 and 12–16. *Journal of Consulting and Clinical Psychology, 47,* 223–233.

Achenbach, T. M., & Edelbrock, C. S. (1981). Behavioral problems and competencies reported by parents of normal and disturbed children aged four through sixteen. *Monographs of the Society for Research in Child Development, 46*(1, Serial No. 188).

Achenbach, T. M., & Edelbrock, C. (1983). *Manual for the Child Behavior*

Checklist and Revised Child Behavior Profile. Burlington: University of Vermont, Department of Psychiatry.

Achenbach, T. M., & Edelbrock, C. (1986). *Manual for the Teacher's Report Form and Teacher Version of the Revised Child Behavior Profile.* Burlington: University of Vermont, Department of Psychiatry.

Achenbach, T. M., Edelbrock, C., & Howell, C. T. (1987). Empirically based assessment of the behavioral/emotional problems of 2- and 3-year-old children. *Journal of Abnormal Child Psychology, 15,* 629–650.

Achenbach, T. M., Howell, C. T., Quay, H. C., & Conners, C. K. (1991). National survey of problems and competencies among four- to sixteen-year-olds. *Monographs of the Society for Research in Child Development, 56*(3, Serial No. 225).

Achenbach, T. M., McConaughy, S. H., & Howell, C. T. (1987). Child/adolescent behavioral and emotional problems: Implications of cross-informant correlations for situational specificity. *Psychological Bulletin, 101,* 213–232.

Adamec, R. G., & Stark-Adamec, C. (1986). Limbic hyperfunction, limbic epilepsy, and interictal behavior. In B. K. Doane & K. E. Livingston (Eds.), *The limbic system* (pp. 129–145). New York: Raven Press.

Adams, K. M., Klinge, V., Vaziri, H., Maczulski, B., & Pasternak, A. (1976). Studies in adolescent transvestism: Life history, psychometric and behavioral descriptors. In D. V. Siva Sankar (Ed.), *Mental health in children* (Vol. 2, pp. 89–112). Westbury, NY: PJD.

Adkins-Regan, E. (1988). Sex hormones and sexual orientation in animals. *Psychobiology, 16,* 335–347.

Ahuja, Y. R., & Plato, C. C. (1990). Effect of environmental pollutants on dermatoglyphic patterns. In N. M. Durham & C. C. Plato (Eds.), *Trends in dermatoglyphic research* (pp. 123–135). Boston: Kluwer Academic.

Ainsworth, M. D. S., Blehar, M. C., Waters, E., & Wall, S. (1978). *Patterns of attachment: A psychological study of the Strange Situation.* Hillsdale, NJ: Erlbaum.

Allen, C. (1949). *The sexual perversions and abnormalities: A study in the psychology of paraphilias* (2nd ed.). London: Oxford University Press.

Allen, C. (1962). *A textbook of psychosexual disorders.* London: Oxford University Press.

Allen, L. S., & Gorski, R. A. (1990). Sex difference in the bed nucleus of the stria terminalis of the human brain. *Journal of Comparative Neurology, 302,* 697–706.

Allen, L. S., & Gorski, R. A. (1991). Sexual dimorphism of the anterior commissure and massa intermedia of the human brain. *Journal of Comparative Neurology, 312,* 97–104.

Allen, L. S., & Gorski, R. A. (1992). Sexual orientation and the size of the anterior commissure in the human brain. *Proceedings of the National Academy of Sciences USA, 89,* 7199–7202.

Allen, L. S., Hines, M., Shryne, J. E., & Gorski, R. A. (1989). Two sexually dimorphic cell groups in the human brain. *Journal of Neuroscience, 9,* 497–506.

Allen, L. S., Richey, M. F., Chai, Y. M., & Gorski, R. A. (1991). Sex differences in the corpus callosum of the living human being. *Journal of Neuroscience, 11,* 933–942.

Alpert-Gillis, L. J., & Connell, J. P. (1989). Gender and sex-role influences on children's self-esteem. *Journal of Personality, 57,* 97–114.

American Psychiatric Association. (1980). *Diagnostic and statistical manual of mental disorders* (3rd ed.). Washington, DC: Author.

American Psychiatric Association. (1987). *Diagnostic and statistical manual of mental disorders* (3rd ed., rev.). Washington, DC: Author.

American Psychiatric Association. (1994). *Diagnostic and statistical manual of mental disorders* (4th ed.). Washington, DC: Author.

Anderson, D. (1987). Family and peer relations of gay adolescents. In S. C. Feinstein (Ed.), *Adolescent psychiatry: Vol. 14. Developmental and clinical studies* (pp. 162–176). Chicago: University of Chicago Press.

Anderson, D. (1990). Adolescent homosexuality. In M. Sugar (Ed.), *Atypical adolescence and sexuality* (pp. 181–200). New York: Norton.

Angier, N. (1991a, August 30). Zone of brain linked to men's sexual orientation. *New York Times,* pp. A1, A18.

Angier, N. (1991b, September 1). The biology of what it means to be gay. *New York Times,* pp. 1, 4.

Annett, M. (1970). A classification of hand preference by association analysis. *British Journal of Psychology, 61,* 303–321.

Antill, J. K. (1987). Parents' beliefs and values about sex roles, sex differences, and sexuality: Their sources and implications. In P. Shaver & C. Hendrick (Eds.), *Sex and gender* (pp. 294–328). Newbury Park, CA: Sage.

Arcostanzo, G., Beglia, G., Lertora, V., & Zecca, G. (1991, June). *The assessment of personality in parents of cross-gender identified children.* Poster presented at the World Congress of Sexology, Amsterdam.

Arnold, A. P., & Breedlove, S. M. (1985). Organizational and activational effects of sex steroids: A reanalysis. *Hormones and Behavior, 19,* 469–498.

Baenninger, M., & Newcombe, N. (1989). The role of experience in spatial test performance: A meta-analysis. *Sex Roles, 20,* 327–344.

Bailey, J. M. (1989). *A test of the maternal stress hypothesis for human male homosexuality.* Unpublished doctoral dissertation, University of Texas at Austin.

Bailey, J. M. (1995, March). Sex differences in the distribution and determinants of sexual orientation. In C. J. Patterson (Chair), *Sexual orientation, children and families: Current issues in research.* Symposium presented at the meeting of the Society for Research in Child Development, Indianapolis.

Bailey, J. M., & Bell, A. P. (1993). Familiality of female and male homosexuality. *Behavior Genetics, 23,* 313–322.

Bailey, J. M., & Benishay, D. S. (1993). Familial aggregation of female sexual orientation. *American Journal of Psychiatry, 150,* 272–277.

Bailey, J. M., & Pillard, R. C. (1991). A genetic study of male sexual orientation. *Archives of General Psychiatry, 48,* 1089–1096.

Bailey, J. M., Pillard, R. C., Neale, M. C., & Agyei, Y. (1993). Heritable factors influence sexual orientation in women. *Archives of General Psychiatry, 50,* 217–223.

Bailey, J. M., Willerman, L., & Parks, C. (1991). A test of the maternal stress theory of human male homosexuality. *Archives of Sexual Behavior, 20,* 277–293.

Bailey, J. M., & Zucker, K. J. (1995). Childhood sex-typed behavior and sexual orientation: A conceptual analysis and quantitative review. *Developmental Psychology, 31,* 43–55.

Bak, R. C. (1953). Fetishism. *Journal of the American Psychoanalytic Association, 1,* 285–298.

Bakker, A., van Kesteren, P. J. M., Gooren, L. J. G., & Bezemer, P. D. (1993). The prevalence of transsexualism in the Netherlands. *Acta Psychiatrica Scandinavica, 87,* 237–238.

Bakker, J., Brand, T., van Ophemert, J., & Slob, A. K. (1993). Hormonal regulation of adult partner preference behavior in neonatally ATD-treated male rats. *Behavioral Neuroscience, 107,* 480–487.

Bakwin, H. (1960). Transvestism in children. *Journal of Pediatrics, 56,* 294–298.

Bakwin, H. (1968). Deviant gender-role behavior in children: Relation to homosexuality. *Pediatrics, 41,* 620–629.

Bakwin, H., & Bakwin, R. M. (1953). Homosexual behavior in children. *Journal of Pediatrics, 43,* 108–111.

Balk, S. J., Dreyfus, N. G., & Harris, P. (1982). Examination of genitals in children: "The remaining taboo." *Pediatrics, 70,* 751–753.

Ball, J. R. B. (1968). A case of hair fetishism, transvestitism, and organic cerebral disorder. *Acta Psychiatrica Scandinavica, 44,* 249–254.

Bancroft, J. (1994). Homosexual orientation: The search for a biological basis. *British Journal of Psychiatry, 164,* 437–440.

Barahal, H. S. (1940). Testosterone in psychotic male homosexuals. *Psychiatric Quarterly, 14,* 319–330.

Barlow, D. H., Abel, G. G., & Blanchard, E. B. (1977). Gender identity change in a transsexual: An exorcism. *Archives of Sexual Behavior, 6,* 387–395.

Barlow, D. H., Abel, G. G., & Blanchard, E. B. (1979). Gender identity change in transsexuals: Follow-up and replications. *Archives of General Psychiatry, 36,* 1001–1007.

Barlow, D. H., Reynolds, E. J., & Agras, W. S. (1973). Gender identity change in a transsexual. *Archives of General Psychiatry, 28,* 569–576.

Baron, M. (1993). Genetic linkage and male homosexual orientation. *British Medical Journal, 307,* 337–338.

Barr, M. L., & Hobbs, G. E. (1954). Chromosomal sex in transvestites. *Lancet, i,* 1109–1110.

Bates, J. E. (1980). The concept of difficult temperament. *Merrill–Palmer Quarterly, 26,* 299–319.

Bates, J. E., & Bentler, P. M. (1973). Play activities of normal and effeminate boys. *Developmental Psychology, 9,* 20–27.

Bates, J. E., Bentler, P. M., & Thompson, S. K. (1973). Measurement of deviant gender development in boys. *Child Development, 44,* 591–598.

Bates, J. E., Bentler, P. M., & Thompson, S. K. (1979). Gender-deviant boys compared with normal and clinical control boys. *Journal of Abnormal Child Psychology, 7,* 243–259.

Bates, J. E., Skilbeck, W. M., Smith, K. V. R., & Bentler, P. M. (1974). Gender role abnormalities in boys: An analysis of clinical ratings. *Journal of Abnormal Child Psychology, 2,* 1–16.

Bates, J. E., Skilbeck, W. M., Smith, K. V. R., & Bentler, P. M. (1975). Intervention with families of gender-disturbed boys. *American Journal of Orthopsychiatry, 45,* 150–157.

Baum, M. J. (1979). Differentiation of coital behavior in mammals: A comparative analysis. *Neuroscience and Biobehavioral Reviews, 3,* 265–284.

Baum, M. J., Carroll, R. S., Erskine, M. S., & Tobet, S. A. (1985). Neuroendocrine response to estrogen and sexual orientation [Letter]. *Science, 230,* 961–962.

Bayer, R. (1981). *Homosexuality and American psychiatry: The politics of diagnosis.* New York: Basic Books.

Bayer, R., & Spitzer, R. L. (1982). Edited correspondence on the status of homosexuality in DSM-III. *Journal of the History of the Behavioral Sciences, 18,* 32–52.

Beach, F. A. (1975). Hormonal modification of sexually dimorphic behavior. *Psychoneuroendocrinology, 1,* 3–23.

Beach, F. A. (1976). Cross-species comparisons and the human heritage. In F. A. Beach (Ed.), *Human sexuality in four perspectives* (pp. 296–316). Baltimore: Johns Hopkins University Press.

Beach, F. A. (1979a). Animal models and psychological inference. In H. A. Katchadourian (Ed.), *Human sexuality: A comparative and developmental perspective* (pp. 98–112). Berkeley: University of California Press.

Beach, F. A. (1979b). Animal models for human sexuality. In *Sex, hormones and behaviour* (Ciba Foundation Symposium No. 62, New Series, pp. 113–143). Amsterdam: Excerpta Medica.

Beach, F. A. (1981). Historical origins of modern research on hormones and behavior. *Hormones and Behavior, 15,* 325–376.

Beatty, W. W. (1979). Gonadal hormones and sex differences in nonreproductive behaviors in rodents: Organizational and activational influences. *Hormones and Behavior, 12,* 112–163.

Beatty, W. W. (1984). Hormonal organization of sex differences in play fighting and spatial behavior. *Progress in Brain Research, 61,* 315–330.

Beatty, W. W. (1992). Gonadal hormones and sex differences in nonreproductive behaviors. In A. A. Gerall, H. Moltz, & I. L. Ward (Eds.), *Handbook of behavioral neurobiology: Vol. 11. Sexual differentiation* (pp. 85–128). New York: Plenum Press.

Beck, A. T., Ward, C. H., Mendelson, M., Mock, J., & Erbaugh, J. (1961). An inventory for measuring depression. *Archives of General Psychiatry, 4,* 561–571.

Becker, J. T., Bass, S. M., Dew, M. A., Kingsley, L., Selnes, O. A., & Sheridan, K. (1992). Hand preference, immune system disorder and cognitive function among gay/bisexual men: The Multicenter AIDS Cohort Study (MACS). *Neuropsychologia, 30,* 229–235.

Begley, S. (1991, September 9). What causes people to be homosexual? *Newsweek,* p. 52.

Bell, A. P., Weinberg, M. S., & Hammersmith, S. K. (1981). *Sexual preference: Its development in men and women.* Bloomington: Indiana University Press.

Bell, R. Q. (1968). A reinterpretation of the direction of effects in studies of socialization. *Psychological Review, 75,* 81–95.

Bell, R. Q., & Harper, L. V. (1977). *Child effects on adults.* Hillsdale, NJ: Erlbaum.

Bell-Dolan, D., & Brazeal, T. J. (1993). Separation anxiety disorder, overanxious disorder, and school refusal. *Child and Adolescent Psychiatric Clinics of North America, 2,* 563–580.

Bem, S. L. (1983). Gender schema theory and its implications for child development: Raising gender-aschematic children in a gender-schematic society. *Signs, 8,* 598–616.

Bem, S. L. (1984). Reply to Morgan and Ayim. *Signs, 10,* 197–199.

Bem, S. L. (1989). Genital knowledge and gender constancy in preschool children. *Child Development, 60,* 649–662.

Bem, S. L. (1993). *The lenses of gender: Transforming the debate on sexual inequality.* New Haven, CT: Yale University Press.

Bender, L., & Paster, S. (1941). Homosexual trends in children. *American Journal of Orthopsychiatry, 11,* 730–743.

Benjamin, H. (1954). Transsexualism and transvestism as psychosomatic somato-psychic syndromes. *American Journal of Psychotherapy, 8,* 219–230.

Benjamin, H. (1966). *The transsexual phenomenon.* New York: Julian Press.

Bentler, P. M. (1976). A typology of transsexualism: Gender identity theory and data. *Archives of Sexual Behavior, 5,* 567–584.

Bentler, P. M., Rekers, G. A., & Rosen, A. C. (1979). Congruence of childhood sex-role identity and behaviour disturbances. *Child: Care, Health, and Development, 5,* 267–283.

Berenbaum, S. A. (1990). Congenital adrenal hyperplasia: Intellectual and psychosexual functioning. In C. S. Holmes (Ed.), *Psychoneuroendocrinology: Brain, behavior, and hormonal interactions* (pp. 227–260). New York: Springer-Verlag.

Berenbaum, S. A., & Hines, M. (1992). Early androgens are related to childhood sex-typed toy preferences. *Psychological Science, 3,* 203–206.

Berenbaum, S. A., & Snyder, E. (1995). Early hormonal influences on childhood sex-typed activity and playmate preferences: Implications for the development of sexual orientation. *Developmental Psychology, 31,* 31–42.

Berger, J. (1994). The psychotherapeutic treatment of male homosexuality. *American Journal of Psychotherapy, 48,* 251–261.

Berman, M. D. (1953). Perception and object relations in a patient with transvestite tendencies. *International Journal of Psycho-Analysis, 34,* 25–39.

Bernstein, G. A., & Borchardt, C. M. (1991). Anxiety disorders of childhood and adolescence: A critical review. *Journal of the American Academy of Child and Adolescent Psychiatry, 30,* 519–532.

Bernstein, P. (1993). Panel report: Gender identity disorder in boys. *Journal of the American Psychoanalytic Association, 41,* 729–742.

Biddle, S., & Armstrong, N. (1992). Children's physical activity: An exploratory study of psychological correlates. *Social Science and Medicine, 34,* 325–331.

Bieber, I., & Bieber, T. B. (1979). Male homosexuality. *Canadian Journal of Psychiatry, 24,* 409–421.

Bieber, I., Dain, H. J., Dince, P. R., Drellich, M. G., Grand, H. G., Gundlach, R. H., Kremer, M. W., Rifkin, A. H., Wilbur, C. B., & Bieber, T. B. (1962). *Homosexuality: A psychoanalytic study of male homosexuals.* New York: Basic Books.

Biller, H. B. (1968). A multiaspect investigation of the masculine development in kindergarten age boys. *Genetic Psychology Monographs, 78,* 89–139.

Biller, H. B. (1969). Father-absence, maternal encouragement, and sex-role development in kindergarten-age boys. *Child Development, 40,* 539–546.

Biller, H. B., & Borstelmann, L. J. (1967). Masculine development: An integrative review. *Merrill–Palmer Quarterly, 13,* 253–294.

Billings, D. B., & Urban, T. (1982). The socio-medical construction of transsexualism. *Social Problems, 29,* 266–282.

Billy, J. O. G., Tanfer, K., Grady, W. R., & Klepinger, D. H. (1993). The sexual behavior of men in the United States. *Family Planning Perspectives, 25,* 52–60.

Birke, L. I. A. (1981). Is homosexuality hormonally determined? *Journal of Homosexuality, 6,* 35–49.

Birken, L. (1988). *Consuming desire: Sexual science and the emergence of the culture of abundance, 1871–1914.* Ithaca, NY: Cornell University Press.

Birkenfeld-Adams, A. (1995). *Quality of attachment in young boys with gender identity disorder.* Doctoral dissertation proposal, York University, Downsview, Ontario.

Birrell, S., & Cole, C. L. (1990). Double fault: Renee Richards and the construction and naturalization of difference. *Sociology of Sport Journal, 7,* 1–21.

Blackwood, E. (1984). Sexuality and gender in certain Native American tribes: The case of cross-gender females. *Signs, 10,* 27–42.

Blakemore, J. E. O., LaRue, A. A., & Olejnik, A. B. (1979). Sex-appropriate toy preference and the ability to conceptualize toys as sex-role related. *Developmental Psychology, 15,* 339–340.

Blanchard, R. (1985a). Typology of male-to-female transsexualism. *Archives of Sexual Behavior, 14,* 247–261.

Blanchard, R. (1985b). Gender dysphoria and gender reorientation. In B. W.

Steiner (Ed.), *Gender dysphoria: Development, research, management* (pp. 365–392). New York: Plenum Press.

Blanchard, R. (1988). Nonhomosexual gender dysphoria. *Journal of Sex Research, 24,* 188–193.

Blanchard, R. (1989). The classification and labeling of nonhomosexual gender dysphorias. *Archives of Sexual Behavior, 18,* 315–334.

Blanchard, R. (1990a). Gender identity disorders in adult women. In R. Blanchard & B. W. Steiner (Eds.), *Clinical management of gender identity disorders in children and adults* (pp. 77–91). Washington, DC: American Psychiatric Press.

Blanchard, R. (1990b). Gender identity disorders in adult men. In R. Blanchard & B. W. Steiner (Eds.), *Clinical management of gender identity disorders in children and adults* (pp. 47–76). Washington, DC: American Psychiatric Press.

Blanchard, R. (1991). Clinical observations and systematic studies of autogynephilia. *Journal of Sex and Marital Therapy, 17,* 235–251.

Blanchard, R. (1994). A structural equation model for age at clinical presentation in nonhomosexual male gender dysphorics. *Archives of Sexual Behavior, 23,* 311–320.

Blanchard, R., & Bogaert, A. F. (1995). *The role of older brothers in the development of male homosexuality.* Manuscript submitted for publication.

Blanchard, R., & Bogaert, A. F. (in press). Biodemographic comparisons of homosexual and heterosexual men in the Kinsey interview data. *Archives of Sexual Behavior.*

Blanchard, R., & Clemmensen, L. H. (1988). A test of the DSM-III-R's implicit assumption that fetishistic arousal and gender dysphoria are mutually exclusive. *Journal of Sex Research, 25,* 426–432.

Blanchard, R., Clemmensen, L. H., & Steiner, B. W. (1987). Heterosexual and homosexual gender dysphoria. *Archives of Sexual Behavior, 16,* 139–152.

Blanchard, R., and Sheridan, P. M. (1990). Gender reorientation and psychosocial adjustment. In R. Blanchard & B. W. Steiner (Eds.), *Clinical management of gender identity disorders in children and adults* (pp. 159–189). Washington, DC: American Psychiatric Press.

Blanchard, R., & Sheridan, P. M. (1992). Sibship size, sibling sex ratio, birth order, and parental age in homosexual and nonhomosexual gender dysphorics. *Journal of Nervous and Mental Disease, 180,* 40–47.

Blanchard, R., & Steiner, B. W. (Eds.). (1990). *Clinical management of gender identity disorders in children and adults.* Washington, DC: American Psychiatric Press.

Blanchard, R., & Zucker, K. J. (1994). Reanalysis of Bell, Weinberg, and Hammersmith's data on birth order, sibling sex ratio, and parental age in homosexual men. *American Journal of Psychiatry, 151,* 1375–1376.

Blanchard, R., Zucker, K. J., Bradley, S. J., & Hume, C. S. (1995). Birth order and sibling sex ratio in homosexual male adolescents and probably prehomosexual feminine boys. *Developmental Psychology, 31,* 22–30.

Blanchard, R., Zucker, K. J., Cohen-Kettenis, P. T., Gooren, L. J. G., & Bailey,

J. M. (in press). Birth order and sibling sex ratio in two samples of Dutch gender-dysphoric homosexual males. *Archives of Sexual Behavior.*

Bleiberg, E., Jackson, L., & Ross, J. L. (1986). Gender identity disorder and object loss. *Journal of the American Academy of Child Psychiatry, 25,* 58–67.

Bleier, R. (1984). *Science and gender: A critique of biology and its theories of women.* Elmsford, NY: Pergamon Press.

Bloch, D. (1976). The threat of infanticide and homosexual identity. *Psychoanalytic Review, 62,* 579–599.

Block, J. H. (1981). *The Child-Rearing Practices Report (CRPR): A set of Q items for the description of parental socialization attitudes and values.* Unpublished manuscript, University of California at Berkeley.

Blount, E. L., & Stokes, T. F. (1984). Self-reinforcement by children. In M. Hersen, R. M. Eisler, & P. M. Miller (Eds.), *Progress in behavior modification* (Vol. 18, pp. 195–225). New York: Academic Press.

Blumer, D., & Walker, A. E. (1975). The neural basis of sexual behavior. In D. F. Benson & D. Blumer (Eds.), *Psychiatric aspects of neurologic disease* (pp. 199–217). New York: Grune & Stratton.

Bogaert, A. F., & Blanchard, R. (in press). Handedness in homosexual and heterosexual men in the Kinsey Interview data. *Archives of Sexual Behavior.*

Bolin, A. (1987). *In search of Eve: Transsexual rites of passage.* South Hadley, MA: Bergin & Garvey.

Boswell, J. (1982–1983). Revolutions, universals and sexual categories. *Salmagundi, 58–59,* 89–113.

Boswell, J. (1990). Sexual and ethical categories in premodern Europe. In D. P. McWhirter, S. A. Sanders, & J. M. Reinisch (Eds.), *Homosexuality/heterosexuality: Concepts of sexual orientation* (pp. 15–31). New York: Oxford University Press.

Boulton, M. J. (1991). A comparison of structural and contextual features of middle school children's playful and aggressive fighting. *Ethology and Sociobiology, 12,* 119–145.

Bowlby, J. (1969). *Attachment and loss: Vol. 1. Attachment.* New York: Basic Books.

Bowler, C., & Collacott, R. A. (1993). Cross-dressing in men with learning disabilities. *British Journal of Psychiatry, 162,* 556–558.

Boyar, R. M., & Aiman, J. (1982). The 24–hour secretory pattern of LH and the response to LHRH in transsexual men. *Archives of Sexual Behavior, 11,* 157–169.

Bradley, S. J. (1980). Female transsexualism: A child and adolescent perspective. *Child Psychiatry and Human Development, 11,* 12–18.

Bradley, S. J. (1985). Gender disorders in childhood: A formulation. In B. W. Steiner (Ed.), *Gender dysphoria: Development, research, management* (pp. 175–188). New York: Plenum Press.

Bradley, S. J. (1990). Gender dysphorias in childhood and adolescence. In B. D. Garfinkel, G. A. Carlson, & E. B. Weller (Eds.), *Psychiatric disorders in children and adolescents* (pp. 121–134). Philadelphia: W. B. Saunders.

Bradley, S. J., Blanchard, R., Coates, S., Green, R., Levine, S. B., Meyer-Bahlburg, H. F. L., Pauly, I. B., & Zucker, K. J. (1991). Interim report of the DSM-IV Subcommittee for Gender Identity Disorders. *Archives of Sexual Behavior, 20,* 333–343.

Bradley, S. J., Steiner, B., Zucker, K., Doering, R. W., Sullivan, J., Finegan, J. K., & Richardson, M. (1978). Gender identity problems of children and adolescents: The establishment of a special clinic. *Canadian Psychiatric Association Journal, 23,* 175–183.

Bradley, S. J., & Zucker, K. J. (1984, October). *Gender-dysphoric adolescents: Presenting and developmental characteristics.* Paper presented at the joint meeting of the Canadian Academy of Child Psychiatry and the American Academy of Child Psychiatry, Toronto.

Bradley, S. J., & Zucker, K. J. (1990). Gender identity disorder and psychosexual problems in children and adolescents. *Canadian Journal of Psychiatry, 35,* 477–486.

Brand, T., Houtsmuller, E. J., & Slob, A. K. (1993). Neonatal programming of adult partner preference in male rats. In M. Haug, R. E. Whalen, C. Aron, & K. L. Olsen (Eds.), *The development of sex differences and similarities in behavior* (pp. 33–49). Dordrecht, The Netherlands: Kluwer Academic.

Breedlove, S. M. (1994). Sexual differentiation of the human nervous system. *Annual Review of Psychology, 45,* 389–418.

Bretherton, I., & Waters, E. (Eds.). (1985). Growing points of attachment theory and research. *Monographs of the Society for Research in Child Development, 50*(1–2, Serial No. 209).

Brooks-Gunn, J. (1986). The relationship of maternal beliefs about sex typing to maternal and young children's behavior. *Sex Roles, 14,* 21–35.

Brown, D. G. (1956). Sex-role preference in young children. *Psychological Monographs, 70*(14, Whole No. 421).

Brown, D. G. (1957). The development of sex-role inversion and homosexuality. *Journal of Pediatrics, 50,* 613–619.

Brown, D. G. (1958). Inversion and homosexuality. *American Journal of Orthopsychiatry, 28,* 424–429.

Brown, E. V. (1979). Sexual self-identification as reflected in children's drawings when asked to "draw-a-person." *Perceptual and Motor Skills, 49,* 35–38.

Bryden, M. P. (1979). Evidence for sex-related differences in cerebral organization. In M. A. Wittig & A. C. Petersen (Eds.), *Sex-related differences in cognitive functioning: Developmental issues* (pp. 121–143). New York: Academic Press.

Bryden, M. P., MacRae, L., & Steenhuis, R. E. (1991). Hand preference in school children. *Developmental Neuropsychology, 7,* 477–486.

Buhrich, N. (1977). A case of familial heterosexual transvestism. *Acta Psychiatrica Scandinavica, 55,* 199–201.

Buhrich, N. (1978). Motivation for cross-dressing in heterosexual transvestism. *Acta Psychiatrica Scandinavica, 57,* 145–152.

Buhrich, N. (1981). Psychological adjustment in transvestism and transsexualism. *Behaviour Research and Therapy, 19,* 407–411.

Buhrich, N. J., Bailey, J. M., & Martin, N. G. (1991). Sexual orientation, sexual identity, and sex-dimorphic behaviors in male twins. *Behavior Genetics, 21, 75–96.*

Buhrich, N. J., & McConaghy, N. (1979). Three clinically discrete categories of fetishistic transvestism. *Archives of Sexual Behavior, 8, 151–157.*

Buhrich, N. J., & Theile, H. (1979). Plasma testosterone, serum FSH, and serum LH levels in transvestism. *Archives of Sexual Behavior, 8, 49–53.*

Bullough, V. L. (1974). Transvestites in the Middle Ages. *American Journal of Sociology, 79, 1381–1394.*

Bullough, V. L. (1975). Transsexualism in history. *Archives of Sexual Behavior, 4, 561–571.*

Bullough, V. L. (1976). *Sexual variance in society and history.* Chicago: University of Chicago Press.

Bullough, V. L. (1985). The Rockefellers and sex research. *Journal of Sex Research, 21, 113–125.*

Bullough, V. L. (1987a). The first clinicians. In L. Diamant (Ed.), *Male and female homosexuality: Psychological approaches* (pp. 21–30). New York: Hemisphere.

Bullough, V. L. (1987b). A nineteenth-century transsexual. *Archives of Sexual Behavior, 16, 81–84.*

Bullough, V. L. (1990). The Kinsey scale in historical perspective. In D. P. McWhirter, S. A. Sanders, & J. M. Reinisch (Eds.), *Homosexuality/heterosexuality: Concepts of sexual orientation* (pp. 3–14). New York: Oxford University Press.

Bullough, V. L. (1994). *Science in the bedroom: A history of sex research.* New York: Basic Books.

Bullough, V. L., & Bullough, B. (1993). *Cross dressing, sex, and gender.* Philadelphia: University of Pennsylvania Press.

Burnham, J. C. (1972). American historians and the subject of sex. *Societas, 2, 307–316.*

Byne, W., & Parsons, B. (1993). Human sexual orientation: The biologic theories reappraised. *Archives of General Psychiatry, 50, 228–239.*

Caldera, Y. M., Huston, A. C., & O'Brien, M. (1989). Social interactions and play patterns of parents and toddlers with feminine, masculine, and neutral toys. *Child Development, 60, 70–76.*

Caplan, P. J., & Hall-McCorquodale, I. (1985a). Mother-blaming in major clinical journals. *American Journal of Orthopsychiatry, 55, 345–353.*

Caplan, P. J., & Hall-McCorquodale, I. (1985b). The scapegoating of mothers: A call for change. *American Journal of Orthopsychiatry, 55, 610–613.*

Carmichael, C. (1977). *Non-sexist childraising.* Boston: Beacon Press.

Caron, C., & Rutter, M. (1991). Comorbidity in child psychopathology: Concepts, issues and research strategies. *Journal of Child Psychology and Psychiatry, 32, 1063–1080.*

Carter, D. B., & Levy, G. D. (1988). Cognitive aspects of early sex-role development: The influence of gender schemas on preschoolers' memories and preferences for sex-typed toys and activities. *Child Development, 59, 782–792.*

Casey, M. B., & Brabeck, M. M. (1990). Women who excel on a spatial task: Proposed genetic and environmental factors. *Brain and Cognition, 12,* 73–84.

Cauldwell, D. O. (1949). Psychopathia transsexualis. *Sexology, 16,* 274–280.

Chahnazarian, A. (1988). Determinants of the sex ratio at birth: Review of recent literature. *Social Biology, 35,* 214–235.

Charatan, F. B., & Galef, H. (1965). A case of transvestism in a six-year-old boy. *Journal of the Hillside Hospital, 14,* 160–177.

Chauncey, G. (1982–1983). From sexual inversion to homosexuality: Medicine and the changing conceptualization of female deviance. *Salmagundi, 58–59,* 114–146.

Chauncey, G. (1994). *Gay New York: Gender, urban culture, and the making of the gay male world, 1890–1940.* New York: Basic Books.

Chazan, S. E. (1995). *The simultaneous treatment of parent and child.* New York: Basic Books.

Chiland, C. (1988). Enfance et transsexualisme. *Psychiatrie de l'Enfant, 31,* 313–373.

Chodorow, N. J. (1992). Heterosexuality as a compromise formation: Reflections on the psychoanalytic theory of sexual development. *Psychoanalysis and Contemporary Thought, 15,* 267–304.

Churchill, W. (1967). *Homosexual behavior among males: A cross-cultural and cross-species investigation.* New York: Hawthorn Books.

Ciccarese, S., Massari, S., & Guanti, G. (1982). Sexual behaviour is independent of H-Y antigen constitution. *Human Genetics, 60,* 371–372.

Cicchetti, D. (1984). The emergence of developmental psychopathology. *Child Development, 55,* 1–7.

Cicchetti, D. (1993). Developmental psychopathology: Reactions, reflections, projections. *Developmental Review, 13,* 471–502.

Cicchetti, D., & Toth, S. L. (Eds.) (1991). *Rochester Symposium on Developmental Psychopathology: Vol. 2. Internalizing and externalizing expressions of dysfunction.* Hillsdale, NJ: Erlbaum.

Clare, D., & Tully, B. (1989). Transhomosexuality, or the dissociation of sexual orientation and sex object choice. *Archives of Sexual Behavior, 18,* 531–536.

Clayton, A. H. (1993). Fetishism and clomiprimine [Letter to the editor]. *American Journal of Psychiatry, 150,* 673–674.

Clemmensen, L. H. (1990). The "real-life test" for surgical candidates. In R. Blanchard & B. W. Steiner (Eds.) , *Clinical management of gender identity disorders in children and adults* (pp. 119–135). Washington, DC: American Psychiatric Press.

Clifft, M. A. (1986). Writing about psychiatric patients: Guidelines for disguising case material. *Bulletin of the Menninger Clinic, 50,* 511–524.

Coates, S. (1985). Extreme boyhood femininity: Overview and new research findings. In Z. DeFries, R. C. Friedman, & R. Corn (Eds.), *Sexuality: New perspectives* (pp. 101–124). Westport, CT: Greenwood.

Coates, S. (1990). Ontogenesis of boyhood gender identity disorder. *Journal of the American Academy of Psychoanalysis, 18,* 414–438.

Coates, S. (1992). The etiology of boyhood gender identity disorder: An integrative model. In J. W. Barron, M. N. Eagle, & D. L. Wolitzky (Eds.), *Interface of psychoanalysis and psychology* (pp. 245–265). Washington, DC: American Psychological Association.

Coates, S., & Friedman, R. C. (1988). *Spatial ability in prepubertal boys with gender identity disorder.* Unpublished manuscript, Roosevelt Hospital, New York.

Coates, S., Friedman, R. C., & Wolfe, S. (1991). The etiology of boyhood gender identity disorder: A model for integrating temperament, development, and psychodynamics. *Psychoanalytic Dialogues, 1,* 481–523.

Coates, S., & Person, E. S. (1985). Extreme boyhood femininity: Isolated behavior or pervasive disorder? *Journal of the American Academy of Child Psychiatry, 24,* 702–709.

Coates, S., & Tuber, S. B. (1988). The representation of object relations in the Rorschachs of extremely feminine boys. In H. Lerner & P. Lerner (Eds.), *Primitive mental states on the Rorschach* (pp. 647–664). New York: International Universities Press.

Coates, S., & Wolfe, S. (in press). Gender identity disorders in toddlers and preschool children. In J. D. Noshpitz, S. Greenspan, J. D. Osofsky, & K. D. Pruett (Eds.), *The handbook of child and adolescent psychiatry.* New York: Wiley.

Coates, S., & Wolfe, S. M. (1995). Gender identity disorder in boys: The interface of constitution and early experience. *Psychoanalytic Inquiry, 15,* 6–38.

Coates, S., Wolfe, S., & Hahn-Burke, S. (1994, June). *Do boys with gender identity disorder have a shy, inhibited temperament?* Poster presented at the meeting of the International Academy of Sex Research, Edinburgh.

Coates, S., & Zucker, K. J. (1988). Gender identity disorders in children. In C. J. Kestenbaum & D. T. Williams (Eds.), *Handbook of clinical assessment of children and adolescents* (Vol. 2, pp. 893–914). New York: New York University Press.

Cohen, F. W. (1976). Art psychotherapy: The treatment of choice for a six-year-old boy with a transsexual syndrome. *Arts in Psychotherapy, 3,* 55–67.

Cohen, J. (1957). The factorial structure of the WAIS between early adulthood and old age. *Journal of Consulting Psychology, 21,* 283–290.

Cohen, J. (1988). *Statistical power analysis for the social sciences* (2nd ed.). Hillsdale, NJ: Erlbaum.

Cohen-Kettenis, P. T., Doorn, C. D., & Gooren, L. J. G. (1992, July). *Cerebral lateralization and spatial ability in transsexuals.* Poster presented at the meeting of the International Academy of Sex Research, Prague.

Cohen-Kettenis, P., & Everaerd, W. (1986). Gender role problems in adolescence. *Advances in Adolescent Mental Health, 1,* 1–28.

Cole, H. J., Zucker, K. J., & Bradley, S. J. (1982). Patterns of gender-role behaviour in children attending traditional and non-traditional day-care centres. *Canadian Journal of Psychiatry, 27,* 410–414.

Coleman, E. (1989). The development of male prostitution activity among gay and bisexual adolescents. In G. Herdt (Ed.), *Gay and lesbian youth* (pp. 131–149). Binghamton, NY: Harrington Park Press.

Coleman, E., Bockting, W. O., & Gooren, L. (1993). Homosexual and bisexual identity in sex-reassigned female-to-male transsexuals. *Archives of Sexual Behavior, 22,* 37–50.

Coleman, M. (1986). Nontraditional boys: A minority in need of reassessment. *Child Welfare, 65,* 252–269.

Collaer, M. L., & Hines, M. (1995). Human behavioral sex differences: A role for gonadal hormones during early development? *Psychological Bulletin, 118,* 55–107.

Commander, M., & Dean, C. (1990). Symptomatic trans-sexualism. *British Journal of Psychiatry, 156,* 894–896.

Connolly, F. H., & Gittleson, N. L. (1971). The relationship between delusions of sexual change and olfactory and gustatory hallucinations in schizophrenia. *British Journal of Psychiatry, 119,* 443–444.

Connor, J. M., & Serbin, L. A. (1977). Behaviorally based masculine- and feminine activity-preference scales for preschoolers: Correlates with other classroom behaviors and cognitive tests. *Child Development, 48,* 1411–1416.

Cooper, A. M. (1991). The unconscious core of perversion. In G. I. Fogel & W. A. Myers (Eds.), *Perversions and near perversions in clinical practice: New psychoanalytic perspectives* (pp. 17–35). New Haven, CT: Yale University Press.

Cordua, G. D., McGraw, K. O., & Drabman, R. S. (1979). Doctor or nurse: Children's perceptions of sex-typed occupations. *Child Development, 50,* 590–593.

Coren, S. (1992). *The left-hander syndrome: The causes and consequences of left-handedness.* New York: Free Press.

Cosentino, C. E., Meyer-Bahlburg, H. F. L., Alpert, J. L., & Gaines, R. (1993). Cross-gender behavior and gender conflict in sexually abused girls. *Journal of the American Academy of Child and Adolescent Psychiatry, 32,* 940–947.

Costabile, A., Smith, P. K., Matheson, L., Aston, J., Hunter, T., & Boulton, M. (1991). Cross-national comparison of how children distinguish serious and playful fighting. *Developmental Psychology, 27,* 881–887.

Cramer, P., & Hogan, K. A. (1975). Sex differences in verbal and play fantasy. *Developmental Psychology, 11,* 145–154.

Croughan, J. L., Saghir, M., Cohen, R., & Robins, E. (1981). A comparison of treated and untreated male cross-dressers. *Archives of Sexual Behavior, 10,* 515–528.

Curtis, R. (1985). Gender identity disorders of boys: A review. *Irish Journal of Psychology, 7,* 50–64.

Dahlgren, I. L., Matuszczyk, J. V., & Hård, E. (1991). Sexual orientation in male rats prenatally exposed to ethanol. *Neurotoxicology and Teratology, 13,* 267–269.

Daniel, W. F., & Yeo, R. A. (1993). Handedness and sexual preference: A reanalysis of data presented by Rosenstein and Bigler. *Perceptual and Motor Skills, 76,* 544–546.

Dank, B. M. (1971). Six homosexual siblings. *Archives of Sexual Behavior, 1,* 193–204.

Davenport, C. W. (1986). A follow-up study of 10 feminine boys. *Archives of Sexual Behavior, 15,* 511–517.

Davenport, C. W., & Harrison, S. I. (1977). Gender identity change in a female adolescent transsexual. *Archives of Sexual Behavior, 6,* 327–341.

Davidson, J. M. (1979). Biological determinants of sex: Their scope and limitations. In H. A. Katchadourian (Ed.), *Human sexuality: A comparative and developmental perspective* (pp. 134–149). Berkeley: University of California Press.

Davies, B. M., & Morgenstern, F. S. (1960). A case of cysticercosis, temporal lobe epilepsy, and transvestism. *Journal of Neurology, Neurosurgery and Psychiatry, 23,* 247–249.

Deaux, K. (1993). Sorry, wrong number—A reply to Gentile's call. *Psychological Science, 4,* 125–126.

De Cecco, J. P. (1987). Homosexuality's brief recovery: From sickness to health and back again. *Journal of Sex Research, 23,* 106–114.

Dekker, R. M., & van de Pol, L. C. (1989). *The tradition of female transvestism in early modern Europe.* New York: St. Martin's Press.

DeKlyen, O. M. (1992). *Childhood psychopathology and intergenerational relations in the representation of attachment: A comparison of normal and clinic-referred disruptive preschoolers and their mothers.* Unpublished doctoral dissertation, University of Washington.

Dellatolas, G., Tubert, P., Castresana, A., Mesbah, M., Giallonardo, T., Lazaratou, H., & Lellouch, J. (1991). Age and cohort effects in adult handedness. *Neuropsychologia, 29,* 255–261.

D'Emilio, J. (1992, January 7). Explain and oppress [Letter to the editor]. *New York Times,* p. A14.

Derogatis, L. (1983). *SCL-90: Administration, scoring and procedures manual for the revised version.* Baltimore: Clinical Psychometric Research.

De Savitsch, E. (1958). *Homosexuality, transvestism, and change of sex.* Springfield, IL: Charles C Thomas.

Devor, H. (1989). *Gender blending: Confronting the limits of duality.* Bloomington: Indiana University Press.

Devor, H. (1993a). Sexual orientation identities, attractions, and practices of female-to-male transsexuals. *Journal of Sex Research, 30,* 303–315.

Devor, H. (1993b). Toward a taxonomy of gendered sexuality. *Journal of Psychology and Human Sexuality, 6*(1), 23–55.

Devor, H. (1994). Transsexualism, dissociation, and child abuse: An initial discussion based on nonclinical data. *Journal of Psychology and Human Sexuality, 6*(3), 49–72.

Diamond, M. (1965). A critical evaluation of the ontogeny of human sexual behavior. *Quarterly Review of Biology, 40,* 147–175.

Diamond, M. (1968). Genetic–endocrine interactions and human psychosexuality. In M. Diamond (Ed.), *Perspectives in reproduction and sexual behavior* (pp. 417–443). Bloomington: Indiana University Press.

Diamond, M. (1976). Human sexual development: Biological foundations for social development. In F. A. Beach (Ed.), *Human sexuality in four perspectives* (pp. 22–61). Baltimore: Johns Hopkins University Press.

Diamond, M. (1982). Sexual identity, monozygotic twins reared in discordant sex roles and a BBC follow-up. *Archives of Sexual Behavior, 11,* 181–186.

Diamond, M. (1993a). Homosexuality and bisexuality in different populations. *Archives of Sexual Behavior, 22,* 291–310.

Diamond, M. (1993b). Some genetic considerations in the development of sexual orientation. In M. Haug, R. E. Whalen, C. Aron, & K. L. Olsen (Eds.), *The development of sex differences and similarities in behavior* (pp. 291–309). Dordrecht, The Netherlands: Kluwer Academic.

Diamond, M. (1994). Bisexualitat aus biologischer Sicht [Bisexuality: Biological aspects]. In E. J. Haeberle & R. Gindorf (Eds.), *Bisexüalitäten: Ideologie und Praxis des Sexualkontaktes mit beiden Geschlechtern [Bisexualities: Ideology and practices of sexual contact with both sexes]* (pp. 41–48). Stuttgart, Germany: Gustav Fischer Verlag.

Di Ceglie, D. (1995). Gender identity disorders in children and adolescents. *British Journal of Hospital Medicine, 53,* 251–256.

Dickey, R. (1990). Gender dysphoria and antisocial behavior. In R. Blanchard & B. W. Steiner (Eds.), *Clinical management of gender identity disorders in children and adults* (pp. 191–199). Washington, DC: American Psychiatric Press.

Dickey, R., & Stephens, J. (1995). Female-to-male transsexualism, heterosexual type: Two cases. *Archives of Sexual Behavior, 24,* 439–445.

Dicks, G. H., & Childers, A. T. (1934). The social transformation of a boy who had lived his first fourteen years as a girl: A case history. *American Journal of Orthopsychiatry, 4,* 508–517.

Dicks, G. H., & Childers, A. T. (1944). The social transformation of a boy who had lived his first fourteen years as a girl: II. Fourteen years later. *American Journal of Orthopsychiatry, 14,* 448–452.

DiPietro, J. A. (1981). Rough and tumble play: A function of gender. *Developmental Psychology, 17,* 50–58.

Dittmann, R. W. (1989). *Pränatal wirksame Hormone und Verhaltensmerkmale von Patientinnen mit den beiden klassichen Varianten des 21-Hydroxylase-Defektes.* New York: Peter Lang.

Dittmann, R. W. (1992). Body positions and movement patterns in female patients with congenital adrenal hyperplasia. *Hormones and Behavior, 26,* 441–456.

Dittmann, R. W., Kappes, M. E., & Kappes, M. H. (1992). Sexual behavior in adolescent and adult females with congenital adrenal hyperplasia. *Psychoneuroendocrinology, 17,* 153–170.

Dittmann, R. W., Kappes, M. H., Kappes, M. E., Börger, D., Meyer-Bahlburg, H. F. L., Stegner, H., Willig, R. H., & Wallis, H. (1990). Congenital adrenal hyperplasia: II. Gender-related behavior and attitudes in female salt-wasting and simple-virilizing patients. *Psychoneuroendocrinology, 15,* 421–434.

Dittmann, R. W., Kappes, M. H., Kappes, M. E., Börger, D., Stegner, H., Willig, R. H., & Wallis, H. (1990). Congenital adrenal hyperplasia: I. Gender-related behavior and attitudes in female patients and sisters. *Psychoneuroendocrinology, 15,* 401–420.

Dixen, J. M., Maddever, H., Van Maasdam, J., & Edwards, P. W. (1984). Psychosocial characteristics of applicants evaluated for surgical gender reassignment. *Archives of Sexual Behavior, 13,* 269–276.

Dodge, K. A. (1980). Social cognition and children's aggressive behavior. *Child Development, 51,* 162–170.

Dodge, K. A. (1993). Social-cognitive mechanisms in the development of conduct disorder and depression. *Annual Review of Psychology, 44,* 559–584.

Doell, R. G., & Longino, H. E. (1988). Sex hormones and human behavior: A critique of the linear model. *Journal of Homosexuality, 15,* 55–78.

Doering, R. W. (1981). *Parental reinforcement of gender-typed behaviors in boys with atypical gender identity.* Unpublished doctoral dissertation, University of Toronto.

Doering, R. W., Zucker, K. J., Bradley, S. J., & MacIntyre, R. B. (1989). Effects of neutral toys on sex-typed play in children with gender identity disorder. *Journal of Abnormal Child Psychology, 17,* 563–574.

Dörner, G. (1976). *Hormones and brain differentiation.* Amsterdam: Elsevier.

Dörner, G. (1988). Neuroendocrine response to estrogen and brain differentiation in heterosexuals, homosexuals, and transsexuals. *Archives of Sexual Behavior, 17,* 57–75.

Dörner, G., Geier, T., Ahrens, L., Krell, L., Münx, G., Sieler, H., Kittner, E., & Müller, H. (1980). Prenatal stress as possible aetiogenic factor of homosexuality in human males. *Endokrinologie, 75,* 365–368.

Dörner, G., Rohde, W., & Krell, L. (1972). Auslösung eines positiven Östrogenfeedback-Effekt bei homosexuellen Männern. *Endokrinologie, 60,* 297–301.

Dörner, G., Rohde, W., & Schnorr, D. (1975). Evocability of a slight positive oestrogen feedback action on LH secretion in castrated and oestrogen-primed men. *Endokrinologie, 66,* 373–376.

Dörner, G., Rohde, W., Schott, G., & Schnabl, C. (1983). On the LH response to oestrogen and LH-RH in transsexual men. *Experimental and Clinical Endocrinology, 82,* 257–267.

Dörner, G., Rohde, W., Seidel, K., Haas, W., & Schott, G. (1976). On the evocability of a positive oestrogen feedback action on LH secretion in transsexual men and women. *Endokrinologie, 67,* 20–25.

Dörner, G., Rohde, W., Stahl, F., Krell, L., & Masius, W. G. (1975). A neuroendocrine predisposition for homosexuality in men. *Archives of Sexual Behavior, 4,* 1–8.

Dörner, G., Schenk, B., Schmiedel, B., & Ahrens, L. (1983). Stressful events in prenatal life of bi- and homosexual men. *Experimental and Clinical Endocrinology, 81,* 83–87.

Douglas, J. W. B. (1975). Early hospital admissions and later disturbances of behaviour and learning. *Developmental Medicine and Child Neurology, 17,* 456–480.

Dowrick, P. W. (1983). Video training of alternatives to cross-gender identity behaviors in a 4-year-old boy. *Child and Family Behavior Therapy, 5,* 59–65.

Duggan, L. (1992). Making it perfectly queer. *Socialist Review, 22,* 11–31.

Dulcan, M. K., & Lee, P. A. (1984). Transsexualism in the adolescent girl. *Journal of the American Academy of Child Psychiatry, 23,* 354–361.

Dull, C. Y., Guiora, A. Z., Paluszny, M., Beit-Hallahmi, B., Catford, J. C., & Cooley, R. E. (1975). The Michigan Gender Identity Test (MIGIT). *Comprehensive Psychiatry, 16,* 581–592.

Dupont, H. (1968). Social learning theory and the treatment of transvestite behavior in an eight year old boy. *Psychotherapy: Theory, Research and Practice, 5,* 44–45.

Eaton, W. O. (1989). Childhood sex differences in motor performance and activity level: Findings and implications. In B. Kirkcaldy (Ed.), *Normalities and abnormalities in human movement* (pp. 58–77). Basel: Karger.

Eaton, W. O., Chipperfield, J. G., & Singbeil, C. E. (1989). Birth order and activity level in children. *Developmental Psychology, 25,* 668–672.

Eaton, W. O., & Enns, L. R (1986). Sex differences in human motor activity level. *Psychological Bulletin, 100,* 19–28.

Eaton, W. O., & Von Bargen, D. (1981). Asynchronous development of gender understanding in preschool children. *Child Development, 52,* 1020–1027.

Eaton, W. O., & Yu, A. P. (1989). Are sex differences in child motor activity level a function of sex differences in maturational status? *Child Development, 60,* 1005–1011.

Eberhart, J. A. (1988). Neural and hormonal correlates of primate sexual behavior. *Comparative Primate Biology: Neurosciences, 4,* 675–705.

Ebers, G. C. (1995, March). *Sib pair studies of MS and sexual orientation.* Paper presented at the Genetics of Human Behavior Conference, Cold Spring Harbor, NY.

Eckert, E. D., Bouchard, T. J., Bohlen, J., & Heston, L. L. (1986). Homosexuality in monozygotic twins reared apart. *British Journal of Psychiatry, 148,* 421–425.

Edelbrock, C., & Achenbach, T. M. (1980). A typology of Child Behavior Profile patterns: Distribution and correlates in disturbed children age 6 to 16. *Journal of Abnormal Child Psychology, 8,* 441–470.

Edelbrock, C., & Achenbach, T. M. (1984). The Teacher Version of the Child Behavior Profile: I. Boys aged 6–11. *Journal of Consulting and Clinical Psychology, 52,* 207–217.

Edelbrock, C., & Costello, A. J. (1988). Convergence between statistically derived behavior problem syndromes and child psychiatric diagnoses. *Journal of Abnormal Child Psychology, 16,* 219–231.

Edelman, M. S., & Omark, D. R. (1973). Dominance hierarchies in young children. *Social Science Information, 12,* 103–110.

Ehrhardt, A. A. (1979). Psychosexual adjustment in adolescence in patients with congenital abnormalities of their sex organs. In H. L. Vallet & I. H. Porter (Eds.), *Genetic mechanisms of sexual development* (pp. 473–483). New York: Academic Press.

Ehrhardt, A. A. (1985). The psychobiology of gender. In A. S. Rossi (Ed.), *Gender and the life course* (pp. 81–96). New York: Aldine.

Ehrhardt, A. A., & Baker, S. W. (1974). Fetal androgens, human central nervous system differentiation, and behavior sex differences. In R. C. Friedman, R. M. Richart, & R. L. Vande Wiele (Eds.), *Sex differences in behavior* (pp. 33–51). New York: Wiley.

Ehrhardt, A. A., Epstein, R., & Money, J. (1968). Fetal androgens and female gender identity in the early-treated adrenogenital syndrome. *Johns Hopkins Medical Journal, 122,* 160–167.

Ehrhardt, A. A., Evers, K., & Money, J. (1968). Influence of androgen and some aspects of sexually dimorphic behavior in women with the late-treated adrenogenital syndrome. *Johns Hopkins Medical Journal, 123,* 115–122.

Ehrhardt, A. A., & Meyer-Bahlburg, H. F. L. (1981). Effects of prenatal sex hormones on gender-related behavior. *Science, 211,* 1312–1318.

Ehrhardt, A. A., Meyer-Bahlburg, H. F. L., Rosen, L. R., Feldman, J. F., Veridiano, N. P., Elkin, E. J., & McEwen, B. S. (1989). The development of gender-related behavior in females following prenatal exposure to diethylstilbestrol (DES). *Hormones and Behavior, 23,* 526–541.

Ehrhardt, A. A., Meyer-Bahlburg, H. F. L., Rosen, L. R., Feldman, J. F., Veridiano, N. P., Zimmerman, I., & McEwen, B. S. (1985). Sexual orientation after prenatal exposure to exogenous estrogen. *Archives of Sexual Behavior, 14,* 57–77.

Eicher, W., Spoljar, M., Cleve, H., Murken, J., Eiermann, W., Richter, K., & Stengel-Rutkowski, S. (1981, June). *H-Y antigen in transsexuality.* Paper presented at the meeting of the World Congress of Sexology, Jerusalem.

Eide-Midtsand, N. (1987). Struggles with the "other one": The reconciliation of a pre-adolescent boy with his masculinity. *Journal of Analytic Psychology, 32,* 157–171.

Eisenberg, N. (1983). Sex-typed toy choices: What do they signify? In M. B. Liss (Ed.), *Social and cognitive skills: Sex roles and children's play* (pp. 45–70). New York: Academic Press.

Eisenberg, N., Murray, E., & Hite, T. (1982). Children's reasoning regarding sex-typed toy choices. *Child Development, 53,* 81–86.

Eisenberg, N., Wolchik, S. A., Hernandez, R., & Pasternack, J. F. (1985). Parental socialization of young children's play: A short-term longitudinal study. *Child Development, 56,* 1506–1513.

Elizabeth, P. H., & Green, R. (1984). Childhood sex-role behaviors: Similarities and differences in twins. *Acta Geneticae Medicae et Gemellologiae, 33,* 173–179.

Ellis, A. (1945). The sexual psychology of human hermaphrodites. *Psychosomatic Medicine, 7,* 108–125.

Ellis, A. (1963). Constitutional factors in homosexuality: A re-examination of the evidence. In H. G. Beigel (Ed.), *Advances in sex research* (pp. 161–186). New York: Harper & Row.

Ellis, H. (1936). *Studies in the psychology of sex* (Vol. 2). New York: Random House. (Original work published 1910)

Ellis, L. (1986). Evidence of neuroandrogenic etiology of sex roles from a combined analysis of human, nonhuman primate and nonprimate mammalian studies. *Personality and Individual Differences, 7,* 519–552.

Ellis, L., & Ames, M. A. (1987). Neurohormonal functioning and sexual orientation: A theory of homosexuality-heterosexuality. *Psychological Bulletin, 101,* 233–258.

Ellis, L., Ames, M. A., Peckham, W., & Burke, D. (1988). Sexual orientation of human offspring may be altered by severe maternal stress during pregnancy. *Journal of Sex Research, 25,* 152–157.

Ellis, L., & Peckham, W. (1991). Prenatal stress and handedness among offspring. *Pre- and Peri-Natal Psychology Journal, 6,* 135–144.

Emmerich, W., Goldman, K. S., Kirsh, B., & Sharabany, R. (1977). Evidence for a transitional phase in the development of gender constancy. *Child Development, 48,* 930–936.

Engel, W., Pfäfflin, F., & Wiedeking, C. (1980). H-Y antigen in transsexuality, and how to explain testis differentiation in H-Y antigen-negative males and ovary differentiation in H-Y antigen-positive females. *Human Genetics, 55,* 313–319.

Epstein, A. W. (1960). Fetishism: A study of its psychopathology with particular reference to a proposed disorder in brain mechanisms as an etiological factor. *Journal of Nervous and Mental Disease, 130,* 107–119.

Epstein, A. W. (1961). Relationship of fetishism and transvestism to brain and particularly to temporal lobe dysfunction. *Journal of Nervous and Mental Disease, 133,* 247–253.

Epstein, A. W. (1969). Fetishism: A comprehensive view. In J. H. Masserman (Ed.), *Science and psychoanalysis: Vol. 15. Dynamics of deviant sexuality* (pp. 81–87). New York: Grune & Stratton.

Epstein, A. W. (1973). The relationship of altered brain states to sexual psychopathology. In J. Zubin & J. Money (Eds.), *Contemporary sexual behavior: Critical issues in the 1970s* (pp. 297–310). Baltimore: Johns Hopkins University Press.

Epstein, S. (1987). Gay politics, ethnic identity: The limits of social constructionism. *Socialist Review, 93–94,* 9–54.

Epstein, S. (1991). Sexuality and identity: The contribution of object relations theory to a constructionist sociology. *Theory and Society, 20,* 825–873.

Erikson, E. H. (1951). Sex differences in the play configurations of preadolescents. *American Journal of Orthopsychiatry, 21,* 667–692.

Erwin, K. (1993). Interpreting the evidence: Competing paradigms and the emergence of lesbian and gay suicide as a "social fact." *International Journal of Health Services, 23,* 437–453.

Escoffier, J. (1985). Sexual revolution and the politics of gay identity. *Socialist Review, 82–83*, 119–153.

Esman, A. H. (1970). Transsexual identification in a three-year-old twin: A brief communication. *Psychosocial Process, 1*, 77–79.

Everitt, B. J., & Bancroft, J. (1991). Of rats and men: The comparative approach to male sexuality. *Annual Review of Sex Research, 2*, 77–117.

Fabrega, H. (1975). The need for an ethnomedical science. *Science, 189*, 969–975.

Fabrega, H. (1994). International systems of diagnosis in psychiatry. *Journal of Nervous and Mental Disease, 182*, 256–263.

Faderman, L. (1992). *Odd girls and twilight lovers: A history of lesbian life in twentieth-century America.* New York: Penguin Books.

Fagan, P. J., Wise, T. N., Derogatis, L. R., & Schmidt, C. W. (1988). Distressed transvestites: Psychometric characteristics. *Journal of Nervous and Mental Disease, 176*, 626–632.

Fagot, B. (1992). [Review of The *"sissy boy syndrome" and the development of homosexuality*]. *Archives of Sexual Behavior, 21*, 327–332.

Fagot, B. I. (1977). Consequences of moderate cross-gender behavior in preschool children. *Child Development, 48*, 902–907.

Fagot, B. I. (1978). The influence of sex of child on parental reactions to toddler children. *Child Development, 49*, 459–465.

Fagot, B. I. (1985a). Changes in thinking about early sex role development. *Developmental Review, 5*, 83–98.

Fagot, B. I. (1985b). Beyond the reinforcement principle: Another step toward understanding sex role development. *Developmental Psychology, 21*, 1097–1104.

Fagot, B. I., & Hagan, R. (1991). Observations of parent reactions to sex-stereotyped behaviors: Age and sex effects. *Child Development, 62*, 617–628.

Fagot, B. I., & Leinbach, M. D. (1985). Gender identity: Some thoughts on an old concept. *Journal of the American Academy of Child Psychiatry, 24*, 684–688.

Fagot, B. I., & Leinbach, M. D. (1989). The young child's gender schema: Environmental input, internal organization. *Child Development, 60*, 663–672.

Fagot, B. I., & Leinbach, M. D. (1993). Gender-role development in young children: From discrimination to labeling. *Developmental Review, 13*, 205–224.

Fagot, B. I., Leinbach, M. D., & Hagan, R. (1986). Gender labeling and the adoption of sex-typed behaviors. *Developmental Psychology, 22*, 440–443.

Fagot, B. I., & O'Brien, M. (1994). Activity level in young children: Cross-age stability, situational influences, correlates with temperament, and the perception of problem behaviors. *Merrill–Palmer Quarterly, 40*, 378–398.

Fairweather, H. (1976). Sex differences in cognition. *Cognition, 4*, 231–280.

Fast, I. (1984). *Gender identity: A differentiation model.* Hillsdale, NJ: Analytic Press.

Fausto-Sterling, A. (1985). *Myths of gender: Biological theories about women and men.* New York: Basic Books.

Fausto-Sterling, A., & Balaban, E. (1993). Genetic and male sexual orientation [Letter]. *Science, 261,* 1257.

Fay, R. E., Turner, C. F., Klassen, A. D., & Gagnon, J. H. (1989). Prevalence and patterns of same-gender sexual contact among men. *Science, 243,* 338–348.

Feder, H. H. (1984). Hormones and sexual behavior. *Annual Review of Psychology, 35,* 165–200.

Fedoroff, J. P. (1988). Buspirone hydrochloride in the treatment of transvestic fetishism. *Journal of Clinical Psychiatry, 49,* 408–409.

Fedoroff, J. P. (1992). Buspirone hydrochloride in the treatment of an atypical paraphilia. *Archives of Sexual Behavior, 21,* 401–406.

Feingold, A. (1988). Cognitive gender differences are disappearing. *American Psychologist, 43,* 95–103.

Feingold, A. (1993). Cognitive gender differences: A developmental perspective. *Sex Roles, 29,* 91–112.

Fenichel, O. (1945). *The psychoanalytic theory of neurosis.* New York: Norton.

Ferenczi, S. (1980). The nosology of male homosexuality (homoeroticism). In S. Ferenczi, *First contributions to psychoanalysis.* New York: Brunner/Mazel. (Original work published 1914)

Finegan, J. K., Niccols, G. A., Zacher, J. E., & Hood, J. E. (1991). The Play Activity Questionnaire: A parent report measure of children's play preferences. *Archives of Sexual Behavior, 20,* 393–408.

Finegan, J. K., Zucker, K. J., Bradley, S. J., & Doering, R. W. (1982). Patterns of intellectual functioning and spatial ability in boys with gender identity disorder. *Canadian Journal of Psychiatry, 27,* 135–139.

Fischhoff, J. (1964). Preoedipal influences in a boy's determination to be "feminine" during the oedipal period. *Journal of the American Academy of Child Psychiatry, 3,* 273–286.

Fisk, N. (1973). Gender dysphoria syndrome (the how, what, and why of a disease). In D. Laub & P. Gandy (Eds.), *Proceedings of the Second Interdisciplinary Symposium on Gender Dysphoria Syndrome* (pp. 7–14). Stanford, CA: Stanford University Press.

Fleminger, J. J., Dalton, R., & Standage, K. F. (1977). Handedness in psychiatric patients. *British Journal of Psychiatry, 131,* 448–452.

Flerx, V. C., Fidler, D. S., & Rogers, R. W. (1976). Sex role stereotypes: Developmental aspects and early intervention. *Child Development, 47,* 998–1007.

Fout, J. C. (1990). A note from the editor. *Journal of the History of Sexuality, 1,* 1–2.

Fraley, M. C., Nelson, E. C., Wolf, A. W., & Lozoff, B. (1991). Early genital naming. *Journal of Developmental and Behavioral Pediatrics, 12,* 301–304.

Frame, C. L., & Matson, J. L. (Eds.). (1987). *Handbook of assessment in childhood psychopathology: Applied issues in differential diagnosis and treatment evaluation*. New York: Plenum Press.

Francis, J. J. (1965). Passivity and homosexual predisposition in latency boys. *Bulletin of the Philadelphia Association of Psychoanalysis, 15*, 160–174.

Frankel, H. (1853). Homo mollis. *Medizinische Zeitung, 22*, 102–103.

Frenkel, R. S. (1993). Problems in female development: Comments on the analysis of an early latency-age girl. *Psychoanalytic Study of the Child, 48*, 171–192.

Freud, S. (1953). Three essays on the theory of sexuality. In J. Strachey (Ed. and Trans.), *The standard edition of the complete psychological works of Sigmund Freud* (Vol. 7, pp. 123–243). London: Hogarth Press. (Original work published 1905)

Freund, K. (1963). A laboratory method for diagnosing predominance of homo- or hetero-erotic interest in the male. *Behaviour Research and Therapy, 1*, 85–93.

Freund, K. (1977). Psychophysiological assessment of change in erotic preference. *Behaviour Research and Therapy, 15*, 297–301.

Freund, K., & Blanchard, R. (1983). Is the distant relationship of fathers and homosexual sons related to the sons' erotic preference for male partners, to the sons' atypical gender identity, or to both? *Journal of Homosexuality, 9*, 7–25.

Freund, K., Watson, R., & Rienzo, D. (1989). Heterosexuality, homosexuality, and erotic age preference. *Journal of Sex Research, 26*, 107–117.

Fridell, S. R., Zucker, K. J., Bradley, S. J., & Maing, D. M. (in press). Physical attractiveness of girls with gender identity disorder. *Archives of Sexual Behavior.*

Friedemann, M. (1966). Reflection on two cases of male transvestism. *American Journal of Psychotherapy, 20*, 270–283.

Friedman, R. C. (1988). *Male homosexuality: A contemporary psychoanalytic perspective*. New Haven, CT: Yale University Press.

Friedman, R. C., & Downey, J. (1993a). Neurobiology and sexual orientation: Current relationships. *Journal of Neuropsychiatry and Clinical Neurosciences, 5*, 131–153.

Friedman, R. C., & Downey, J. (1993b). Psychoanalysis, psychobiology, and homosexuality. *Journal of the American Psychoanalytic Association, 41*, 1159–1198.

Friedman, R. C., & Downey, J. I. (1994). Homosexuality. *New England Journal of Medicine, 331*, 923–930.

Friedman, R. C., Wollesen, F., & Tendler, R. (1976). Psychological development and blood levels of sex steroids in male identical twins of divergent sexual orientation. *Journal of Nervous and Mental Disease, 163*, 282–288.

Friend, M. R., Schiddel, L., Klein, B., & Dunaeff, D. (1954). Observations on the development of transvestitism in boys. *American Journal of Orthopsychiatry, 24*, 563–575.

Gadpaille, W. J. (1972). Research into the physiology of maleness and femaleness: Its contribution to the etiology and psychodynamics of homosexuality. *Archives of General Psychiatry, 26,* 193–206.

Gadpaille, W. J. (1980). Cross-species and cross-cultural contributions to understanding homosexual activity. *Archives of General Psychiatry, 37,* 349–356.

Gagnon, J. H. (1990). The explicit and implicit use of the scripting perspective in sex research. *Annual Review of Sex Research, 1,* 1–43.

Gagnon, J. H., & Simon, W. (1973). *Sexual conduct.* Chicago: Aldine.

Garber, J., & Hollon, S. D. (1991). What can specificity designs say about causality in psychopathology research? *Psychological Bulletin, 110,* 129–136.

Garber, M. (1989). Spare parts: The surgical construction of gender. *differences: A Journal of Feminist Cultural Studies, 1,* 137–159.

Garden, G. M. F., & Rothery, D. J. (1992). A female monozygotic twin pair discordant for transsexualism: Some theoretical implications. *British Journal of Psychiatry, 161,* 852–854.

Gardner, W., & Wilcox, B. L. (1993). Political intervention in scientific peer review: Research on adolescent sexual behavior. *American Psychologist, 48,* 972–983.

Garfinkel, B. D., Carlson, G. A., & Weller, E. B. (Eds.). (1990). *Psychiatric disorders in children and adolescents.* Philadelphia: W. B. Saunders.

Gebhard, P. H. (1972). Incidence of overt homosexuality in the United States and Western Europe. In J. Livingood (Ed.), *NIMH Task Force on Homosexuality: Final report and background papers* (DHEW Publication No. HSM 72-9116, pp. 22–29). Rockville, MD: National Institute of Mental Health.

Gebhard, P. H., & Johnson, A. B. (1979). *The Kinsey data: Marginal tabulations of the 1938–1963 interviews conducted by the Institute for Sex Research.* Philadelphia: W. B. Saunders.

Gelder, M. (1979). Behaviour therapy for sexual deviations. In I. Rosen (Ed.), *Sexual deviation* (2nd ed., pp. 351–375). New York: Oxford University Press.

Gelder, M. G., & Marks, I. M. (1969). Aversion treatment in transvestism and transsexualism. In R. Green & J. Money (Eds.), *Transsexualism and sex reassignment* (pp. 383–413). Baltimore: Johns Hopkins University Press.

Gelman, D. (1992, February 24). Born or bred? *Newsweek,* pp. 46–53.

Gelman, S. A., Collman, P., & Maccoby, E. E. (1986). Inferring properties from categories versus inferring categories from properties: The case of gender. *Child Development, 57,* 396–404.

Gentile, D. A. (1993). Just what are sex and gender, anyway? A call for a new terminological standard. *Psychological Science, 4,* 120–122.

Gerall, A. A., Moltz, H., & Ward, I. L. (Eds.). (1992). *Handbook of behavioral neurobiology: Vol. 11. Sexual differentiation.* New York: Plenum Press.

Gert, B. (1992). A sex caused inconsistency in DSM-III-R: The definition of mental disorder and the definition of paraphilias. *Journal of Medicine and Philosophy, 17,* 155–171.

Geschwind, N., & Galaburda, A. M. (1985a). Cerebral lateralization. Biological mechanisms, associations, and pathology: I. A hypothesis and a program for research. *Archives of Neurology, 42,* 428–459.

Geschwind, N., & Galaburda, A. M. (1985b). Cerebral lateralization. Biological mechanisms, associations, and pathology: II. A hypothesis and a program for research. *Archives of Neurology, 42,* 521–552.

Geschwind, N., & Galaburda, A. M. (1985c). Cerebral lateralization. Biological mechanisms, associations, and pathology: III. A hypothesis and a program for research. *Archives of Neurology, 42,* 634–654.

Gewirtz, J. L., & Hernandez, J. P. (1984, August). *Gender can be determined from the baby's face.* Paper presented at the meetings of the American Psychological Association, Toronto.

Gewirtz, J. L., & Hernandez, J. P. (1985, August). *Gender can be determined from the baby's live face and from slide photographs of the baby's face.* Paper presented at the meetings of the American Psychological Association, Los Angeles.

Gewirtz, J. L., Weber, R. A., & Nogueras, M. (1990, April). *The role of facial characteristics in neonatal-gender discrimination from photographs.* Paper presented at the meeting of the International Conference on Infant Studies, Montreal.

Gilbert, A. N., & Wysocki, C. J. (1992). Hand preference and age in the United States. *Neuropsychologia, 30,* 601–608.

Gilligan, C. (1982). *In a different voice: Psychological theory and women's development.* Cambridge, MA: Harvard University Press.

Gilmore, K. (1995). Gender identity disorder in a girl: Insights from adoption. *Journal of the American Psychoanalytic Association, 43,* 39–59.

Gilpin, D. C., Raza, S., & Gilpin, D. (1979). Transsexual symptoms in a male child treated by a female therapist. *American Journal of Psychotherapy, 33,* 453–463.

Gittleson, N. L., & Dawson-Butterworth, K. (1967). Subjective ideas of sexual change in female schizophrenics. *British Journal of Psychiatry, 113,* 491–494.

Gittleson, N. L., & Levine, S. (1966). Subjective ideas of sexual change in male schizophrenics. *British Journal of Psychiatry, 112,* 779–782.

Gladue, B. A. (1985). Neuroendocrine response to estrogen and sexual orientation [Letter]. *Science, 230,* 962.

Gladue, B. A. (1988). Hormones in relationship to homosexual/bisexual/heterosexual gender orientation. In J. M. A. Sitsen (Ed.), *Handbook of sexology: Vol. 6. The pharmacology and endocrinology of sexual function* (pp. 388–409). Amsterdam: Elsevier.

Gladue, B. A. (1990). Hormones and neuroendocrine factors in atypical human sexual behavior. In J. R. Feierman (Ed.), *Pedophilia: Biosocial dimensions* (pp. 274–298). New York: Springer-Verlag.

Gladue, B. A., & Bailey, J. M. (1995). Spatial ability, handedness, and human sexual orientation. *Psychoneuroendocrinology, 20,* 487–497.

Gladue, B. A., Beatty, W. W., Larson, J., & Staton, R. D. (1990). Sexual orientation and spatial ability in men and women. *Psychobiology, 18,* 101–108.

Gladue, B. A., Green, R., & Hellman, R. E. (1984). Neuroendocrine response to estrogen and sexual orientation. *Science, 225,* 1496–1499.

Glasser, M. (1979). Some aspects of the role of aggression in the perversions. In I. Rosen (Ed.), *Sexual deviation* (2nd ed., pp. 278–305). New York: Oxford University Press.

Goddard, R. (1986). *Gender and non gender disturbed boyhood separation anxiety disorder: The role of aggression and object relations as manifested in Rorschach imagery.* Unpublished doctoral dissertation, City University of New York.

Goddard, R., & Tuber, S. (1989). Boyhood separation anxiety disorder: Thought disorder and object relations psychopathology as manifested in Rorschach imagery. *Journal of Personality Assessment, 53,* 239–252.

Gonsiorek, J. C. (1991). The empirical basis for the demise of the illness model of homosexuality. In J. C. Gonsiorek & J. D. Weinrich (Eds.), *Homosexuality: Research implications for public policy* (pp. 115–136). Newbury Park, CA: Sage.

Goodman, R. E., Anderson, D. C., Bulock, D. E., Sheffield, B., Lynch, S. S., & Butt, W. R. (1985). Study on the effect of estradiol on gonadotrophin levels in untreated male-to-female transsexuals. *Archives of Sexual Behavior, 14,* 141–146.

Gooren, L. (1986a). The neuroendocrine response of luteinizing hormone to estrogen administration in heterosexual, homosexual, and transsexual subjects. *Journal of Clinical Endocrinology and Metabolism, 63,* 583–588.

Gooren, L. (1986b). The neuroendocrine response of luteinizing hormone to estrogen administration in the human is not sex specific but dependent on the hormonal environment. *Journal of Clinical Endocrinology and Metabolism, 63,* 589–593.

Gooren, L. (1990a). Biomedical theories of sexual orientation: A critical examination. In D. P. McWhirter, S. A. Sanders, & J. M. Reinisch (Eds.), *Homosexuality/heterosexuality: Concepts of sexual orientation* (pp. 71–87). New York: Oxford University Press.

Gooren, L. (1990b). The endocrinology of transsexualism: A review and commentary. *Psychoneuroendocrinology, 15,* 3–14.

Gooren, L., Frants, R. R., Ericksson, A. W., & Rao, B. R. (1989). *Transsexualism in twins.* Paper presented at the International Conference on Twin Studies, Rome.

Gooren, L. J. G. (1988). An appraisal of endocrine theories of homosexuality and gender dysphoria. In J. M. A. Sitsen (Ed.), *Handbook of sexology: Vol. 6. The pharmacology and endocrinology of sexual function* (pp. 410–424). Amsterdam: Elsevier.

Gooren, L. J. G., Rao, B. R., van Kessel, H., & Harmsen-Louman, W. (1984). Estrogen positive feedback on LH secretion in transsexuality. *Psychoneuroendocrinology, 9,* 249–259.

Gorski, R. A., Gordon, J. H., Shryne, J. E., & Southam, A. M. (1978). Evidence for a morphological sex difference within the medial preoptic area of the rat brain. *Brain Research, 148,* 333–346.

Götestam, K. O., Coates, T. J., & Ekstrand, M. (1992). Handedness, dyslexia and twinning in homosexual men. *International Journal of Neuroscience, 63,* 179–186.

Goy, R. W., Bercovitch, F. B., & McBrair, M. C. (1988). Behavioral masculinization is independent of genital masculinization in prenatally androgenized female rhesus macaques. *Hormones and Behavior, 22,* 552–571.

Goy, R. W., & Goldfoot, D. A. (1975). Neuroendocrinology: Animal models and problems of human sexuality. *Archives of Sexual Behavior, 4,* 405–418.

Goy, R. W., & McEwen, B. S. (1980). *Sexual differentiation of the brain.* Cambridge, MA: MIT Press.

Goy, R. W., & Wallen, K. (1979). Experiential variables influencing play, footclasp mounting and adult sexual competence in male rhesus monkeys. *Psychoneuroendocrinology, 4,* 1–12.

Green, R. (1968). Childhood cross-gender identification. *Journal of Nervous and Mental Disease, 147,* 500–509.

Green, R. (1969). Mythological, historical, and cross-cultural aspects of transsexualism. In R. Green & J. Money (Eds.), *Transsexualism and sex reassignment* (pp. 13–22). Baltimore: The Johns Hopkins Press.

Green, R. (1970). Little boys who behave as girls. *California Medicine, 113,* 12–16.

Green, R. (1971). Diagnosis and treatment of gender identity disorders during childhood. *Archives of Sexual Behavior, 1,* 167–174.

Green, R. (1972). Homosexuality as a mental illness. *International Journal of Psychiatry, 10,* 77–98.

Green, R. (1974). *Sexual identity conflict in children and adults.* New York: Basic Books.

Green, R. (1976). One-hundred ten feminine and masculine boys: Behavioral contrasts and demographic similarities. *Archives of Sexual Behavior, 5,* 425–446.

Green, R. (1980). Patterns of sexual identity development in childhood: Relationship to subsequent sexual partner preference. In J. Marmor (Ed.), *Homosexual behavior: A modern reappraisal* (pp. 255–266). New York: Basic Books.

Green, R. (1987). *The "sissy boy syndrome" and the development of homosexuality.* New Haven, CT: Yale University Press.

Green, R. (1993). Dimensions of human sexual identity: Transsexuals, homosexuals, fetishists, cross-gendered children and animal models. In M. Haug, R. E. Whalen, C. Aron, & K. L. Olsen (Eds.), *The development of sex differences and similarities in behavior* (pp. 477–486). Dordrecht, The Netherlands: Kluwer Academic.

Green, R. (1994a). Atypical psychosexual development. In M. Rutter, E. Taylor, & L. Hersov (Eds.), *Child and adolescent psychiatry: Modern ap-*

proaches (3rd ed., pp. 749–758). Oxford: Blackwell Scientific.

Green, R. (1994b). Sexual problems and therapies: A quarter century of developments and changes. In A. S. Rossi (Ed.), *Sexuality and the life course* (pp. 341–361). Chicago: University of Chicago Press.

Green, R., & Fuller, M. (1973a). Family doll play and female identity in preadolescent males. *American Journal of Orthopsychiatry, 43,* 123–127.

Green, R., & Fuller, M. (1973b). Group therapy with feminine boys and their parents. *International Journal of Group Psychotherapy, 23,* 54–68.

Green, R., Fuller, M., & Rutley, B. (1972). It-Scale for Children and Draw-a-Person test: 30 feminine vs. 25 masculine boys. *Journal of Personality Assessment, 36,* 349–352.

Green, R., Fuller, M., Rutley, B., & Hendler, J. (1972). Playroom toy preferences of fifteen masculine and fifteen feminine boys. *Behaviour Research and Therapy, 3,* 425–429.

Green, R., & Money, J. (1960). Incongruous gender role: Nongenital manifestations in prepubertal boys. *Journal of Nervous and Mental Disease, 131,* 160–168.

Green, R., & Money, J. (1961a). Effeminacy in prepubertal boys: Summary of eleven cases and recommendations for case management. *Pediatrics, 27,* 286–291.

Green, R., & Money, J. (1961b). "Tomboys" and "sissies." *Sexology, 28,* 2–5.

Green, R., & Money, J. (Eds.). (1969). *Transsexualism and sex reassignment.* Baltimore: The Johns Hopkins Press.

Green, R., Neuberg, D. S., & Finch, S. J. (1983). Sex-typed motor behaviors of "feminine" boys, conventionally masculine boys, and conventionally feminine girls. *Sex Roles, 9,* 571–579.

Green, R., Newman, L. E., & Stoller, R. J. (1972). Treatment of boyhood "transsexualism": An interim report of four years' experience. *Archives of General Psychiatry, 26,* 213–217.

Green, R., Roberts, C. W., Williams, K., Goodman, M., & Mixon, A. (1987). Specific cross-gender behaviour in boyhood and later homosexual orientation. *British Journal of Psychiatry, 151,* 84–88.

Green, R., & Stoller, R. J. (1971). Two monozygotic (identical) twin pairs discordant for gender identity. *Archives of Sexual Behavior, 1,* 321–327.

Green, R., Williams, K., & Goodman, M. (1982). Ninety-nine "tomboys" and "non-tomboys": Behavioral contrasts and demographic similarities. *Archives of Sexual Behavior, 11,* 247–266.

Green, R., Williams, K., & Goodman, M. (1985). Masculine or feminine gender identity in boys: Developmental differences between two diverse family groups. *Sex Roles, 12,* 1155–1162.

Green, R., Williams, K., & Harper, J. (1980). Cross-sex identity: Peer group integration and the double standard of childhood sex-typing. In J. Samson (Ed.), *Childhood and sexuality* (pp. 542–548). Montreal: Editions Etudes Vivantes.

Greenacre, P. (1955). Further considerations regarding fetishism. *Psychoanalytic Study of the Child, 10,* 187–194.

Greenacre, P. (1968). Perversions: General considerations regarding their genetic and dynamic background. *Psychoanalytic Study of the Child, 23,* 47–62.

Greenberg, D. F. (1989). *The construction of homosexuality.* Chicago: University of Chicago Press.

Greenberg, M. T., Cicchetti, D., & Cummings, E. M. (Eds.). (1990). *Attachment in the preschool years: Theory, research, and intervention.* Chicago: University of Chicago Press.

Greenberg, M. T., Speltz, M. L., & DeKlyen, M. (1993). The role of attachment in the early development of disruptive behavior problems. *Development and Psychopathology, 5,* 191–213.

Greenberg, M. T., Speltz, M. L., DeKlyen, M., & Endriga, M. C. (1991). Attachment security in preschoolers with and without externalizing behavior problems: A replication. *Development and Psychopathology, 3,* 413–430.

Greenson, R. R. (1966). A transvestite boy and a hypothesis. *International Journal of Psycho-Analysis, 47,* 396–403.

Grimshaw, G. M. (1993). *Relations between prenatal testosterone and cerebral lateralization: A test of three hypotheses.* Unpublished master's thesis, University of Waterloo, Waterloo, Ontario.

Grimshaw, G. M., Zucker, K. J., Bradley, S. J., Lowry, C. B., & Mitchell, J. N. (1991, August). *Verbal and spatial ability in boys with gender identity disorder.* Poster presented at the meeting of the International Academy of Sex Research, Barrie, Ontario.

Gross, D. J., Landau, H., Kohn, G., Farkas, A., Elrayyes, E., El-Shawwa, R., Lasch, E. E., & Rösler, A. (1986). Male pseudohermaphroditism due to 17-beta-hydroxysteroid dehydrogenase deficiency: Gender reassignment in early infancy. *Acta Endocrinologica, 112,* 238–246.

Gunderson, J. G., & Kolb, J. E. (1978). Discriminating features of borderline patients. *American Journal of Psychiatry, 135,* 792–796.

Gunderson, J. G., Kolb, J. E., & Austin, V. (1981). The Diagnostic Interview for Borderline Patients. *American Journal of Psychiatry, 138,* 896–903.

Gutheil, E. (1930). Analysis of a case of transvestitism. In W. Stekel (Ed.), *Sexual aberrations* (pp. 281–318). New York: Liveright.

Gutterman, E. M., O'Brien, J. D., & Young, J. G. (1987). Structured diagnostic interviews for children and adolescents: Current status and future directions. *Journal of the American Academy of Child and Adolescent Psychiatry, 26,* 621–630.

Haber, C. H. (1991a). The psychoanalytic treatment of a preschool boy with a gender identity disorder. *Journal of the American Psychoanalytic Association, 39,* 107–129.

Haber, C. H. (1991b). The reorganization of a cross-gender symptom. In A. G. Schmuckler (Ed.), *Saying goodbye: A casebook of termination in child and adolescent analysis and therapy* (pp. 29–50). Hillsdale, NJ: Analytic Press.

Haeberle, E. J. (1982). The Jewish contribution to the development of sexology. *Journal of Sex Research, 18,* 305–323.

Halbreich, U., Segal, S., & Chowers, I. (1978). Day-to-day variations in serum levels of follicle-stimulating hormone and luteinizing hormone in homosexual males. *Biological Psychiatry, 13,* 541–549.

Hall, J. A., & Halberstadt, A. G. (1980). Masculinity and femininity in children: Development of the Children's Personal Attributes Questionnaire. *Developmental Psychology, 16,* 270–280.

Hall, J. A. Y., & Kimura, D. (1994). Dermatoglyphic asymmetry and sexual orientation in men. *Behavioral Neuroscience, 108,* 1203–1206.

Hall, J. A. Y., & Kimura, D. (1995). Sexual orientation and performance on sexually dimorphic motor tasks. *Archives of Sexual Behavior, 24,* 395–407.

Halperin, D. M. (1989). Is there a history of sexuality? *History and Theory, 28,* 257–274.

Halpern, D. F. (1992). *Sex differences in cognitive abilities* (2nd ed.). Hillsdale, NJ: Erlbaum.

Halpern, D. F., & Cass, M. (1994). Laterality, sexual orientation, and immune system functioning: Is there a relationship? *International Journal of Neuroscience, 77,* 167–180.

Halpern, D. F., & Coren, S. (1993). Left-handedness and life span: A reply to Harris. *Psychological Bulletin, 114,* 235–241.

Hamburger, C. (1953). The desire for change of sex as shown by personal letters from 465 men and women. *Acta Endocrinologica, 14,* 361–375.

Hamburger, C., Sturup, G. K., & Dahl-Iverson, E. (1953). Transvestism: Hormonal, psychiatric, and surgical treatment. *Journal of the American Medical Association, 152,* 391–396.

Hamer, D. (1995, May). *The role of genes in sexual orientation and sex-typical behavior.* Paper presented at the International Behavioral Development Symposium: Biological Basis of Sexual Orientation and Sex-Typical Behavior, Minot State University, Minot, ND.

Hamer, D., & Copeland, P. (1994). *The science of desire: The search for the gay gene and the biology of behavior.* New York: Simon & Schuster.

Hamer, D. H., Hu, S., Magnuson, V. L., Hu, N., & Pattatucci, A. M. L. (1993a). A linkage between DNA markers on the X chromosome and male sexual orientation. *Science, 261,* 321–327.

Hamer, D. H., Hu, S., Magnuson, V. L., Hu, N., & Pattatucci, A. M. L. (1993b). [Response to "Genetics and male sexual orientation"]. *Science, 261,* 1259.

Hamer, D. H., Hu, S., Magnuson, V. L., Hu, N., & Pattatucci, A. M. L. (1993c). [Response to "Male sexual orientation and genetic evidence"]. *Science, 262,* 2065.

Hamer, D. H., Hu, S., Magnuson, V. L., Hu, N., & Pattatucci, A. M. L. (1993d, June). *Molecular genetic studies of sexual orientation.* Paper presented at the meeting of the International Academy of Sex Research, Pacific Grove, CA.

Hampson, J. G. (1955). Hermaphroditic genital appearance, rearing and eroticism in hyperadrenocorticism. *Bulletin of the Johns Hopkins Hospital, 96,* 265–273.

Hansen, B. (1989). American physicians' earliest writings about homosexuals, 1880–1900. *Milbank Quarterly, 67,* 92–108.

Hare, E. H., & Moran, P. A. P. (1979). Parent age and birth order in homosexual patients: A replication of Slater's study. *British Journal of Psychiatry, 134,* 178–182.

Harlow, H. F., & Harlow, M. K. (1965). The affectional systems. In A. M. Schrier, H. F. Harlow, & F. Stollnitz (Eds.), *Behavior of nonhuman primates: Modern research trends* (Vol. 2, pp. 287–334). New York: Academic Press.

Harris, L. J. (1978). Sex differences in spatial ability: Possible environmental, genetic, and neurological factors. In M. Kinsbourne (Ed.), *Asymmetrical functions of the brain* (pp. 405–522). Cambridge, England: Cambridge University Press.

Harrison, P. J., Everall, I. P., & Catalan, J. (1994). Is homosexual behaviour hard-wired?: Sexual orientation and brain structure. *Psychological Medicine, 24,* 811–816.

Harry, J. (1982). *Gay children grown up: Gender culture and gender deviance.* New York: Praeger.

Harry, J. (1983). Parasuicide, gender, and gender deviance. *Journal of Health and Social Behavior, 24,* 350–361.

Hauser, R. E. (1990). The *berdache* and the Illinois Indian tribe during the last half of the seventeenth century. *Ethnohistory, 37,* 45–65.

Hausman, B. L. (1992). Demanding subjectivity: Transsexualism, medicine, and the technologies of gender. *Journal of the History of Sexuality, 3,* 270–302.

Hay, D. F. (1980). Multiple functions of proximity seeking in infancy. *Child Development, 51,* 636–645.

Hay, W. M., Barlow, D. H., & Hay, L. R. (1981). Treatment of stereotypic cross-gender motor behavior using covert modeling in a boy with gender identity confusion. *Journal of Consulting and Clinical Psychology, 49,* 388–394.

Hazell, P. L. (1992). Clinical continuity [Letter to the editor]. *Journal of the American Academy of Child and Adolescent Psychiatry, 31,* 172–173.

Heinrich, P., & Triebe, J. K. (1972). Sex preferences in children's human figure drawings. *Journal of Personality Assessment, 36,* 263–267.

Helleday, J., Siwers, B., Ritzen, E. M., & Hugdahl, K. (1994). Normal lateralization for handedness and ear advantage in a verbal dichotic listening task in women with congenital adrenal hyperplasia (CAH). *Neuropsychologia, 32,* 875–880.

Hendricks, S. E., Graber, B., & Rodriguez-Sierra, J. F. (1989). Neuroendocrine responses to exogenous estrogen: No differences between heterosexual and homosexual men. *Psychoneuroendocrinology, 14,* 177–185.

Herbst, A. L., Ulfelder, H., & Poskanzer, D. C. (1971). Adenocarcinoma of the vagina: Association of maternal stilbestrol therapy with tumor appearance in young women. *New England Journal of Medicine, 284,* 878–881.

Herdt, G. (Ed.). (1989). *Gay and lesbian youth.* Binghamton, NY: Harrington Park Press.

Herdt, G. (1990a). Developmental discontinuities and sexual orientation across cultures. In D. P. McWhirter, S. A. Sanders, & J. M. Reinisch (Eds.), *Homosexuality/heterosexuality: Concepts of sexual orientation* (pp. 208–236). New York: Oxford University Press.

Herdt, G. (1990b). Mistaken gender: 5-alpha reductase hermaphroditism and biological reductionism in sexual identity reconsidered. *American Anthropologist, 92,* 433–446.

Herdt, G. (Ed.). (1994). *Third sex, third gender: Beyond sexual dimorphism in culture and history.* New York: Zone Books.

Herdt, G., & Stoller, R. J. (1990). *Intimate communications: Erotics and the study of culture.* New York: Columbia University Press.

Herdt, G. H. (1980). Semen depletion and the sense of maleness. *Ethnopsychiatrica, 3,* 79–116.

Herdt, G. H. (1981). *Guardians of the flute: Idioms of masculinity.* New York: McGraw-Hill.

Herdt, G. H. (Ed.). (1984). *Ritualized homosexuality in Melanesia.* Berkeley: University of California Press.

Herdt, G. H., & Davidson, J. (1988). The Sambia "Turnim-man": Sociocultural and clinical aspects of gender formation in male pseudohermaphrodites with 5-alpha reductase deficiency in Papua New Guinea. *Archives of Sexual Behavior, 17,* 33–56.

Herjanic, B., & Reich, W. (1982). Development of a structured psychiatric interview for children: Agreement between child and parent on individual symptoms. *Journal of Abnormal Child Psychology, 10,* 307–324.

Herman, A., Grabowska, A., & Dulko, S. (1993). Transsexualism and sex-related differences in hemispheric asymmetry. *Acta Neurobiologiae Experimentalis, 53,* 269–274.

Herman, S. P. (1983). Gender identity disorder in a five-year-old boy. *Yale Journal of Biology and Medicine, 56,* 15–22.

Herzer, M. (1985). Kertbeny and the nameless love. *Journal of Homosexuality, 12,* 1–26.

Hetherington, E. M. (1966). Effects of paternal absence on sex-typed behaviors in Negro and white preadolescent males. *Journal of Personality and Social Psychology, 4,* 87–91.

Hier, D. B., & Crowley, W. F. (1982). Spatial ability in androgen-deficient men. *New England Journal of Medicine, 306,* 1202–1205.

Higham, E. (1976). Case management of the gender incongruity syndrome in childhood and adolescence. *Journal of Homosexuality, 2,* 49–57.

Hildebrandt, K. A., & Fitzgerald, H. E. (1979). Facial feature determinants of perceived infant attractiveness. *Infant Behavior and Development, 2,* 329–339.

Hines, M. (1982). Prenatal gonadal hormones and sex differences in human behavior. *Psychological Bulletin, 92,* 56–80.

Hines, M., & Collaer, M. L. (1993). Gonadal hormones and sexual differentiation of human behavior: Developments from research on endocrine syndromes and studies of brain structure. *Annual Review of Sex Research, 4,* 1–48.

Hines, M., & Kaufman, F. R. (1994). Androgen and the development of human sex-typical behavior: Rough-and-tumble play and sex of preferred playmates in children with congenital adrenal hyperplasia (CAH). *Child Development, 65,* 1042–1053.

Hines, M., & Shipley, C. (1984). Prenatal exposure to diethylstilbestrol (DES) and the development of sexually dimorphic cognitive abilities and cerebral lateralization. *Developmental Psychology, 20,* 81–94.

Hirschfeld, M. (1910). *Die Transvestiten: Eine Untersuchung über den erotischen Verkleidungstrieb.* Berlin: Pulvermacher.

Hirschfeld, M. (1923). Die intersexuelle konstitution. *Jahrbuch für Sexuelle Zwischenstufen, 23,* 3–27.

Hirschfeld, M. (1991). *Transvestites: The erotic drive to cross-dress* (M. A. Lombardi-Nash, Trans.). Buffalo, NY: Prometheus Books. (Original work published 1910)

Hiscock, M., Inch, R., Jacek, C., Hiscock-Kalil, C., & Kalil, K. M. (1994). Is there a sex difference in human laterality?: I. An exhaustive survey of auditory laterality studies from six neuropsychology journals. *Journal of Clinical and Experimental Neuropsychology, 16,* 423–435.

Hodges, J. K. (1980). Regulation of oestrogen-induced LH release in male and female marmoset monkeys *(Callithrix jacchus). Journal of Reproduction and Fertility, 60,* 389–398.

Hoenig, J. (1977a). The development of sexology during the second half of the 19th century. In J. Money & H. Musaph (Eds.), *Handbook of sexology* (Vol. I, pp. 5–20). Amsterdam: Elsevier.

Hoenig, J. (1977b). Dramatis personae: Selected biographical sketches of 19th century pioneers in sexology. In J. Money & H. Musaph (Eds.), *Handbook of sexology* (Vol. I, pp. 21–43). Amsterdam: Elsevier.

Hoenig, J. (1981). Etiological research in transsexualism. *Psychiatric Journal of the University of Ottawa, 6,* 184–189.

Hoenig, J. (1982). Transsexualism. In K. L. Granville-Grossman (Ed.), *Recent advances in clinical psychiatry* (pp. 171–199). London: Churchill Livingstone.

Hoenig, J. (1985a). Etiology of transsexualism. In B. W. Steiner (Ed.), *Gender dysphoria: Development, research, management* (pp. 33–73). New York: Plenum Press.

Hoenig, J. (1985b). The origin of gender identity. In B. W. Steiner (Ed.), *Gender dysphoria: Development, research, management* (pp. 11–32). New York: Plenum Press.

Hoenig, J., & Torr, J. B. D. (1964). Karyotyping of transexualists. *Journal of Psychosomatic Research, 8,* 157–159.

Hofman, M. A., Fliers, E., Goudsmit, E., & Swaab, D. F. (1988). Morphometric analysis of the suprachiasmatic and paraventricular nuclei in the human brain. *Journal of Anatomy, 160,* 127–143.

Hofman, M. A., & Swaab, D. F. (1989). The sexually dimorphic nucleus of the preoptic area in the human brain: A comparative morphometric study. *Journal of Anatomy, 164,* 55–72.

Holder, E. (1982). A latency girl's struggle towards femininity. *Bulletin of the Hampstead Clinic, 5,* 55–70.

Hollingshead, A. B. (1975). *Four factor index of social status.* Unpublished manuscript, Department of Sociology, Yale University, New Haven, CT.

Holtzen, D. W. (1994). Handedness and sexual orientation. *Journal of Clinical and Experimental Neuropsychology, 16,* 702–712.

Hooper, S. R., Hynd, G. W., & Mattison, R. E. (Eds.). (1992). *Child psychopathology: Diagnostic criteria and clinical assessment.* Hillsdale, NJ: Erlbaum.

Hopkins, J. (1984). The probable role of trauma in a case of foot and shoe fetishism: Aspects of the psychotherapy of a 6-year-old girl. *International Review of Psychoanalysis, 11,* 79–91.

Hora, T. (1953). The structural analysis of transvestitism. *Psychoanalytic Review, 40,* 268–274.

Horton, A. M. (1980). Behavioral treatment of childhood gender role confusion. *Child Behavior Therapy, 2,* 82–83.

Housden, J. (1965). An examination of the biological etiology of transvestism. *International Journal of Social Psychiatry, 11,* 301–305.

Hoyer, N. (1933). *Man into woman.* New York: Dutton.

Hubert, N. C., Wachs, T. D., Peters-Martin, P., & Gandour, S. (1982). The study of early temperament: Measurement and conceptual issues. *Child Development, 53,* 571–600.

Hunt, D. D., Carr, J. E., & Hampson, J. L. (1981). Cognitive correlates of biologic sex and gender identity in transsexualism. *Archives of Sexual Behavior, 10,* 65–77.

Hunter, R., Logue, V., & McMenemy, W. H. (1963). Temporal lobe epilepsy supervening on longstanding transvestism and fetishism. *Epilepsia, 4,* 60–65.

Hurtig, A. L. (1992). The psychosocial effects of ambiguous genitalia. *Comprehensive Therapy, 18,* 22–25.

Hurtig, A. L., & Rosenthal, I. M. (1987). Psychological findings in early treated cases of female pseudohermaphroditism caused by virilizing congenital adrenal hyperplasia. *Archives of Sexual Behavior, 16,* 209–223.

Huston, A. C. (1983). Sex-typing. In E. M. Hetherington (Vol. Ed.), *Handbook of child psychology* (4th ed.): *Vol. 4. Socialization, personality, and social development* (pp. 387–467). New York: Wiley.

Hutter, J. (1993). The social construction of homosexuals in the nineteenth century: The shift from the sin to the influence of medicine on criminalizing sodomy in Germany. *Journal of Homosexuality, 24,* 73–93.

Hyde, J. S. (1981). How large are cognitive gender differences? A meta-analysis using w^2 and d. *American Psychologist, 36,* 892–901.

Hyde, J. S., & Linn, M. C. (1988). Gender differences in verbal ability: A meta-analysis. *Psychological Bulletin, 104,* 53–69.

Ignico, A. A. (1990). The influence of gender-role perception on activity preferences of children. *Play and Culture, 3,* 302–310.

Imperato-McGinley, J. (1983). Sexual differentiation: Normal and abnormal. In L. Martini & V. H. T. James (Eds.), *Current topics in endocrinology: Vol. 5. Fetal endocrinology and metabolism* (pp. 231–307). New York: Academic Press.

Imperato-McGinley, J., Guerrero, L., Gautier, T., & Peterson, R. E. (1974). Steroid 5-alpha-reductase deficiency in man: An inherited form of male pseudohermaphroditism. *Science, 186,* 1213–1215.

Imperato-McGinley, J., Peterson, R. E., & Gautier, T. (1976). Gender identity and hermaphroditism [Letter]. *Science, 191,* 872.

Imperato-McGinley, J., Peterson, R. E., Gautier, T., & Sturla, E. (1979a). Androgens and the evolution of male-gender identity among male pseudohermaphrodites with 5-alpha-reductase deficiency. *New England Journal of Medicine, 300,* 1233–1237.

Imperato-McGinley, J., Peterson, R. E., Gautier, T., & Sturla, E. (1979b). Androgens and the evolution of male-gender identity among male pseudohermaphrodites with 5-alpha-reductase deficiency. *Obstetrical and Gynecological Survey, 34,* 769–770.

Imperato-McGinley, J., Peterson, R. E., Gautier, T., & Sturla, E. (1979c). Male pseudohermaphroditism secondary to 5-alpha-reductase deficiency: A model for the role of androgens in both the development of the male phenotype and the evolution of a male gender identity. *Journal of Steroid Biochemistry, 11,* 637–645.

Imperato-McGinley, J., Peterson, R. E., Gautier, T., & Sturla, E. (1985). The impact of androgens on the evolution of male gender identity. In Z. De-Fries, R. C. Friedman, & R. Corn (Eds.), *Sexuality: New perspectives* (pp. 125–140). Westport, CT: Greenwood.

Imperato-McGinley, J., Peterson, R. E., Stoller, R., & Goodwin, W. E. (1979). Male pseudohermaphroditism secondary to 17 beta-hydroxysteroid dehydrogenase deficiency: Gender role change with puberty. *Journal of Clinical Endocrinology and Metabolism, 49,* 391–395.

Interdisciplinary Centre for the Study of Science, Society, and Religion, Free University of Amsterdam and the Schorer Foundation. (1989). *Homosexuality, which homosexuality? Essays from the International Scientific Conference on Lesbian and Gay Studies.* London: GMP.

Intons-Peterson, M. J. (1988). *Children's concepts of gender.* Norwood, NJ: Ablex.

Ipp, H. R. (1986). *Object relations of feminine boys: A Rorschach assessment.* Unpublished doctoral dissertation, York University, Downsview, Ontario.

Irvine, J. M. (1990). *Disorders of desire: Sex and gender in modern American sexology.* Philadelphia: Temple University Press.

Isay, R. A. (1989). *Being homosexual: Gay men and their development.* New York: Farrar Straus Giroux.

Jacklin, C. N., DiPietro, J. A., & Maccoby, E. E. (1984). Sex-typing behavior and sex-typing pressure in child/parent interaction. *Archives of Sexual Behavior, 13,* 413–425.

James, S., Orwin, A., & Davies, D. W. (1972). Sex chromosome abnormality in a patient with transsexualism. *British Medical Journal, iii,* 29.

James, W. H. (1987). The human sex ratio: Part I. A review of the literature. *Human Biology, 59,* 721–752.

James, W. H. (1989). Foetal testosterone levels, homosexuality and handedness: A research proposal for jointly testing Geschwind's and Dörner's hypotheses. *Journal of Theoretical Biology, 136,* 177–180.

Jamison, C. S., Jamison, P. L., & Meier, R. J. (1994). Effect of prenatal testosterone administration on palmar dermatoglyphic intercore ridge counts of rhesus monkeys (*Macaca mulatta*). *American Journal of Physical Anthropology, 94,* 409–419.

Jensch, K. (1941). Weiterer Beitrag zur Genealogie der Homosexualität. *Archiv für Psychiatrie und Nervenkrankheiten, 112,* 679–696.

Johnson, J. (1973). 'Psychopathia sexualis.' *British Journal of Psychiatry, 122,* 211–218.

Jolles, I. (1952). A study of validity of some hypotheses for the qualitative interpretation of the H-T-P for children of elementary school age: I. Sexual identification. *Journal of Clinical Psychology, 8,* 113–118.

Joyce, P. R., & Ding, L. (1985). Transsexual sisters. *Australian and New Zealand Journal of Psychiatry, 19,* 188–189.

Junginger, J. (1988). Summation of arousal in partial fetishism. *Journal of Behaviour Therapy and Experimental Psychiatry, 19,* 297–300.

Kagan, J. (1958). The concept of identification. *Psychological Review, 65,* 295–305.

Kagan, J. (1989). *Unstable ideas: Temperament, cognition and self.* Cambridge, MA: Harvard University Press.

Kagan, J., Reznick, J. S., & Snidman, N. (1987). The physiology and psychology of behavioral inhibition in children. *Child Development, 58,* 1459–1473.

Kallmann, F. J. (1952a). Comparative twin study on the genetic aspects of male homosexuality. *Journal of Nervous and Mental Disease, 115,* 283–298.

Kallmann, F. J. (1952b). Twin and sibship study of overt male homosexuality. *American Journal of Human Genetics, 4,* 136–146.

Kalter, N. (1977). Children of divorce in an out-patient psychiatric population. *American Journal of Orthopsychiatry, 47,* 40–51.

Kando, T. (1973). *Sex change: The achievement of gender identity among feminized transsexuals.* Springfield, IL: Charles C Thomas.

Kaplan, A. G. (1980). Human sex-hormone abnormalities viewed from an androgynous perspective: A reconsideration of the work of John Money. In J. E. Parsons (Ed.), *The psychobiology of sex differences and sex roles* (pp. 81–91). Washington, DC: Hemisphere.

Karush, R. K. (1993). Sam: A child analysis. *Journal of Clinical Psychoanalysis, 2,* 43–62.

Katcher, A. (1955). The discrimination of sex differences by young children. *Journal of Genetic Psychology, 87,* 131–143.

Katz, P. A. (1986). Modification of children's gender-stereotyped behavior: General issues and research considerations. *Sex Roles, 14,* 591–602.

Katz, P. A. (1987). Variations in family constellation: Effects on gender schemata. In L. S. Liben & M. L. Signorella (Eds.), *Children's gender schemata* (pp. 39–56). San Francisco: Jossey-Bass.

Katz, P. A., & Boswell, S. (1986). Flexibility and traditionality in children's gender roles. *Genetic, Social, and General Psychology Monographs, 112,* 105–147.

Katz, P. A., & Walsh, P. V. (1991). Modification of children's gender-stereotyped behavior. *Child Development, 62,* 338–351.

Kaufman, A. S. (1975). Factor analysis of the WISC-R at 11 age levels between 6½ and 16½ years. *Journal of Consulting and Clinical Psychology, 43,* 135–147.

Kaufman, M. (1991). Answering parents' questions about homosexuality. *Canadian Family Physician, 37,* 1197–1201.

Kelley, D. B. (1988). Sexually dimorphic behaviors. *Annual Review of Neuroscience, 11,* 225–251.

Kendler, K. S. (1993). Twin studies of psychiatric illness: Current status and future directions. *Archives of General Psychiatry, 50,* 905–915.

Kenna, J. C., & Hoenig, J. (1978). Verbal characteristics of male and female transsexuals. *Psychiatria Clinica, 11,* 233–236.

Kenna, J. C., & Hoenig, J. (1979). Verbal tests and transsexualism. *Acta Psychiatrica Scandinavica, 59,* 80–86.

Kennedy, H. (1988). *Ulrichs: The life and work of Karl Heinrich Ulrichs, pioneer of the modern gay movement.* Boston: Alyson.

Kenrick, D. T. (1987). Gender, genes, and the social environment: A biosocial interactionist perspective. In P. Shaver & C. Hendrick (Eds.), *Sex and gender* (pp. 14–43). Newbury Park, CA: Sage.

Kerbeshian, J., & Burd, L. (1991). Tourette syndrome and recurrent paraphilic masturbatory fantasy. *Canadian Journal of Psychiatry, 36,* 155–157.

Kerns, K. A., & Berenbaum, S. A. (1991). Sex differences in spatial ability in children. *Behavior Genetics, 21,* 383–396.

Kessler, S. J. (1990). The medical construction of gender: Case management of intersexed infants. *Signs, 16,* 3–26.

Kestenbaum, C. J., & Williams, D. T. (Eds.). (1988). *Handbook of clinical assessment of children and adolescents* (Vol. 2). New York: New York University Press.

Kimura, D., & Carson, M. W. (1993). Cognitive pattern and finger ridge asymmetry. *Society for Neuroscience Abstracts, 19,* 560.

Kimura, D., & Harshman, R. A. (1984). Sex differences in brain organization for verbal and nonverbal functions. *Progress in Brain Research, 61,* 423–441.

King, C. D. (1945). The meaning of normal. *Yale Journal of Biology and Medicine, 18,* 493–501.

King, D. (1984). Condition, orientation, role or false consciousness? Models of homosexuality and transsexualism. *Sociological Review, 32,* 38–56.

King, D. (1993) *The transvestite and the transsexual: Public categories and private identities.* Aldershot, England: Avebury.

King, M. (1993). Sexual orientation and the X. *Nature, 364,* 288–289.

King, M., & McDonald, E. (1992). Homosexuals who are twins: A study of 46 probands. *British Journal of Psychiatry, 160,* 407–409.

Kinsey, A. C., Pomeroy, W. B., & Martin, C. E. (1948). *Sexual behavior in the human male.* Philadelphia: W. B. Saunders.

Kirk, S. A., & Kutchins, H. (1992). *The selling of DSM: The rhetoric of science in psychiatry.* New York: Aldine/De Gruyter.

Kirkpatrick, M., & Friedman, C. T. H. (1976). Treatment of requests for sex-change surgery with psychotherapy. *American Journal of Psychiatry, 133,* 1194–1196.

Kirsch, J. A. W., & Weinrich, J. D. (1991). Homosexuality, nature, and biology: Is homosexuality natural? Does it matter? In J. C. Gonsiorek & J. D. Weinrich (Eds.), *Homosexuality: Research implications for public policy* (pp. 13–31). Newbury Park, CA: Sage.

Klein, A. R., & Bates, J. E. (1980). Gender-typing of game choices and qualities of boys' play behavior. *Journal of Abnormal Child Psychology, 8,* 201–212.

Klein, R. G., & Last, C. G. (1989). *Anxiety disorders in children.* Newbury Park, CA: Sage.

Köckott, G., & Fahrner, E. M. (1988). Male-to-female and female-to-male transsexuals: A comparison. *Archives of Sexual Behavior, 17,* 539–546.

Kohlberg, L. (1966). A cognitive-developmental analysis of children's sex-role concepts and attitudes. In E. E. Maccoby (Ed.), *The development of sex differences* (pp. 82–173). Stanford, CA: Stanford University Press.

Kohnstamm, G. A., Bates, J. E., & Rothbart, M. K. (Eds.). (1989). *Temperament in childhood.* New York: Wiley.

Kohut, H. (1984). *How does analysis cure?* Chicago: University of Chicago Press.

Kolarsky, A., Freund, K., Machek, J., & Polak, O. (1967). Male sexual deviation: Association with early temporal lobe damage. *Archives of General Psychiatry, 17,* 735–743.

Kolers, N. (1986). *Some ego functions in boys with gender identity disturbance.* Unpublished doctoral dissertation, York University, Downsview, Ontario.

Komisaruk, B. R. (1978). The nature of the neural substrate of female sexual behaviour in mammals and its hormonal sensitivity: Review and speculations. In J. B. Hutchison (Ed.), *Biological determinants of sexual behavior* (pp. 349–393). New York: Wiley.

Konstantareas, M. M., & Homatidis, S. (1985). Dominance hierarchies in normal and conduct-disordered children. *Journal of Abnormal Child Psychology, 13,* 259–268.

Koranyi, E. K. (1980). *Transsexuality in the male: The spectrum of gender dysphoria.* Springfield, IL: Charles C Thomas.

Kosky, R. J. (1987). Gender-disordered children: Does inpatient treatment help? *Medical Journal of Australia, 146,* 565–569.

Kotelchuck, M., Zelazo, P. R., Kagan, J., & Spelke, E. (1975). Infant reaction to parental separations when left with familiar and unfamiliar adults. *Journal of Genetic Psychology, 126,* 255–262.

Kourany, R. F. C. (1987). Suicide among homosexual adolescents. *Journal of Homosexuality, 13*, 111–117.

Kovacs, M. (1983). *The Interview Schedule for Children (ISC): Interrater and parent–child agreement.* Unpublished manuscript, University of Pittsburgh School of Medicine.

Krafft-Ebing, R. V. (1886). *Psychopathia sexualis.* Stuttgart: Ferdinand Enke.

Krasnoff, A. G., Walker, J. T., & Howard, M. (1989). Early sex-linked activities and interests related to spatial abilities. *Personality and Individual Differences, 10*, 81–85.

Krekling, S., & Nordvik, H. (1992). Observational training improves adult women's performance on Piaget's water-level task. *Scandinavian Journal of Psychology, 33*, 117–124.

Kronberg, J., Tyano, S., Apter, A., & Wijsenbeek, H. (1981). Treatment of transsexualism in adolescence. *Journal of Adolescence, 4*, 177–185.

Krueger, D. W. (1978). Symptom passing in a transvestite father and three sons. *American Journal of Psychiatry, 135*, 739–742.

Kruesi, M. J. P., Fine, S., Valladares, L., Phillips, R. A., & Rapoport, J. L. (1992). Paraphilias: A double-blind crossover comparison of clomipramine versus desipramine. *Archives of Sexual Behavior, 21*, 587–593.

Kujawski, J. H., & Bower, T. G. R. (1993). Same-sex preferential looking during infancy as a function of abstract representation. *British Journal of Developmental Psychology, 11*, 201–209.

Kula, K., Dulko, S. Pawlikowski, M., Imieliński, K., & Slowikowska, J. (1986). A nonspecific disturbance of the gonadostat in women with transsexualism and isolated hypergonadotropism in the male-to-female disturbance of gender identity. *Experimental and Clinical Endocrinology, 87*, 8–14.

Kula, K., & Pawlikowski, M. (1986). Gonadotropins and gonadal function in transsexualism and hypospadias. *Monographs in Neural Sciences, 12*, 69–74.

La Freniere, P., Strayer, F. F., & Gauthier, R. (1984). The emergence of same-sex affiliative preferences among preschool peers: A developmental/ethological perspective. *Child Development, 55*, 1958–1965.

Lang, T. (1940). Studies in the genetic determination of homosexuality. *Journal of Nervous and Mental Disease, 92*, 55–64.

Lang, T. (1960). Die Homosexualität als genetisches Problem. *Acta Geneticae Medicae et Gemellologiae, 9*, 370–381.

Langevin, R. (1983). *Sexual strands: Understanding and treating sexual anomalies in men.* Hillsdale, NJ: Erlbaum.

Langevin, R., & Martin, M. (1975). Can erotic responses be classically conditioned? *Behavior Therapy, 6*, 350–355.

Langevin, R., Paitich, D., & Russon, A. E. (1985). Are rapists sexually anomalous, aggressive, or both? In R. Langevin (Ed.), *Erotic preference, gender identity and aggression in men: New research studies* (pp. 17–38). Hillsdale, NJ: Erlbaum.

Langlois, J. H., & Downs, A. C. (1980). Mothers, fathers, and peers as socialization agents of sex-typed play behaviors in young children. *Child Development, 51*, 1237–1247.

Langlois, J. H., & Roggman, L. A. (1990). Attractive faces are only average. *Psychological Science, 1*, 115–121.

Lansky, L. M., Feinstein, H., & Peterson, J. (1988). Demography of handedness in two samples of randomly selected adults (*N* = 2083). *Neuropsychologia, 26*, 465–477.

Last, C. G., & Hersen, M. (Eds.). (1989). *Handbook of child psychiatric diagnosis.* New York: Wiley.

La Torre, R. A., Gossmann, I., & Piper, W. E. (1976). Cognitive style, hemispheric specialization, and tested abilities of transsexuals and nontranssexuals. *Perceptual and Motor Skills, 43*, 719–722.

Laumann, E. O., Gagnon, J. H., Michael, R. T., & Michaels, S. (1994). *The social organization of sexuality: Sexual practices in the United States.* Chicago: University of Chicago Press.

Laws, D. R., & Marshall, W. L. (1991). Masturbatory reconditioning with sexual deviates: An evaluative review. *Advances in Behaviour Research and Therapy, 13*, 13–25.

Leaper, C. (Ed.). (1994). *Childhood gender segregation: Causes and consequences.* San Francisco: Jossey-Bass.

Lebovitz, P. S. (1972). Feminine behavior in boys: Aspects of its outcome. *American Journal of Psychiatry, 128*, 1283–1289.

Lee, A. C. (1985). Normal and pathological gender-role development in children. In G. Stricker & R. H. Keisner (Eds.), *From research to clinical practice: The implications of social and developmental research for psychotherapy* (pp. 287–312). New York: Plenum Press.

Leigh, B. C., Temple, M. T., & Trocki, K. F. (1993). The sexual behavior of US adults: Results from a national survey. *American Journal of Public Health, 83*, 1400–1408.

Leinbach, M. D., & Fagot, B. I. (1986). Acquisition of gender labels: A test for toddlers. *Sex Roles, 15*, 655–666.

Leinbach, M. D., & Fagot, B. I. (1993). Categorical habituation to male and female faces: Gender schematic processing in infancy. *Infant Behavior and Development, 16*, 317–332.

LeVay, S. (1991). A difference in hypothalamic structure between heterosexual and homosexual men. *Science, 253*, 1034–1037.

LeVay, S. (1993). *The sexual brain.* Cambridge, MA: MIT Press.

Levin, J. S., & DeFrank, R. S. (1988). Maternal stress and pregnancy outcomes: A review of the psychosocial literature. *Journal of Psychosomatic Obstetrics and Gynaecology, 9*, 3–16.

Levin, S. M., Balistrier, J., & Schukit, M. (1972). The development of sexual discrimination in children. *Journal of Child Psychology and Psychiatry, 13*, 47–53.

Levine, S. B. (1980). Psychiatric diagnosis of patients requesting sex reassignment surgery. *Journal of Sex and Marital Therapy, 6*, 164–173.

Levine, S. B. (1993). Gender-disturbed males. *Journal of Sex and Marital Therapy, 19*, 131–141.

Levine, S. B., & Lothstein, L. M. (1981). Transsexualism or the gender dysphoria syndromes. *Journal of Sex and Marital Therapy, 7,* 85–113.

Lev-Ran, A. (1974). Sexuality and educational levels of women with the late-treated adrenogenital syndrome. *Archives of Sexual Behavior, 3,* 27–32.

Levy, G. D. (1994). High and low gender schematic children's release from proactive interference. *Sex Roles, 30,* 93–108.

Levy, G. D., & Haaf, R. A. (1994). Detection of gender-related categories by 10-month-old infants. *Infant Behavior and Development, 17,* 457–459.

Levy, J., & Heller, W. (1992). Gender differences in human neuropsychological function. In A. A. Gerall, H. Moltz, & I. L. Ward (Eds.), *Handbook of behavioral neurobiology: Vol. 11. Sexual differentiation* (pp. 245–274). New York: Plenum Press.

Lewes, K. (1988). *The psychoanalytic theory of male homosexuality.* New York: Simon & Schuster.

Leyendecker, G., Wardlaw, S., Leffek, B., & Nocke, W. (1971). Studies on the function of the hypothalamic sexual centre in the human: Presence of a cyclic centre in a genetic male. *Acta Endocrinologica, 155*(Suppl.), 36.

Liakos, A. (1967). Familial transvestism. *British Journal of Psychiatry, 113,* 49–51.

Liben, L. S. (1991). The Piagetian water-level task: Looking beneath the surface. *Annals of Child Development, 8,* 81–144.

Liben, L. S., & Bigler, R. S. (1987). Reformulating children's gender schemata. In L. S. Liben & M. L. Signorella (Eds.), *Children's gender schemata* (pp. 89–105). San Francisco: Jossey-Bass.

Liben, L. S., & Signorella, M. L. (Eds.). (1987). *Children's gender schemata.* San Francisco: Jossey-Bass.

Lieberson, S., & Bell, E. O. (1992). Children's first names: An empirical study of social taste. *American Journal of Sociology, 98,* 511–554.

Lihn, H. (1970). Fetishism: A case report. *International Journal of Psycho-Analysis, 51,* 351–358.

Lim, M. H., & Bottomley, V. (1983). A combined approach to the treatment of effeminate behaviour in a boy: A case study. *Journal of Child Psychology and Psychiatry, 24,* 469–479.

Linday, L. A. (1994). Maternal reports of pregnancy, genital, and related fantasies in preschool and kindergarten children. *Journal of the American Academy of Child and Adolescent Psychiatry, 33,* 416–423.

Lindesay, J. (1987). Laterality shift in homosexual men. *Neuropsychologia, 25,* 965–969.

Linn, M. C., & Petersen, A. C. (1985). Emergence and characterization of sex differences in spatial ability: A meta-analysis. *Child Development, 56,* 1479–1498.

Linn, M. C., & Petersen, A. C. (1986). A meta-analysis of gender differences in spatial ability: Implications for mathematics and science achievement. In J. S. Hyde & M. C. Linn (Eds.), *The psychology of gender: Advances through meta-analysis* (pp. 67–101). Baltimore: Johns Hopkins University Press.

Lish, J. D., Ehrhardt, A. A., Meyer-Bahlburg, H. F. L., Rosen, L. R., Gruen, R.

S., & Veridiano, N. P. (1991). Gender-related behavior development in females exposed to diethylstilbestrol (DES) in utero: An attempted replication. *Journal of the American Academy of Child and Adolescent Psychiatry, 30*, 29–37.

Lish, J. D., Meyer-Bahlburg, H. F. L., Ehrhardt, A. A., Travis, B. G., & Veridiano, N. P. (1992). Prenatal exposure to diethylstilbestrol (DES): Childhood play behavior and adult gender-role behavior in women. *Archives of Sexual Behavior, 21*, 423–441.

Livingstone, I. R., Sagel, J., Distiller, L. A., Morley, J., & Katz, M. (1978). The effect of luteinizing hormone releasing hormone (LRH) on pituitary gonadotropins in male homosexuals. *Hormones and Metabolism Research, 10*, 248–249.

Lobel, M. (1994). Conceptualizations, measurement, and effects of prenatal maternal stress on birth outcomes. *Journal of Behavioral Medicine, 17*, 225–272.

Loeb, L., & Shane, M. (1982). The resolution of a transsexual wish in a five-year-old boy. *Journal of the American Psychoanalytic Association, 30*, 419–434.

Loeb, L. R. (1992). Analysis of the transference neurosis in a child with transsexual symptoms. *Journal of the American Psychoanalytic Association, 40*, 587–605.

Loehlin, J. C., & Nichols, R. C. (1976). *Heredity, environment, and personality: A study of 850 sets of twins.* Austin: University of Texas Press.

Lothstein, L. M. (1980). The adolescent gender dysphoric patient: An approach to treatment and management. *Journal of Pediatric Psychology, 5*, 93–109.

Lothstein, L. M. (1982). Sex reassignment surgery: Historical, bioethical, and theoretical issues. *American Journal of Psychiatry, 139*, 417–426.

Lothstein, L. M. (1983). *Female-to-male transsexualism: Historical, clinical, and theoretical issues.* Boston: Routledge & Kegan Paul

Lothstein, L. M. (1988). Selfobject failure and gender identity. In A. Goldberg (Ed.), *Frontiers in self psychology* (Vol. 3, pp. 213–235). Hillsdale, NJ: Analytic Press.

Lothstein, L. M. (1992). Clinical management of gender dysphoria in young boys: Genital mutilation and DSM IV implications. *Journal of Psychology and Human Sexuality, 5*, 87–106.

Lothstein, L. M., & Levine, S. B. (1981). Expressive psychotherapy with gender dysphoric patients. *Archives of General Psychiatry, 38*, 924–929.

Lovejoy, J., & Wallen, K. (1988). Sexually dimorphic behavior in group-housed rhesus monkeys *(Macaca mulatta)* at 1 year of age. *Psychobiology, 16*, 348–356.

Lowry, C. B., & Zucker, K. J. (1991, June). *Is there an association between separation anxiety disorder and gender identity disorder in boys?* Poster presented at the meeting of the Society for Research in Child and Adolescent Psychopathology, Zandvoort, The Netherlands.

Lowry Sullivan, C. B., Zucker, K. J., & Bradley, S. J. (1995). [Traits of separation anxiety in boys with gender identity disorder]. Unpublished raw data.

Lukianowicz, N. (1959). Survey of various aspects of transvestism in the light of our present knowledge. *Journal of Nervous and Mental Disease, 128,* 36–64.

Lukianowicz, N. (1962). A rudimentary form of transvestism. *American Journal of Psychotherapy, 16,* 665–675.

Lykken, D. T., McGue, M., & Tellegen, A. (1987). Recruitment bias in twin research: The rule of two-thirds reconsidered. *Behavior Genetics, 17,* 343–362.

Lynn, D. B. (1974). *The father: His role in child development.* Monterey, CA: Brooks/Cole.

Lytton, H., & Romney, D. M. (1991). Parents' differential socialization of boys and girls: A meta-analysis. *Psychological Bulletin, 109,* 267–296.

Maccoby, E. E. (1988). Gender as a social category. *Developmental Psychology, 24,* 755–765.

Maccoby, E. E. (1992). The role of parents in the socialization of children: An historical overview. *Developmental Psychology, 28,* 1006–1017.

Maccoby, E. E., & Jacklin, C. N. (1974). *The psychology of sex differences.* Stanford, CA: Stanford University Press.

Maccoby, E. E., & Jacklin, C. N. (1987). Gender segregation in childhood. *Advances in Child Development and Behavior, 20,* 239–287.

MacCulloch, M. J., & Waddington, J. L. (1981). Neuroendocrine mechanisms and the aetiology of male and female homosexuality. *British Journal of Psychiatry, 139,* 341–345.

MacDonald, M. W. (1938). Criminally aggressive behavior in passive, effeminate boys. *American Journal of Orthopsychiatry, 8,* 70–78.

Macke, J. P., Hu, N., Hu, S., Bailey, M., King, V. L., Brown, T., Hamer, D., & Nathans, J. (1993). Sequence variation in the androgen receptor gene is not a common determinant of male sexual orientation. *American Journal of Human Genetics, 53,* 844–852.

MacLean, P. D. (1962). New findings relevant to the evolution of psychosexual functions of the brain. *Journal of Nervous and Mental Disease, 135,* 289–301.

MacLean, P. D. (1965). New findings relevant to the evolution of psychosexual functions of the brain. In J. Money (Ed.), *Sex research: New developments* (pp. 197–218). New York: Holt, Rinehart & Winston.

MacLean, P. D., & Ploog, D. W. (1962). Cerebral representation of penile erection. *Journal of Neurophysiology, 25,* 29–55.

Maing, D. M. (1991). *Patterns of psychopathology in sexually abused girls.* Unpublished doctoral dissertation, University of Windsor, Windsor, Ontario.

Malitz, S. (1966). Another report on the wearing of diapers and rubber pants by an adult male. *American Journal of Psychiatry, 122,* 1435–1437.

Malyon, A. K. (1981). The homosexual adolescent: Developmental issues and social bias. *Child Welfare, 60,* 321–330.

Mann, V. A., Sasanuma, S., Sakuma, N., & Masaki, S. (1990). Sex differences in cognitive abilities: A cross-cultural perspective. *Neuropsychologia, 28,* 1063–1077.

Marantz, S. A. (1984). *Mothers of extremely feminine boys: Psychopathology and childrearing patterns.* Unpublished doctoral dissertation, New York University.

Marantz, S., & Coates, S. (1991). Mothers of boys with gender identity disorder: A comparison of matched controls. *Journal of the American Academy of Child and Adolescent Psychiatry, 30,* 310–315.

Marchant-Haycox, S. E., McManus, I. C., & Wilson, G. D. (1991). Left-handedness, homosexuality, HIV infection and AIDS. *Cortex, 27,* 49–56.

Marcus, D. E., & Overton, W. F. (1978). The development of cognitive gender constancy and sex role preferences. *Child Development, 49,* 434–444.

Marshall, E. (1995). NIH's "gay gene" study questioned. *Science, 268,* 1841.

Martin, A. D. (1982). Learning to hide: The socialization of the gay adolescent. In S. C. Feinstein (Ed.), *Adolescent psychiatry: Vol. 9. Developmental and clinical studies* (pp. 52–65). Chicago: University of Chicago Press.

Martin, C. L. (1990). Attitudes and expectations about children with nontraditional and traditional gender roles. *Sex Roles, 22,* 151–165.

Martin, C. L. (1991). The role of cognition in understanding gender effects. *Advances in Child Development and Behavior, 23,* 113–149.

Martin, C. L., & Halverson, C. F. (1981). A schematic processing model of sex typing and stereotyping in children. *Child Development, 52,* 1119–1134.

Martin, C. L., & Halverson, C. F. (1987). The role of cognition in sex role acquisition. In D. B. Carter (Ed.), *Current conceptions of sex roles and sex typing: Theory and research* (pp. 123–137). New York: Praeger.

Martin, K. A. (1993). Gender and sexuality: Medical opinion on homosexuality, 1900–1950. *Gender and Society, 7,* 246–260.

Masand, P. S. (1993). Successful treatment of sexual masochism and transvestic fetishism associated with depression with fluoxetine hydrochloride. *Depression, 1,* 50–52.

Masters, M. S., & Sanders, B. (1993). Is the gender difference in mental rotation disappearing? *Behavior Genetics, 23,* 337–341.

Masters, W. H., & Johnson, V. E. (1979). *Homosexuality in perspective.* Boston: Little, Brown.

Matlock, J. (1993). Masquerading women, pathologized men: Cross-dressing, fetishism, and the theory of perversion, 1882–1935. In E. Apter & W. Pietz (Eds.), *Fetishism as cultural discourse* (pp. 31–61). Ithaca, NY: Cornell University Press.

McCauley, E., & Ehrhardt, A. A. (1984). Follow-up of females with gender identity disorders. *Journal of Nervous and Mental Disease, 172,* 353–358.

McConaghy, M. (1979). Gender permanence and the genital basis of gender: Stages in the development of constancy of gender identity. *Child Development, 50,* 1223–1226.

McConaghy, N. (1967). Penile volume change to moving pictures of male and female nudes in heterosexual and homosexual males. *Behaviour Research and Therapy, 5,* 43–48.

McConaghy, N., Armstrong, M. S., Birrell, P. C., & Buhrich, N. (1979). The incidence of bisexual feelings and opposite sex behavior in medical students. *Journal of Nervous and Mental Disease, 167,* 685–688.

McConaghy, N., & Blaszczynski, A. (1980). A pair of monozygotic twins discordant for homosexuality: Sex-dimorphic behavior and penile volume responses. *Archives of Sexual Behavior, 9,* 123–131.

McConaghy, N., & Silove, D. (1991). Opposite sex behaviours correlate with degree of homosexual feelings in the predominantly heterosexual. *Australian and New Zealand Journal of Psychiatry, 25,* 77–83.

McCord, J., McCord, W., & Thurber, E. (1962). Some effects of paternal absence on male children. *Journal of Abnormal and Social Psychology, 64,* 361–369.

McCormick, C. (1990). *A neuropsychological study of sexual orientation: Neurobiological implications.* Unpublished doctoral dissertation, McMaster University, Hamilton, Ontario.

McCormick, C. M., & Witelson, S. F. (1991). A cognitive profile of homosexual men compared to heterosexual men and women. *Psychoneuroendocrinology, 16,* 459–473.

McCormick, C. M., & Witelson, S. F. (1994). Functional cerebral asymmetry and sexual orientation in men and women. *Behavioral Neuroscience, 108,* 525–531.

McCormick, C. M., Witelson, S. F., & Kingstone, E. (1990). Left-handedness in homosexual men and women: Neuroendocrine implications. *Psychoneuroendocrinology, 15,* 69–76.

McDevitt, J. B. (1985, November). *Pre-oedipal determinants of an infantile gender disorder.* Paper presented at the International Symposium on Separation–Individuation and the Roots of Internalization and Identification, Paris.

McGivern, R. F., Raum, W. J., Salido, E., & Redei, E. (1988). Lack of prenatal testosterone surge in fetal rats exposed to alcohol: Alterations in testicular morphology and physiology. *Alcoholism: Clinical and Experimental Research, 12,* 243–247.

McGlone, J. (1980). Sex differences in human brain asymmetry: A critical survey. *Behavioral and Brain Sciences, 3,* 215–263.

McGuire, R. J., Carlisle, J. M., & Young, B. G. (1965). Sexual deviations as conditioned behaviour: A hypothesis. *Behaviour Research and Therapy, 2,* 185–190.

McIntosh, M. (1968). The homosexual role. *Social Problems, 16,* 182–192.

McManus, I. C., Naylor, J., & Booker, B. L. (1990). Left-handedness and myasthenia gravis. *Neuropsychologia, 28,* 947–955.

McNeil, T. F., & Kaij, L. (1979). Etiological relevance of comparisons of high-risk and low-risk groups. *Acta Psychiatrica Scandinavica, 59,* 545–560.

Meaney, M. J., Stewart, J., & Beatty, W. W. (1985). Sex differences in social play: The socialization of sex roles. *Advances in the Study of Behavior, 15,* 1–58.

Memorial for Harry Benjamin. (1988). *Archives of Sexual Behavior, 17,* 1–31.

Mendonica, B. B., Bloise, W., Arnhold, I. J. P., Batista, M. C., de Almeida Toledo, S. P., Drummond, M. C. F., Nicolau, W., & Mattar, E. (1987). Male pseudohermaphroditism due to nonsalt-losing 3-beta-hydroxysteroid dehydrogenase deficiency: Gender role change and absence of gynecomastia at puberty. *Journal of Steroid Biochemistry, 28,* 669–675.

Metcalf, S., & Williams, W. (1977). A case of male childhood transsexualism and its management. *Australian and New Zealand Journal of Psychiatry, 11,* 53–59.

Meulenberg, P. M. M., & Hofman, J. A. (1991). Maternal testosterone and fetal sex. *Journal of Steroid Biochemistry and Molecular Biology, 39,* 51–54.

Meyer, J. K. (1982). The theory of gender identity disorders. *Journal of the American Psychoanalytic Association, 30,* 381–418.

Meyer, J. K., & Dupkin, C. (1985). Gender disturbance in children: An interim clinical report. *Bulletin of the Menninger Clinic, 49,* 236–269.

Meyer, J. K., & Sohmer, B. H. (1983). Gender problems in children. *Drug Therapy, 13,* 43–56.

Meyer, L. S., & Riley, E. P. (1986). Social play in juvenile rats prenatally exposed to alcohol. *Teratology, 34,* 1–7.

Meyer-Bahlburg, H. F. L. (1977). Sex hormones and male homosexuality in comparative perspective. *Archives of Sexual Behavior, 6,* 297–325.

Meyer-Bahlburg, H. F. L. (1979). Sex hormones and female homosexuality: A critical examination. *Archives of Sexual Behavior, 8,* 101–119.

Meyer-Bahlburg, H. F. L. (1982). Hormones and psychosexual differentiation: Implications for the management of intersexuality, homosexuality and transsexuality. *Clinics in Endocrinology and Metabolism, 11,* 681–701.

Meyer-Bahlburg, H. F. L. (1984). Psychoendocrine research on sexual orientation: Current status and future options. *Progress in Brain Research, 61,* 375–398.

Meyer-Bahlburg, H. F. L. (1985). Gender identity disorder of childhood: Introduction. *Journal of the American Academy of Child Psychiatry, 24,* 681–683.

Meyer-Bahlburg, H. F. L. (1990–1991). Can homosexuality in adolescents be "treated" by sex hormones? *Journal of Child and Adolescent Psychopharmacology, 1,* 231–235.

Meyer-Bahlburg, H. F. L. (1993a). Gender identity development in intersex patients. *Child and Adolescent Psychiatric Clinics of North America, 2,* 501–512.

Meyer-Bahlburg, H. F. L. (1993b). Psychobiologic research on homosexuality. *Child and Adolescent Psychiatric Clinics of North America, 2,* 489–500.

Meyer-Bahlburg, H. F. L. (1993c, November). *Gender identity disorder in young boys: A treatment protocol.* Paper presented at the XIII International Symposium on Gender Dysphoria, New York.

Meyer-Bahlburg, H. F. L. (1994). Intersexuality and the diagnosis of gender identity disorder. *Archives of Sexual Behavior, 23,* 21–40.

Meyer-Bahlburg, H. F. L. (1995). Psychoneuroendocrinology and sexual pleasure: The aspect of sexual orientation. In P. R. Abramson & S. D. Pinkerton (Eds.)., *Sexual nature, sexual culture* (pp. 135–153). Chicago: University of Chicago Press.

Meyer-Bahlburg, H. F. L., & Ehrhardt, A. A. (1986). Prenatal diethylstilbestrol exposure: Behavioral consequences in humans. *Monographs in Neural Sciences, 12,* 90–95.

Meyer-Bahlburg, H. F. L., Ehrhardt, A. A., Feldman, J. F., Rosen, L. R., Veridiano, N. P., & Zimmerman, I. (1985). Sexual activity level and sexual functioning in women prenatally exposed to diethylstilbestrol. *Psychosomatic Medicine, 47,* 497–511.

Meyer-Bahlburg, H. F. L., Ehrhardt, A. A., Rosen, L. R., Gruen, R. S., Veridiano, N. P., Vann, P. H., & Neuwalder, H. F. (1995). Prenatal estrogens and the development of homosexual orientation. *Developmental Psychology, 31,* 12–21.

Meyer-Bahlburg, H. F. L., Feldman, J. F., & Ehrhardt, A. A. (1985). Questionnaires for the assessment of atypical gender role behavior: A methodological study. *Journal of the American Academy of Child Psychiatry, 24,* 695–701.

Meyer-Bahlburg, H. F. L., Rotheram-Borus, M. J., Dolezal, C., Rosario, M., Exner, T. M., Gruen, R. S., & Ehrhardt, A. A. (1992, July). *Sexual identity vs. sexual orientation vs. gender of partner among New York City adolescent males.* Paper presented at the meeting of the International Academy of Sex Research, Prague.

Meyer-Bahlburg, H. F. L., Sandberg, D. E., Dolezal, C. L., & Yager, T. J. (1994). Gender-related assessment of childhood play. *Journal of Abnormal Child Psychology, 22,* 643–660.

Meyer-Bahlburg, H. F. L., Sandberg, D. E., Yager, T. J., Dolezal, C. L., & Ehrhardt, A. A. (1994). Questionnaire scales for the assessment of atypical gender development in girls and boys. *Journal of Psychology and Human Sexuality, 6*(4), 19–39.

Miller, B. L., Cummings, J. L., McIntyre, H., Ebers, G., & Grode, M. (1986). Hypersexuality or altered sexual preference following brain injury. *Journal of Neurology, Neurosurgery and Psychiatry, 49,* 867–873.

Minton, H. L. (1986). Femininity in men and masculinity in women: American psychiatry and psychology portray homosexuality in the 1930's. *Journal of Homosexuality, 13,* 1–21.

Minton, H. L. (1988). American psychology and the study of human sexuality. *Journal of Psychology and Human Sexuality, 1,* 17–34.

Mischel, W. (1966). A social-learning view of sex differences in behavior. In E. E. Maccoby (Ed.), *The development of sex differences* (pp. 56–81). Stanford, CA: Stanford University Press.

Mitchell, J. N. (1991). *Maternal influences on gender identity disorder in boys: Searching for specificity.* Unpublished doctoral dissertation, York University, Downsview, Ontario.

Mitchell, J. N., & Zucker, K. J. (1991, August). *The Recalled Childhood Gender Identity Scale: Psychometric properties.* Poster presented at the meeting of the International Academy of Sex Research, Barrie, Ontario.

Mitchell, J. N., Zucker, K. J., Bradley, S. J., & Lowry Sullivan, C. B. (1995). [Maternal influences on boys with gender identity disorder]. Unpublished raw data.

Mitchell, S. A. (1981). The psychoanalytic treatment of homosexuality: Some technical considerations. *International Review of Psychoanalysis, 8,* 63–80.

Mitchell, W., Falconer, M. A., & Hill, D. (1954). Epilepsy with fetishism relieved by temporal lobectomy. *Lancet, ii,* 626–630.

Moll, A. (1891). *Die konträre sexualempfindung.* Berlin: Fischers Medicinische Buchhandlung.

Moll, A. (1919). *The sexual life of the child* (E. Paul, Trans.). New York: Macmillan. (Original work published 1907)

Moller, L. C., Hymel, S., & Rubin, K. H. (1992). Sex typing in play and popularity in middle childhood. *Sex Roles, 26,* 331–353.

Money, J. (1952). *Hermaphroditism: An inquiry into the nature of a human paradox.* Unpublished doctoral dissertation, Harvard University.

Money, J. (1955). Hermaphroditism, gender and precocity in hyperadrenocorticism: Psychologic findings. *Bulletin of the Johns Hopkins Hospital, 96,* 253–264.

Money, J. (1965). Psychologic evaluation of the child with intersex problems. *Pediatrics, 36,* 51–55.

Money, J. (1968). Psychologic approach to psychosexual misidentity with elective mutism: Sex reassignment in two cases of hyperadrenocortical hermaphroditism. *Clinical Pediatrics, 7,* 331–339.

Money, J. (1969). Sex assignment as related to hermaphroditism and transsexualism. In R. Green & J. Money (Eds.), *Transsexualism and sex reassignment* (pp. 91–113). Baltimore: The Johns Hopkins Press.

Money, J. (1970a). Sexual dimorphism and homosexual gender identity. *Psychological Bulletin, 74,* 425–440.

Money, J. (1970b). Matched pairs of hermaphrodites: Behavioral biology of sexual differentiation from chromosomes to gender identity. *Engineering and Science, 33,* 34–39.

Money, J. (1973). Gender role, gender identity, core gender identity: Usage and definition of terms. *Journal of the American Academy of Psychoanalysis, 1,* 397–403.

Money, J. (1975). Ablatio penis: Normal male infant sex-reassigned as a girl. *Archives of Sexual Behavior, 4,* 65–71.

Money, J. (1976a). The development of sexology as a discipline. *Journal of Sex Research, 12,* 83–87.

Money, J. (1976b). Gender identity and hermaphroditism [Letter]. *Science, 191,* 872.

Money, J. (1979). [Letter to the editor]. *Obstetrical and Gynecological Survey, 34,* 770–771.

Money, J. (1981). The development of sexuality and eroticism in humankind. *Quarterly Review of Biology, 56,* 379–404.

Money, J. (1984). Paraphilias: Phenomenology and classification. *American Journal of Psychotherapy, 38,* 164–179.

Money, J. (1985). The conceptual neutering of gender and the criminalization of sex. *Archives of Sexual Behavior, 14,* 279–290.

Money, J. (1987a). Sin, sickness, or status? Homosexual gender identity and psychoneuroendocrinology. *American Psychologist, 42,* 384–399.

Money, J. (1987b). Psychologic considerations in patients with ambisexual development. *Seminars in Reproductive Endocrinology, 5,* 307–313.

Money, J. (1988). *Gay, straight, and in-between: The sexology of erotic orientation.* New York: Oxford University Press.

Money, J. (1991). *Biographies of gender and hermaphroditism in paired comparisons.* Amsterdam: Elsevier.

Money, J. (1993). *The Adam principle. Genes, genitals, hormones, & gender: Selected readings in sexology.* Buffalo, NY: Prometheus Books.

Money, J. (1994a). *Sex errors of the body and related syndromes: A guide to counseling children, adolescents, and their families* (2nd ed.). Baltimore: Paul H. Brookes.

Money, J. (1994b). The concept of gender identity disorder in childhood and adolescence after 39 years. *Journal of Sex and Marital Therapy, 20,* 163–177.

Money, J., & Dalery, J. (1976). Iatrogenic homosexuality: Gender identity in seven 46,XX chromosomal females with hyperadrenocortical hermaphroditism born with a penis, three reared as boys, four reared as girls. *Journal of Homosexuality, 1,* 357–371.

Money, J., Devore, H., & Norman, B. F. (1986). Gender identity and gender transposition: Longitudinal outcome study of 32 male hermaphrodites assigned as girls. *Journal of Sex and Marital Therapy, 12,* 165–181.

Money, J., & Ehrhardt, A. A. (1972). *Man and woman, boy and girl: The differentiation and dimorphism of gender identity from conception to maturity.* Baltimore: The Johns Hopkins Press.

Money, J., & Epstein, R. (1967). Verbal aptitude in eonism and prepubertal effeminacy: A feminine trait. *Transactions of the New York Academy of Sciences, 29,* 448–454.

Money, J., Hampson, J. G., & Hampson, J. L. (1955a). Hermaphroditism: Recommendations concerning assignment of sex, change of sex, and psychologic management. *Bulletin of the Johns Hopkins Hospital, 97,* 284–300.

Money, J., Hampson, J. G., & Hampson, J. L. (1955b). An examination of some basic sexual concepts: The evidence of human hermaphroditism. *Bulletin of the Johns Hopkins Hospital, 97,* 301–319.

Money, J., Hampson, J. G., & Hampson, J. L. (1956). Sexual incongruities and psychopathology: The evidence of human hermaphroditism. *Bulletin of the Johns Hopkins Hospital, 98,* 43–57.

Money, J., Hampson, J. G., & Hampson, J. L. (1957). Imprinting and the establishment of gender role. *Archives of Neurology and Psychiatry, 77,* 333–336.

Money, J., & Lehne, G. K. (1993). Gender-identity disorders. In R. T. Ammerman, C. G. Last, & M. Hersen (Eds.), *Handbook of prescriptive treatments for children and adolescents* (pp. 240–253). Boston: Allyn & Bacon.

Money, J., & Lewis, V. G. (1987). Bisexually concordant, heterosexually and homosexually discordant: A matched-pair comparison of male and female adrenogenital syndrome. *Psychiatry, 50,* 97–111.

Money, J., & Russo, A. J. (1979). Homosexual outcome of discordant gender identity/role in childhood: Longitudinal follow-up. *Journal of Pediatric Psychology, 4,* 29–41.

Money, J., Schwartz, M., & Lewis, V. G. (1984). Adult erotosexual status and fetal hormonal masculinization and demasculinization: 46,XX congenital virilizing adrenal hyperplasia and 46,XY androgen-insensitivity syndrome compared. *Psychoneuroendocrinology, 9,* 405–414.

Moore, K. L., & Barr, M. L. (1955). Smears from the oral mucosa in the detection of chromosomal sex. *Lancet, ii,* 57–58.

Moose, B. J. (1993). *Spatial ability, sexual orientation, self esteem and sexual satisfaction measures in bisexuals, heterosexuals and homosexuals.* Unpublished master's thesis, California State University, Stanislaus, Turlock, CA.

Morgan, K. P., & Ayim, M. (1984). Comment on Bem's "Gender schema theory and its implications for child development: Raising gender-aschematic children in a gender-schematic society." *Signs, 10,* 188–196.

Morin, S., & Schultz, P. (1978). The gay movement and the rights of children. *Journal of Social Issues, 34,* 137–148.

Mowry, B. J., & Levinson, D. F. (1993). Genetic linkage and schizophrenia: Methods, recent findings and future directions. *Australian and New Zealand Journal of Psychiatry, 27,* 200–218.

Mühsam, E. (1921). Der einflusz der kastration der sexualneurotiker. *Deutsche Medizinische Wochenschrift, 6,* 155–156.

Mulaikal, R. M., Migeon, C. J., & Rock, J. A. (1987). Fertility rates in female patients with congenital adrenal hyperplasia due to 21–hydroxylase deficiency. *New England Journal of Medicine, 316,* 178–182.

Müller, M., Kraus-Orlitta, U., Dirlich-Wilhelm, H., & Förster, C. (1983). Motorisches Geschlechtsrollenverhalten bei Mädchen mit adrenogenitalem Syndrom: Eine Beobachtungsstudie zur geschlechtstypischen Körperhaltung [Sex role motor behavior in girls with the adrenogenital syndrome: An observational study on sex-typed posture]. *Zeitschrift für Kinder- und Jugendpsychiatrie, 11,* 100–115.

Myers, M. F. (1982). Counseling the parents of young homosexual male patients. *Journal of Homosexuality, 8,* 131–143.

Myrick, R. D. (1970). The counsellor-consultant and the effeminate boy. *Personnel and Guidance Journal, 48,* 355–361.

Nadler, R. D. (1990). Homosexual behavior in nonhuman primates. In D. P. McWhirter, S. A. Sanders, & J. M. Reinisch (Eds.), *Homosexuality/heterosexuality: Concepts of sexual orientation* (pp. 138–170). New York: Oxford University Press.

Nanda, S. (1990). *Neither man nor woman: The Hijras of India.* Belmont, CA: Wadsworth.

Nash, J. (1965). The father in contemporary culture and current psychological literature. *Child Development, 36,* 261–297.

Nass, R., Baker, S., Speiser, P., Virdis, R., Balsamo, A., Cacciari, E., Loche, A., Dumic, M., & New, M. (1987). Hormones and handedness: Left-hand bias in female congenital adrenal hyperplasia patients. *Neurology, 37,* 711–715.

Neisen, J. (1992). Gender identity disorder of childhood: By whose standard and for what purpose? A response to Rekers and Morey. *Journal of Psychology and Human Sexuality, 5,* 65–67.

Newell-Morris, L. L., Fahrenbruch, C. E., & Sackett, G. P. (1989). Prenatal psychological stress, dermatoglyphic asymmetry and pregnancy outcome in the pigtailed macaque *(Macaca nemestrina)*. *Biology of the Neonate, 56,* 61–75.

Newman, B. S., & Muzzonigro, P. G. (1993). The effects of traditional family values on the coming out process of gay male adolescents. *Adolescence, 28,* 213–226.

Newman, L. E. (1970). Transsexualism in adolescence: Problems in evaluation and treatment. *Archives of General Psychiatry, 23,* 112–121.

Newman, L. E. (1976). Treatment for the parents of feminine boys. *American Journal of Psychiatry, 133,* 683–687.

Nicolosi, J. (1991). *Reparative therapy of male homosexuality: A new clinical approach.* Northvale, NJ: Jason Aronson.

Nieuwenhuijsen, K., Slob, A. K., & van der Werff ten Bosch, J. J. (1988). Gender-related behaviors in group-living stumptail macaques. *Psychobiology, 16,* 357–371.

Nordyke, N. S., Baer, D. M., Etzel, B. C., & LeBlanc, J. M. (1977). Implications of the stereotyping and modification of sex role. *Journal of Applied Behavior Analysis, 10,* 553–557.

Nyborg, H. (1983). Spatial ability in men and women: Review and new theory. *Advances in Behaviour Research and Therapy, 5,* 89–140.

Nyborg, H. (1984). Performance and intelligence in hormonally-different groups. *Progress in Brain Research, 61,* 491–508.

Nye, R. A. (1989a). Sex difference and male homosexuality in French medical discourse, 1830–1930. *Bulletin of the History of Medicine, 63,* 32–51.

Nye, R. A. (1989b). Honor, impotence, and male sexuality in nineteenth-century French medicine. *French Historical Studies, 16,* 48–71.

Nye, R. A. (1991). The history of sexuality in context: National sexological traditions. *Science in Context, 4,* 387–406.

Nye, R. A. (1993). The medical origins of sexual fetishism. In E. Apter & W. Pietz (Eds.), *Fetishism as cultural discourse* (pp. 13–30). Ithaca, NY: Cornell University Press.

O'Brien, M., & Huston, A. C. (1985). Activity level and sex-stereotyped toy choice in toddler boys and girls. *Journal of Genetic Psychology, 146,* 527–533.

O'Donohue, W., & Paud, J. J. (1994). The conditioning of human sexual arousal. *Archives of Sexual Behavior, 23,* 321–344.

Oldfield, R. C. (1971). The assessment and analysis of handedness: The Edinburgh Inventory. *Neuropsychologia, 9,* 97–113.

Ollendick, T. H., & Hersen, M. (Eds.). (1983). *Handbook of child psychopathology.* New York: Plenum Press.

Olsen, K. L. (1992). Genetic influences on sexual behavior differentiation. In A. A. Gerall, H. Moltz, & I. L. Ward (Eds.), *Handbook of behavioral neurobiology: Vol. 11. Sexual differentiation* (pp. 1–40). New York: Plenum Press.

Oomura, Y., Yoshimatsu, H., & Aou, S. (1983). Medial preoptic and hypothalamic neuronal activity during sexual behavior of the male monkey. *Brain Research, 266,* 340–343.

Oppenheimer, A. (1991). The wish for a sex change: A challenge to psychoanalysis? *International Journal of Psycho-Analysis, 72,* 221–231.

Orlebeke, J. F., Boomsma, D. I., Gooren, L. J. G., Verschoor, A. M., & van den Bree, M. J. M. (1992). Elevated sinistrality in transsexuals. *Neuropsychology, 6,* 351–355.

Orvaschel, H. (1989). Diagnostic interviews for children and adolescents. In C. G. Last & M. Hersen (Eds.), *Handbook of child psychiatric diagnosis* (pp. 483–495). New York: Wiley.

Ovesey, L., & Person, E. (1976). Transvestism: A disorder of the sense of self. *International Journal of Psychoanalytic Psychotherapy, 5,* 219–235.

Owen, W. F. (1985). Medical problems of the homosexual adolescent. *Journal of Adolescent Health Care, 6,* 178–185.

Padgug, R. A. (1979). Sexual matters: On conceptualizing sexuality in history. *Radical History Review, 20,* 3–23.

Pagon, R. A. (1987). Diagnostic approach to the newborn with ambiguous genitalia. *Pediatric Clinics of North America, 34,* 1019–1031.

Paluszny, M., Beit-Hallahmi, B., Catford, J. C., Cooley, R. E., Dull, C. Y., & Guiora, A. Z. (1973). Gender identity and its measurement in children. *Comprehensive Psychiatry, 14,* 281–290.

Pandita-Gunawardena, R. (1990). Paraphilic infantilism: A rare case of fetishistic behaviour. *British Journal of Psychiatry, 157,* 767–770.

Paoletti, J. B. (1983). Clothes make the boy, 1860–1910. *Dress, 9,* 16–20.

Paoletti, J. B. (1987). Clothing and gender in America: Children's fashions, 1890–1920. *Signs, 13,* 136–143.

Paoletti, J. B., & Thompson, S. (1987, May). *Gender differences in infants' rompers, 1910–1930.* Paper presented at the meeting of the Costume Society of America, Richmond, VA.

Pare, C. M. B. (1956). Homosexuality and chromosomal sex. *Journal of Psychosomatic Research, 1,* 247–251.

Pare, C. M. B. (1965). Etiology of homosexuality: Genetic and chromosomal aspects. In J. Marmor (Ed.), *Sexual inversion: The multiple roots of homosexuality* (pp. 70–80). New York: Basic Books.

Parkes, C. M. (1975). *Bereavement: Studies of grief in adult life.* Harmondsworth, England: Penguin Books.

Pascual-Leone, J., & Morra, S. (1991). Horizontality of water level: A neo-Piagetian developmental review. *Advances in Child Development and Behavior, 23,* 231–276.

Pattatucci, A. M. L., & Hamer, D. H. (in press). Development and familiality of sexual orientation in females. *Behavior Genetics.*

Pattatucci, A. M. L., Patterson, C., Benjamin, J., & Hamer, D. H. (1995). *A re-*

ciprocal interaction between sex, sexual orientation and handedness. Manuscript submitted for publication.

Patterson, C. J. (1992). Children of lesbian and gay parents. *Child Development, 63,* 1025–1042.

Paul, J. P. (1993). Childhood cross-gender behavior and adult homosexuality: The resurgence of biological models of sexuality. *Journal of Homosexuality, 24,* 41–54.

Pauly, I. B. (1974). Female transsexualism: Part I. *Archives of Sexual Behavior, 3,* 487–507.

Pauly, I. B. (1992). Terminology and classification of gender identity disorders. *Journal of Psychology and Human Sexuality, 5,* 1–14.

Pauly, I. B., & Edgerton, M. T. (1986). The gender identity movement: A growing surgical–psychiatric liaison. *Archives of Sexual Behavior, 15,* 315–329.

Pellegrini, A. D. (1989). What is a category? The case of rough-and-tumble play. *Ethology and Sociobiology, 10,* 331–341.

Pellett, T. L., & Harrison, J. M. (1992). Children's perceptions of the gender appropriateness of physical activities: A further analysis. *Play and Culture, 5,* 305–313.

Perachio, A. A., Marr, L. D., & Alexander, M. (1979). Sexual behavior in male rhesus monkeys elicited by electrical stimulation of preoptic and hypothalamic areas. *Brain Research, 177,* 127–144.

Perelle, I. B., & Ehrman, L. (1994). An international study of human handedness: The data. *Behavior Genetics, 24,* 217–227.

Pérez-Palacios, G., Chávez, B., Méndez, J. P., Imperato-McGinley, J., & Ulloa-Aguirre, A. (1987). The syndromes of androgen resistance revisited. *Journal of Steroid Biochemistry, 27,* 1101–1108.

Perilstein, R. D., Lipper, S., & Friedman, L. J. (1991). Three cases of paraphilias responsive to fluoxetine treatment. *Journal of Clinical Psychiatry, 52,* 169–170.

Perry, M. E. (1987). The manly woman: A historical case study. *American Behavioral Scientist, 31,* 86–100.

Person, E., & Ovesey, L. (1974a). The transsexual syndrome in males: I. Primary transsexualism. *American Journal of Psychotherapy, 28,* 4–20.

Person, E., & Ovesey, L. (1974b). The transsexual syndrome in males: II. Secondary transsexualism. *American Journal of Psychotherapy, 28,* 174–193.

Person, E., & Ovesey, L. (1978). Transvestism: New perspectives. *Journal of the American Academy of Psychoanalysis, 6,* 301–323.

Person, E. S., & Ovesey, L. (1983). Psychoanalytic theories of gender identity. *Journal of the American Academy of Psychoanalysis, 11,* 203–226.

Person, E. S., & Ovesey, L. (1984). Homosexual cross-dressers. *Journal of the American Academy of Psychoanalysis, 12,* 167–186.

Peterson, M. E., & Dickey, R. (1995). Surgical sex reassignment: A comparative survey of international centers. *Archives of Sexual Behavior, 24,* 135–156.

Pfäfflin, F., & Junge, A. (1992). *Geschlechts-umwandlung: Abhandlungen zur transsexualität.* New York: Schattauer.

Philippopoulos, G. S. (1964). A case of transvestism in a 17-year-old girl: Psychopathology–psychodynamics. *Acta Psychotherapeutica, 12,* 29–37.

Phoenix, C. H., Goy, R. W., Gerall, A. A., & Young, W. C. (1959). Organizing action of prenatally administered testosterone propionate on the tissues mediating mating behavior in the female guinea pig. *Endocrinology, 65,* 369–382.

Picariello, M. L., Greenberg, D. N., & Pillemer, D. B. (1990). Children's sex-related stereotyping of colors. *Child Development, 61,* 1453–1460.

Pillard, R. C. (1990). The Kinsey scale: Is it familial? In D. P. McWhirter, S. A. Sanders, & J. M. Reinisch (Eds.), *Homosexuality/heterosexuality: Concepts of sexual orientation* (pp. 88–100). New York: Oxford University Press.

Pillard, R. C., Poumadere, J., & Carretta, R. A. (1982). A family study of sexual orientation. *Archives of Sexual Behavior, 11,* 511–520.

Pillard, R. C., & Weinrich, J. D. (1986). Evidence of familial nature of male homosexuality. *Archives of General Psychiatry, 43,* 808–812.

Pleak, R. R. (1991, October). *Treating gender-disturbed children: Ethical issues.* Paper presented at the meeting of the American Academy of Child and Adolescent Psychiatry, San Francisco.

Pleak, R. R., & Anderson, D. A. (1993, June). *Group psychotherapy for parents of boys with gender identity disorder of childhood.* Poster presented at the meeting of the International Academy of Sex Research, Pacific Grove, CA.

Pleak, R. R., Meyer-Bahlburg, H. F. L., O'Brien, J. D., Bowen, H. A., & Morganstein, A. (1989). Cross-gender behavior and psychopathology in boy psychiatric outpatients. *Journal of the American Academy of Child and Adolescent Psychiatry, 28,* 385–393.

Pleak, R. R., Sandberg, D. E., Hirsch, G. S., & Anderson, D. A. (1991, October). *Cross-gender behavior in boy psychiatric patients: Replication and reinterpretation.* Paper presented at the meeting of the American Academy of Child and Adolescent Psychiatry, San Francisco.

Plomin, R. (1983). Childhood temperament. In B. B. Lahey & A. E. Kazdin (Eds.), *Advances in clinical child psychology* (Vol. 6, pp. 45–92). New York: Plenum Press.

Plomin, R. (1994). *Genetics and experience: The interplay between nature and nurture.* Thousand Oaks, CA: Sage.

Plomin, R., & Daniels, D. (1987). Why are children in the same family so different from one another? *Behavioral and Brain Sciences, 10,* 1–60.

Plomin, R., & Rende, R. (1991). Human behavioral genetics. *Annual Review of Psychology, 42,* 161–190.

Polani, P. E., & Adinolfi, M. (1983). The H-Y antigen and its functions: A review and a hypothesis. *Journal of Immunogenetics, 10,* 85–102.

Pomerantz, S. M., Roy, M. M., & Goy, R. W. (1988). Social and hormonal influences on behavior of adult male, female, and pseudohermaphroditic rhesus monkeys. *Hormones and Behavior, 22,* 219–230.

Post, R. M., Weiss, S. R. B., Uhde, T. W., Clark, M., & Rosen, J. B. (1993). Implications of cocaine kindling, induction of the proto-oncogene c-fos, and contingent tolerance. In H. Hoehn-Saric & D. R. McLeod (Eds.), *Progress in psychiatry: Biology of anxiety disorders* (pp. 121–175). Washington, DC: American Psychiatric Press.

Poulin-Dubois, D., Serbin, L. A., Kenyon, B., & Derbyshire, A. (1994). Infants' intermodal knowledge about gender. *Developmental Psychology, 30,* 436–442.

Power, T. G. (1981). Sex-typing in infancy: The role of the father. *Infant Mental Health Journal, 2,* 226–240.

Prenzlauer, S., Drescher, J., & Winchel, R. (1992). Suicide among homosexual youth [Letter to the editor]. *American Journal of Psychiatry, 149,* 1416.

Prior, M. (1992). Childhood temperament. *Journal of Child Psychology and Psychiatry, 33,* 249–279.

Prince, V., & Bentler, P. M. (1972). Survey of 504 cases of transvestism. *Psychological Reports, 31,* 903–917.

Pritchard, M. (1962). Homosexuality and genetic sex. *Journal of Mental Science, 108,* 616–623.

Pruett, K. D., & Dahl, E. K. (1982). Psychotherapy of gender identity conflict in young boys. *Journal of the American Academy of Child Psychiatry, 21,* 65–70.

Quadagno, D. M., Briscoe, R., & Quadagno, J. S. (1977). Effects of perinatal gonadal hormones on selected nonsexual behavior patterns: A critical assessment of the nonhuman and human literature. *Psychological Bulletin, 84,* 62–80.

Quinton, D., & Rutter, M. (1975). Early hospital admissions and later disturbances of behaviour: An attempted replication of Douglas' findings. *Developmental Medicine and Child Neurology, 18,* 447–459.

Rachman, S. (1966). Sexual fetishism: An experimental analog. *Psychological Record, 16,* 293–296.

Rainbow, S. (1986). *Male childhood gender identity disorder and separation anxiety disorder: An initial comparison.* Unpublished doctoral dissertation, Yeshiva University.

Randell, J. B. (1959). Transvestitism and trans-sexualism: A study of 50 cases. *British Medical Journal, ii,* 1448–1452.

Raymond, J. G. (1979). *The transsexual empire: The making of the she-male.* Boston: Beacon Press.

Reinisch, J. M., Rosenblum, L. A., & Sanders, S. A. (Eds.). (1987). *Masculinity/femininity: Basic perspectives.* New York: Oxford University Press.

Reinisch, J. M., & Sanders, S. A. (1992). Prenatal hormonal contributions to sex differences in human cognitive and personality development. In A. A. Gerall, H. Moltz, & I. L. Ward (Eds.), *Handbook of behavioral neurobiology: Vol. 11. Sexual differentiation* (pp. 221–243). New York: Plenum Press.

Reinisch, J. M., Ziemba-Davis, M., & Sanders, S. A. (1991). Hormonal contributions to sexually dimorphic behavioral development in humans. *Psychoneuroendocrinology, 16,* 213–278.

Reiss, D., Plomin, R., & Hetherington, E. M. (1991). Genetics and psychiatry: An unheralded window on the environment. *American Journal of Psychiatry, 148,* 283–291.

Rekers, G. A. (1972). *Pathological sex-role development in boys: Behavioral treatment and assessment.* Unpublished doctoral dissertation, University of California at Los Angeles.

Rekers, G. A. (1975). Stimulus control over sex-typed play in cross-gender identified boys. *Journal of Experimental Child Psychology, 20,* 136–148.

Rekers, G. A. (1977a). Assessment and treatment of childhood gender problems. In B. B. Lahey & A. E. Kazdin (Eds.), *Advances in clinical child psychology* (Vol. 1, pp. 267–306). New York: Plenum Press.

Rekers, G. A. (1977b). Atypical gender development and psychosocial adjustment. *Journal of Applied Behavior Analysis, 10,* 559–571.

Rekers, G. A. (1979). Sex-role behavior change: Intrasubject studies of boyhood gender disturbance. *Journal of Psychology, 103,* 255–269.

Rekers, G. A. (1982a). *Growing up straight: What every family should know about homosexuality.* Chicago: Moody Press.

Rekers, G. A. (1982b). *Shaping your child's sexual identity.* Grand Rapids, MI: Baker Book House.

Rekers, G. A. (1985). Gender identity problems. In P. A. Bornstein & A. E. Kazdin (Eds.), *Handbook of clinical behavior therapy with children* (pp. 658–699). Homewood, IL: Dorsey Press.

Rekers, G. A. (1986). Inadequate sex role differentiation in childhood: The family and gender identity disorders. *Journal of Family and Culture, 2,* 8–37.

Rekers, G. A., Amaro-Plotkin, H. D., & Low, B. P. (1977). Sex-typed mannerisms in normal boys and girls as a function of sex and age. *Child Development, 48,* 275–278.

Rekers, G. A., Bentler, P. M., Rosen, A. C., & Lovaas, O. I. (1977). Child gender disturbances: A clinical rationale for intervention. *Psychotherapy: Theory, Research, and Practice 14,* 2–11.

Rekers, G. A., Crandall, B. F., Rosen, A. C., & Bentler, P. M. (1979). Genetic and physical studies of male children with psychological gender disturbances. *Psychological Medicine, 9,* 373–375.

Rekers, G. A., & Kilgus, M. D. (1995). Differential diagnosis and rationale for treatment of gender identity disorders and transvestism. In G. A. Rekers (Ed.), *Handbood of child and adolescent sexual problems* (pp. 255–271). New York: Lexington Books.

Rekers, G. A., Kilgus, M., & Rosen, A. C. (1990). Long-term effects of treatment for gender identity disorder of childhood. *Journal of Psychology and Human Sexuality, 3,* 121–153.

Rekers, G. A., & Lovaas, O. I. (1974). Behavioral treatment of deviant sex-role behaviors in a male child. *Journal of Applied Behavior Analysis, 7,* 173–190.

Rekers, G. A., Lovaas, O. I., & Low, B. (1974). The behavioral treatment of a "transsexual" preadolescent boy. *Journal of Abnormal Child Psychology, 2,* 99–116.

Rekers, G. A., & Mead, S. (1979). Early intervention for female sexual identity disturbance: Self-monitoring of play behavior. *Journal of Abnormal Child Psychology, 7,* 405–423.

Rekers, G. A., Mead, S. L., Rosen, A. C., & Brigham, S. L. (1983). Family correlates of male childhood gender disturbance. *Journal of Genetic Psychology, 142,* 31–42.

Rekers, G. A., & Morey, S. M. (1989a). Sex-typed body movements as a function of severity of gender disturbance in boys. *Journal of Psychology and Human Sexuality, 2,* 183–196.

Rekers, G. A., & Morey, S. M. (1989b). Relationship of maternal report of feminine behaviors and extraversion to clinician's rating of gender disturbance. *Perceptual and Motor Skills, 69,* 387–394.

Rekers, G. A., & Morey, S. M. (1989c). Personality problems associated with childhood gender disturbance. *Italian Journal of Clinical and Cultural Psychology, 1,* 85–90.

Rekers, G. A., & Morey, S. M. (1990). The relationship of measures of sex-typed play with clinician ratings of degree of gender disturbance. *Journal of Clinical Psychology, 46,* 28–34.

Rekers, G. A., Rosen, A. C., & Morey, S. M. (1990). Projective test findings for boys with gender disturbance: Draw-a-Person test, IT scale, and Make-a-Picture Story test. *Perceptual and Motor Skills, 71,* 771–779.

Rekers, G. A., & Swihart, J. J. (1989). The association of gender identity disorder with parental separation. *Psychological Reports, 65,* 1272–1274.

Rekers, G. A., & Varni, J. W. (1977a). Self-monitoring and self-reinforcement processes in a pre-transsexual boy. *Behaviour Research and Therapy, 15,* 177–180.

Rekers, G. A., & Varni, J. W. (1977b). Self-regulation of gender-role behaviors: A case study. *Journal of Behavior Therapy and Experimental Psychiatry, 8,* 427–432.

Rekers, G. A., Willis, T. J., Yates, C. E., Rosen, A. C., & Low, B. P. (1977). Assessment of childhood gender behavior change. *Journal of Child Psychology and Psychiatry, 18,* 53–65.

Rekers, G. A., & Yates, C. E. (1976). Sex-typed play in feminoid boys vs. normal boys and girls. *Journal of Abnormal Child Psychology, 4,* 1–8.

Rekers, G. A., Yates, C. E., Willis, T. J., Rosen, A. C., & Taubman, M. (1976). Childhood gender identity change: Operant control over sex-typed play and mannerisms. *Journal of Behavior Therapy and Experimental Psychiatry, 7,* 51–57.

Remafedi, G. (1987a). Adolescent homosexuality: Psychosocial and medical implications. *Pediatrics, 79,* 331–337.

Remafedi, G. (1987b). Male homosexuality: The adolescent's perspective. *Pediatrics, 79,* 326–330.

Remafedi, G., Farrow, J. A., & Deisher, R. W. (1991). Risk factors for attempted suicide in gay and bisexual youth. *Pediatrics, 87,* 869–875.

Remafedi, G., Resnick, M., Blum, R., & Harris, L. (1992). Demography of sexual orientation in adolescents. *Pediatrics, 89,* 714–721.

Rembar, J., Novick, J., & Kalter, N. (1982). Attrition among families of divorce: Patterns in an outpatient psychiatric population. *Journal of the American Academy of Child Psychiatry, 21,* 409–413.

Renik, O., Spielman, P., & Afterman, J. (1978). Bamboo phobia in an eighteen-month-old boy. *Journal of the American Psychoanalytic Association, 26,* 255–282.

Resnick, S. M., Berenbaum, S. A., Gottesman, I. I., & Bouchard, T. J. (1986). Early hormonal influences on cognitive functioning in congenital adrenal hyperplasia. *Developmental Psychology, 22,* 191–198.

Rich, C. L., Fowler, R. C., Young, D., & Blankush, M. (1986). San Diego Suicide Study: Comparison of gay to straight males. *Suicide and Life-Threatening Behavior, 16,* 448–457.

Richters, J. E. (1992). Depressed mothers as informants about their children: A critical review of the evidence for distortion. *Psychological Bulletin, 112,* 485–499.

Rigg, C. A. (1982). Homosexuality in adolescence. *Pediatric Annals, 11,* 826–829.

Risch, N., Squires-Wheeler, E., & Keats, B. J. B. (1993). Male sexual orientation and genetic evidence. *Science, 262,* 2063–2065.

Risman, B. J. (1982). The (mis)acquisition of gender identity among transsexuals. *Qualitative Sociology, 5,* 312–325.

Roberts, C. W., Green, R., Williams, K., & Goodman, M. (1987). Boyhood gender identity development: A statistical contrast of two family groups. *Developmental Psychology, 23,* 544–557.

Robins, L. N., Helzer, J. E., Croughan, J., & Ratcliff, K. S. (1981). National Institute of Mental Health Diagnostic Interview Schedule. *Archives of General Psychiatry, 38,* 381–389.

Robinson, B. E., Walters, L. H., & Skeen, P. (1989). Response of parents to learning that their child is homosexual and concern over AIDS: A national study. In F. W. Bozett (Ed.), *Homosexuality and the family* (pp. 59–80). New York: Haworth Press.

Roesler, T., & Deisher, R. W. (1972). Youthful male homosexuality. *Journal of the American Medical Association, 219,* 1018–1023.

Rogers, L., & Walsh, J. (1982). Shortcomings of the psychomedical research of John Money and co-workers into sex differences in behavior: Social and political implications. *Sex Roles, 8,* 269–281.

Rogers, S. M., & Turner, C. F. (1991). Male-male sexual contact in the U.S.A.: Findings from five sample surveys, 1970–1990. *Journal of Sex Research, 28,* 491–519.

Rohde, W., Uebelhack, R., & Dörner, G. (1986). Neuroendocrine response to oestrogen in transsexual men. *Monographs in Neural Sciences, 12,* 75–78.

Roiphe, H., & Galenson, E. (1981). *Infantile origins of sexual identity.* New York: International Universities Press.

Roiphe, H., & Spira, N. (1991). Object loss, aggression, and gender identity. *Psychoanalytic Study of the Child, 46,* 37–50.

Roscoe, W. (1991). *The Zuni man–woman.* Albuquerque: University of New Mexico Press.

Rosen, A. C., & Rekers, G. A. (1980). Toward a taxonomic framework for variables of sex and gender. *Genetic Psychology Monographs, 102,* 191–218.

Rosen, A. C., Rekers, G. A., & Brigham, S. L. (1982). Gender stereotypy in gender-dysphoric young boys. *Psychological Reports, 51,* 371–374.

Rosen, A. C., Rekers, G. A., & Friar, L. R. (1977). Theoretical and diagnostic issues in child gender disturbances. *Journal of Sex Research, 13,* 89–103.

Rosen, A. C., & Teague, J. (1974). Case studies in the development of masculinity and femininity in male children. *Psychological Reports, 34,* 971–983.

Rosen, R. C., & Beck, J. G. (1988). *Patterns of sexual arousal: Psychophysiological processes and clinical applications.* New York: Guilford Press.

Rosenblum, L. A. (1990). Primates, homo sapiens, and homosexuality. In D. P. McWhirter, S. A. Sanders, & J. M. Reinisch (Eds.), *Homosexuality/heterosexuality: Concepts of sexual orientation* (pp. 171–174). New York: Oxford University Press.

Rosenstein, L. D., & Bigler, E. D. (1987). No relationship between handedness and sexual preference. *Psychological Reports, 60,* 704–706.

Rosenthal, D. (1970). *Genetic theory and abnormal behavior.* New York: McGraw-Hill.

Rösler, A., & Kohn, G. (1983). Male pseudohermaphroditism due to 17-beta-hydroxysteroid dehydrogenase deficiency: Studies on the natural history of the defect and effect of androgens on gender role. *Journal of Steroid Biochemistry, 19,* 663–674.

Ross, M. W. (1983). *The married homosexual man: A psychological study.* Boston: Routledge & Kegan Paul.

Rotheram-Borus, M. J., Rosario, M, & Hunter, J. (in press). Suicidal behavior and gay-related stress among gay and bisexual male adolescents in New York City. *Journal of Adolescent Research.*

Routh, D. K., Walton, M. D., & Padan-Belkin, E. (1978). Development of activity level in children revisited: Effects of mother presence. *Developmental Psychology, 14,* 571–581.

Rowe, D. C., & Plomin, R. (1977). Temperament in early childhood. *Journal of Personality Assessment, 41,* 150–156.

Ruan, F., & Bullough, V. L. (1988). The first case of transsexual surgery in mainland China. *Journal of Sex Research, 25,* 546–547.

Ruan, F., Bullough, V. L., & Tsai, Y. (1989). Male transsexualism in mainland China. *Archives of Sexual Behavior, 18,* 517–522.

Rubin, R. T., Reinisch, J. M., & Haskett, R. F. (1981). Postnatal gonadal steroid effects on human behavior. *Science, 211,* 1318–1324.

Ruse, M. (1981). Are there gay genes?: Sociobiology and homosexuality. *Journal of Homosexuality, 6,* 5–34.

Rutter, M. (1978). Diagnostic validity in child psychiatry. *Advances in Biological Psychiatry, 2,* 2–22.

Sack, W. H. (1985). Gender identity conflict in young boys following divorce. *Journal of Divorce, 9,* 47–59.

Sackin, H. D. (1985). *Cross-dressing and fetishism in childhood: The analysis of a five-year-old magician.* Unpublished manuscript, Hospital for Sick Children, Toronto.

Sagarin, E. (1975). Sex rearing and sexual orientation: The reconciliation of apparently contradictory data. *Journal of Sex Research, 11,* 329–334.

Saghir, M. T., & Robins, E. (1973). *Male and female homosexuality: A comprehensive investigation.* Baltimore: Williams & Wilkins.

Salessi, J. (1994). The Argentine dissemination of homosexuality, 1890–1914. *Journal of the History of Sexuality, 4,* 337–368.

Sameroff, A. (1975). Transactional models in early social relations. *Human Development, 18,* 65–79.

Sandberg, D. E., & Meyer-Bahlburg, H. F. L. (1994). Variability in middle childhood play behavior: Effects of gender, age, and family background. *Archives of Sexual Behavior, 23,* 645–663.

Sandberg, D. E., Meyer-Bahlburg, H. F. L., Ehrhardt, A. A., & Yager, T. J. (1993). The prevalence of gender-atypical behavior in elementary school children. *Journal of the American Academy of Child and Adolescent Psychiatry, 32,* 306–314.

Sanders, G., & Ross-Field, L. (1986a). Sexual orientation and visuo-spatial ability. *Brain and Cognition, 5,* 280–290.

Sanders, G., & Ross-Field, L. (1986b). Sexual orientation, cognitive abilities and cerebral asymmetry: A review and a hypothesis tested. *Italian Journal of Zoology, 20,* 459–470.

Sanders, G., & Wright, M. (1993, June). *Sexual orientation differences in targeted throwing and manual dexterity tasks.* Poster presented at the meeting of the International Academy of Sex Research, Pacific Grove, CA.

Satz, P., Miller, E. N., Selnes, O., Van Gorp, W., D'Elia, L. F., & Visscher, B. (1991). Hand preference in homosexual men. *Cortex, 27,* 295–306.

Saudino, K. J., & Eaton, W. O. (1991). Infant temperament and genetics: An objective twin study of motor activity level. *Child Development, 62,* 1167–1174.

Saudino, K. J., & Eaton, W. O. (1995). Continuity and change in objectively assessed temperament: A longitudinal twin study of activity level. *British Journal of Developmental Psychology, 13,* 81–85.

Saunders, J. M., & Valente, S. M. (1987). Suicide risk among gay men and lesbians: A review. *Death Studies, 11,* 1–23.

Savin-Williams, R. C. (1989). Coming out to parents and self-esteem among gay and lesbian youth. In F. W. Bozett (Ed.), *Homosexuality and the family* (pp. 1–35). New York: Haworth Press.

Savin-Williams, R. C. (1990). *Gay and lesbian youth: Expressions of identity.* New York: Hemisphere.

Schachter, S. C. (1994). Handedness in women with intrauterine exposure to diethylstilbestrol. *Neuropsychologia, 32,* 619–623.

Scharfman, M. A. (1976). Perverse development in a young boy. *Journal of the American Psychoanalytic Association, 24,* 499–524.

Schlegel, W. S. (1962). Die konstitutionsbiologischen Grundlagen der Homosexualität. *Zeitschrift für Menschlich Vererbungsforschung und Konstitutionslehre, 36,* 341–364.

Schmidt, G., & Clement, U. (1990). Does peace prevent homosexuality? [Letter to the editor]. *Archives of Sexual Behavior, 19,* 183–187.

Schneider, M. L. (1992). The effect of mild stress during pregnancy on birthweight and neuromotor maturation in rhesus monkey infants *(Macaca mulatta). Infant Behavior and Development, 15,* 389–403.

Schneider, M. S. (1988). *Often invisible: Counselling gay and lesbian youth.* Toronto: Central Toronto Youth Services.

Schneider, S. G., Farberow, N. L., & Kruks, G. (1989). Suicidal behavior in adolescent and adult gay men. *Suicide and Life-Threatening Behavior, 19,* 381–394.

Schoettle, U. C., & Cantwell, D. P. (1980). Children of divorce: Demographic variables, symptoms, and diagnoses. *Journal of the American Academy of Child Psychiatry, 19,* 453–475.

Schrut, A. (1987, December). *Parent–child interaction and the development of gender identity and sexual partner choice.* Paper presented at the meeting of the American Academy of Psychoanalysis, Phoenix, AZ.

Schultz, N. M. (1979). *Severe gender identity confusion in an eight-year-old boy.* Unpublished doctoral dissertation, Yeshiva University.

Scott, W. A. (1958). Research definitions of mental health and mental illness. *Psychological Bulletin, 55,* 29–45.

Sears, R. R., Maccoby, E. E., & Levin, H. (1957). *Patterns of child rearing.* Stanford, CA: Stanford University Press.

Sears, R. R., Rau, L., & Alpert, R. (1965). *Identification and child rearing.* Stanford, CA: Stanford University Press.

Sedgwick, E. K. (1991). How to bring your kids up gay. *Social Text, 9,* 18–27.

Serbin, L. A. (1980). Sex-role socialization: A field in transition. In B. B. Lahey & A. E. Kazdin (Eds.), *Advances in clinical child psychology* (Vol. 3, pp. 41–96). New York: Plenum Press.

Serbin, L. A., & Connor, J. M. (1979). Sex-typing of children's play preferences and patterns of cognitive performance. *Journal of Genetic Psychology, 134,* 315–316.

Serbin, L. A., Powlishta, K. K., & Gulko, J. (1993). The development of sex typing in middle childhood. *Monographs of the Society for Research in Child Development, 58*(2, Serial No. 232).

Serbin, L. A., Zelkowitz, P., Doyle, A., Gold, D., & Wheaton, B. (1990). The socialization of sex-differentiated skills and academic performance: A mediational model. *Sex Roles, 23,* 613–628.

Seyler, L. E., Canalis E., Spare, S., & Reichlin, S. (1978). Abnormal gonadotropin secretory responses to LRH in transsexual women after diethylstilbestrol priming. *Journal of Clinical Endocrinology and Metabolism, 47,* 176–183.

Shaffer, D., Schwab-Stone, M., Fisher, P., Cohen, P., Piacentini, J., Davies, M., Conners, C. K., & Regier, D. (1993). The Diagnostic Interview Schedule for Children–Revised Version (DISC-R): I. Preparation, field testing, interrater reliability, and acceptability. *Journal of the American Academy of Child and Adolescent Psychiatry, 32,* 643–650.

Shakin, M., Shakin, D., & Sternglanz, S. H. (1985). Infant clothing: Sex labeling for strangers. *Sex Roles, 12,* 955–964.

Shane, M., & Shane, E. (1995). Clinical perspectives on gender role/identity disorder. *Psychoanalytic Inquiry, 15,* 39–59.

Shankel, L. W., & Carr, A. C. (1956). Transvestism and hanging episodes in a male adolescent. *Psychiatric Quarterly, 30,* 478–493.

Shearman, R. P. (1982). Intersexuality. In P. J. V. Beumont & G. D. Burrows (Eds.), *Handbook of psychiatry and endocrinology* (pp. 325–354). Amsterdam: Elsevier.

Sherman, J. A. (1978). *Sex-related cognitive differences.* Springfield, IL: Charles C Thomas.

Sherman, R. F. (1985). *Separation conflict as a component of severe gender identity confusion in schoolage boys.* Unpublished doctoral dissertation, Adelphi University.

Siegel, E. V. (1988). *Female homosexuality: Choice without volition.* Hillsdale, NJ: Analytic Press.

Siegel, E. V. (1991). *Middle-class waifs: The psychodynamic treatment of affectively disturbed children.* Hillsdale, NJ: Analytic Press.

Siegelman, M. (1974). Parental backgrounds of male homosexuals and heterosexuals. *Archives of Sexual Behavior, 3,* 3–19.

Siegelman, M. (1981). Parental backgrounds of homosexual and heterosexual men: A cross national replication. *Archives of Sexual Behavior, 10,* 506–512.

Signorella, M., & Jamison, W. (1986). Masculinity, femininity, androgyny, and cognitive performance: A meta-analysis. *Psychological Bulletin, 100,* 207–228.

Signorella, M. L. (1987). Gender schemata: Individual differences and contextual effects. In L. S. Liben & M. L. Signorella (Eds.). *Children's gender schemata* (pp. 23–27). San Francisco: Jossey-Bass.

Signorella, M. L., Bigler, R. S., & Liben, L. S. (1993). Developmental differences in children's gender schemata about others: A meta-analytic review. *Developmental Review, 13,* 147–183.

Silverman, M. A. (1990). The prehomosexual boy in treatment. In C. W. Socarides & V. D. Volkan (Eds.), *The homosexualities: Reality, fantasy, and the arts* (pp. 177–197). Madison, CT: International Universities Press.

Silverman, W. K. (1991). Diagnostic reliability of anxiety disorders in children using structured interviews. *Journal of Anxiety Disorders, 5,* 105–124.

Skilbeck, W. M., Bates, J. E., & Bentler, P. M. (1975). Human figure drawings of gender-problem and school-problem boys. *Journal of Abnormal Child Psychology, 3,* 191–199.

Slaby, R. G., & Frey, K. S. (1975). Development of gender constancy and selective attention to same-sex models. *Child Development, 46,* 849–856.

Slater, E. (1958). The sibs and children of homosexuals. In D. R. Smith & W. M. Davidson (Eds.), *Symposium on nuclear sex* (pp. 79–83). London: Heinemann Medical Books.

Slater, E. (1962). Birth order and maternal age of homosexuals. *Lancet, i,* 69–71.

Slijper, F. M. E. (1984). Androgens and gender role behaviour in girls with congenital adrenal hyperplasia (CAH). *Progress in Brain Research, 61,* 417–422.

Slijper, F. M. E., van der Kamp, H. J., Brandenburg, H., de Muinck Keizer-Schrama, S. M. P. F., Drop, S. L. S., & Molenaar, J. C. (1992). Evaluation of psychosexual development of young women with CAH: A pilot study. In W. Bezemer, P. Cohen-Kettenis, K. Slob, & N. van Son-Schoones (Eds.), *Sex matters* (pp. 47–50). Amsterdam: Elsevier.

Slimp, J. C., Hart, B. L., & Goy, R. W. (1978). Heterosexual, autosexual and social behavior of adult male rhesus monkeys with medial preoptic–anterior hypothalamic lesions. *Brain Research, 142,* 105–122.

Slob, A. K., & Schenck, P. E. (1986). Heterosexual experiences and isosexual behavior in laboratory-housed male stump-tailed macaques *(M. arctoides). Archives of Sexual Behavior, 15,* 261–268.

Sloman, S. S. (1948). Emotional problems in "planned for" children. *American Journal of Orthopsychiatry, 18,* 523–528.

Smith, P. K., & Boulton, M. (1990). Rough-and-tumble play, aggression and dominance: Perception and behaviour in children's encounters. *Human Development, 33,* 271–282.

Smith, P. K., & Daglish, L. (1977). Sex differences in parent and infant behavior in the home. *Child Development, 48,* 1250–1254.

Smith, P. K., & Lewis, K. (1985). Rough-and-tumble play, fighting, and chasing in nursery school children. *Ethology and Sociobiology, 6,* 175–181.

Snow, E., & Bluestone, H. (1969). Fetishism and murder. In J. H. Masserman (Ed.), *Science and psychoanalysis: Vol. 15. Dynamics of deviant sexuality* (pp. 88–97). New York: Grune & Stratton.

Snow, M. E., Jacklin, C. N., & Maccoby, E. E. (1983). Sex-of-child differences in father–child interaction at one year of age. *Child Development, 54,* 227–232.

Snow, W. G., & Weinstock, J. (1990). Sex differences among non-brain-damaged adults on the Wechsler Adult Intelligence Scales: A review of the literature. *Journal of Clinical and Experimental Neuropsychology, 12,* 873–886.

Socarides, C. W. (1978). *Homosexuality.* New York: Jason Aronson.

Socarides, C. W. (1982). Abdicating fathers, homosexual sons: Psychoanalytic observations on the contribution of the father to the development of male homosexuality. In S. H. Cath (Ed.), *Father and child: Developmental and clinical perspectives* (pp. 509–521). Boston: Little, Brown.

Socarides, C. W. (1988). *The preoedipal origin and psychoanalytic therapy of sexual perversions.* Madison, CT: International Universities Press.

Socarides, C. W. (1990). The homosexualities: A psychoanalytic classification. In C. W. Socarides & V. D. Volkan (Eds.), *The homosexualities: Reality, fantasy, and the arts* (pp. 9–46). Madison, CT: International Universities Press.

Socarides, C. W., & Volkan, V. D. (Eds.). (1991). *The homosexualities and the therapeutic process.* Madison, CT: International Universities Press.

Spanier, G. B. (1976). Measuring dyadic adjustment: New scales for assessing the quality of marriage and similar dyads. *Journal of Marriage and the Family, 38,* 15–28.

Speltz, M. L., Greenberg, M. T., & DeKlyen, M. (1990). Attachment in preschoolers with disruptive behavior: A comparison of clinic-referred and nonproblem children. *Development and Psychopathology, 2,* 31–46.

Spensley, J., & Barter, J. T. (1971). The adolescent transvestite on a psychiatric service: Family patterns. *Archives of Sexual Behavior, 1,* 347–356.

Sperling, M. (1964). The analysis of a boy with transvestite tendencies: A contribution to the genesis and dynamics of transvestism. *Psychoanalytic Study of the Child, 19,* 470–493.

Spijkstra, J. J., Spinder, T., & Gooren, L. J. G. (1988). Short-term patterns of pulsatile LH secretion do not differ between male-to-female transsexuals and heterosexual men. *Psychoneuroendocrinology, 13,* 279–283.

Spinder, T., Spijkstra, J. J., Gooren, L. J. G., & Burger, C. W. (1989). Pulsatile luteinizing hormone release and ovarian steroid levels in female-to-male transsexuals compared to heterosexual women. *Psychoneuroendocrinology, 14,* 97–102.

Spira, A., Bajos, N., and the ACSF Group. (1994). *Sexual behaviour and AIDS.* Ashgate, England: Avebury.

Spitzer, R. L. (1981). The diagnostic status of homosexuality in DSM-III: A reformulation of the issues. *American Journal of Psychiatry, 138,* 210–215.

Spitzer, R. L., & Endicott, J. (1978). Medical and mental disorder: Proposed definition and criteria. In R. L. Spitzer & D. F. Klein (Eds.), *Critical issues in psychiatric diagnosis* (pp. 15–39). New York: Raven Press.

Spitzer, R. L., Williams, J. B. W., Gibbon, M., & First, M. B. (1992). The Structured Clinical Interview for DSM-III-R (SCID): I. History, rationale, and description. *Archives of General Psychiatry, 49,* 624–629.

Sreenivasan, U. (1985). Effeminate boys in a child psychiatric clinic: Prevalence and associated factors. *Journal of the American Academy of Child Psychiatry, 24,* 689–694.

Sroufe, L. A., & Rutter, M. (1984). The domain of developmental psychopathology. *Child Development, 55,* 17–29.

Sroufe, L. A., & Waters, E. (1977). Attachment as an organizational construct. *Child Development, 48,* 1184–1199.

Standards of care: The hormonal and surgical sex reassignment of gender dysphoric persons. (1985). *Archives of Sexual Behavior, 14,* 79–90.

Stattin, H., & Klackenberg-Larsson, I. (1991). The short- and long-term implications for parent–child relations of parents' prenatal preferences for their child's gender. *Developmental Psychology, 27,* 141–147.

Steenhuis, R. E., Bryden, M. P., Schwartz, M., & Lawson, S. (1990). Reliability of hand preference items and factors. *Journal of Clinical and Experimental Neuropsychology, 12,* 921–930.

Stein, D. J. (1993). Cross-cultural psychiatry and the DSM-IV. *Comprehensive Psychiatry, 34,* 322–329.

Steiner, B. W. (1985a). A personal perspective. In B. W. Steiner (Ed.), *Gender dysphoria: Development, research, management* (pp. 417–421). New York: Plenum Press.

Steiner, B. W. (Ed.). (1985b). *Gender dysphoria: Development, research, management.* New York: Plenum Press.

Steiner, B. W., Sanders, R. M., & Langevin, R. (1985). Crossdressing, erotic preference, and aggression: A comparison of male transvestites and transsexuals. In R. Langevin (Ed.), *Erotic preference, gender identity and aggression in men: New research studies* (pp. 261–275). Hillsdale, NJ: Erlbaum.

Steiner, B. W., Zajac, A. S., & Mohr, J. W. (1974). A gender identity project: The organization of a multidisciplinary study. *Canadian Psychiatric Association Journal, 19,* 7–12.

Stevenson, I. (1977). The Southeast Asian interpretation of gender dysphoria: An illustrative case report. *Journal of Nervous and Mental Disease, 165,* 201–208.

Stevenson, J. (1992). Evidence for a genetic etiology in hyperactivity in children. *Behavior Genetics, 22,* 337–344.

Stevenson, M. R., & Black, K. N. (1988). Paternal absence and sex-role development: A meta-analysis. *Child Development, 59,* 793–814.

Stirtzinger, R., & Mishna, F. (1994). The borderline family in the borderline child: Understanding and managing the noise. *Canadian Journal of Psychiatry, 39,* 333–340.

Stoller, R. J. (1964a). The hermaphroditic identity of hermaphrodites. *Journal of Nervous and Mental Disease, 139,* 453–457.

Stoller, R. J. (1964b). A contribution to the study of gender identity. *International Journal of Psycho-Analysis, 45,* 220–226.

Stoller, R. J. (1965). The sense of maleness. *Psychoanalytic Quarterly, 34,* 207–218.

Stoller, R. J. (1966). The mother's contribution to infantile transvestic behavior. *International Journal of Psycho-Analysis, 47,* 384–395.

Stoller, R. J. (1967). "It's only a phase": Femininity in boys. *Journal of the American Medical Association, 201,* 314–315.

Stoller, R. J. (1968a). The sense of femaleness. *Psychoanalytic Quarterly, 37,* 42–55.

Stoller, R. J. (1968b). Male childhood transsexualism. *Journal of the American Academy of Child Psychiatry, 7,* 193–209.

Stoller, R. J. (1968c). *Sex and gender: Vol. 1. The development of masculinity and femininity.* New York: Jason Aronson.

Stoller, R. J. (1970). Psychotherapy of extremely feminine boys. *International Journal of Psychiatry, 9,* 278–281.

Stoller, R. J. (1971). The term "transvestism." *Archives of General Psychiatry, 24,* 230–237.

Stoller, R. J. (1972). The "bedrock" of masculinity and femininity: Bisexuality. *Archives of General Psychiatry, 26,* 207–212.

Stoller, R. J. (1975). *Sex and gender: Vol. 2. The transsexual experiment.* London: Hogarth Press.

Stoller, R. J. (1978). Boyhood gender aberrations: Treatment issues. *Journal of the American Psychoanalytic Association, 26*, 541–558.

Stoller, R. J. (1979). Fathers of transsexual children. *Journal of the American Psychoanalytic Association, 27*, 837–866.

Stoller, R. J. (1980). Problems with the term "homosexuality." *Hillside Journal of Clinical Psychiatry, 2*, 3–25.

Stoller, R. J. (1982). Transvestism in women. *Archives of Sexual Behavior, 11*, 99–115.

Stoller, R. J. (1985a). Maternal influences in the precocious emergence of fetishism in a two-year-old boy. In E. J. Anthony & G. H. Pollock (Eds.), *Parental influences in health and disease* (pp. 427–475). Boston: Little, Brown.

Stoller, R. J. (1985b). *Presentations of gender.* New Haven, CT: Yale University Press.

Stoller, R. J., & Newman, L. E. (1971). The bisexual identity of transsexuals: Two case reports. *Archives of Sexual Behavior, 1*, 17–28.

Stone, C., & Bernstein, L. (1980). Case management with borderline children: Theory and practice. *Clinical Social Work Journal, 8*, 147–160.

Sulcov, M. B. (1973). *Transsexualism: Its social reality.* Unpublished doctoral dissertation, Indiana University.

Sullivan, C. B. L., Bradley, S. J., & Zucker, K. J. (1995). Gender identity disorder (transsexualism) and transvestic fetishism. In V. B. Van Hasselt & M. Hersen (Eds.), *Handbook of adolescent psychopathology: A guide to diagnosis and treatment* (pp. 525–558). New York: Lexington Books.

Sullivan, L. (1990). *From female to male: The life of Jack Bee Garland.* Boston: Alyson.

Suomi, S. J. (1991). Early stress and adult emotional reactivity in rhesus monkeys. In *The childhood environment and adult disease* (Ciba Foundation Symposium No. 156, New Series, pp. 171–188). New York: Wiley.

Swaab, D. F., & Fliers, E. (1985). A sexually dimorphic nucleus in the human brain. *Science, 228*, 1112–1115.

Swaab, D. F., Fliers, E., & Partiman, T. S. (1985). The suprachiasmatic nucleus of the human brain in relation to sex, age and senile dementia. *Brain Research, 342*, 37–44.

Swaab, D. F., Gooren, L. J. G., & Hofman, M. A. (1992a). The human hypothalamus in relation to gender and sexual orientation. *Progress in Brain Research, 93*, 205–217.

Swaab, D. F., Gooren, L. J. G., & Hofman, M. A. (1992b). Gender and sexual orientation in relation to hypothalamic structures. *Hormone Research, 38*(Suppl. 2), 51–61.

Swaab, D. F., & Hofman, M. A. (1984). Sexual differentiation of the human brain: A historical perspective. *Progress in Brain Research, 61*, 361–373.

Swaab, D. F., & Hofman, M. A. (1990). An enlarged suprachiasmatic nucleus in homosexual men. *Brain Research, 537*, 141–148.

Swaab, D. F., & Hofman, M. A. (1995). Sexual differentiation of the human hypothalamus in relation to gender and sexual orientation. *Trends in Neurosciences, 18*, 264–270.

Swan, S. (1993). *The wives of Bath*. Toronto: Alfred A. Knopf.

Sweet, M. J., & Zwilling, L. (1993). The first medicalization: The taxonomy and etiology of queerness in classical Indian medicine. *Journal of the History of Sexuality, 3,* 590–607.

Szasz, T. S. (1961). *The myth of mental illness*. New York: Hoeber-Harper.

Taneja, N., Ammini, A. C., Mohapatra, I., Saxena, S., & Kucheria, K. (1992). A transsexual male with 47,XYY karyotype. *British Journal of Psychiatry, 161,* 698–699.

Taylor, P. J., Dalton, R., Fleminger, J. J., & Lishman, W. A. (1982). Differences between two studies of hand preference in psychiatric patients. *British Journal of Psychiatry, 140,* 166–173.

Thacher, B. (1985, April). *A mother's role in the evolution of gender dysphoria: The initial phase of joint treatment in the psychotherapy of a 4-year-old boy who wanted to be a girl.* Paper presented at the meeting of the Division of Psychoanalysis, American Psychological Association, New York.

Thomas, H., & Turner, G. F. W. (1991). Individual differences and development in water-level task performance. *Journal of Experimental Child Psychology, 51,* 171–194.

Thomas, J. R., & French, K. E. (1985). Gender differences across age in motor performance: A meta-analysis. *Psychological Bulletin, 98,* 260–282.

Thompson, S. K. (1975). Gender labels and early sex role development. *Child Development, 46,* 339–347.

Thompson, S. K., Bates, J. E., & Bentler, P. M. (1977, March). *Testing assumptions of gender identification by comparing gender problem and normal groups of boys and their parents.* Paper presented at the meeting of the Society for Research in Child Development, New Orleans.

Thorne, B. (1986). *Crossing the gender divide: What "tomboys" can teach us about processes of gender separation among children.* Unpublished manuscript, Michigan State University.

Thorne, B. (1993). *Gender play: Girls and boys in school.* New Brunswick, NJ: Rutgers University Press.

Tkachuk, J., & Zucker, K. J. (1991, August). *The relation among sexual orientation, spatial ability, handedness, and recalled childhood gender identity in women and men.* Poster presented at the meeting of the International Academy of Sex Research, Barrie, Ontario.

Tolor, A., & Tolor, B. (1974). Children's figure drawings and changing attitudes toward sex roles. *Psychological Reports, 34,* 343–349.

Torgersen, S. (1987). Sampling problems in twin research. *Journal of Psychiatric Research, 21,* 385–390.

Tremble, B., Schneider, M., & Appathurai, C. (1989). Growing up gay or lesbian in a multicultural context. In G. Herdt (Ed.), *Gay and lesbian youth* (pp. 253–267). Binghamton, NY: Harrington Park Press.

Trickett, P. K., & Susman, E. J. (1988). Parental perceptions of child-rearing practices in physically abusive and nonabusive families. *Developmental Psychology, 24,* 270–276.

Troiden, R. R. (1979). Becoming homosexual: A model of gay identity acquisition. *Psychiatry, 42,* 362–373.

Troiden, R. R. (1988). Homosexual identity development. *Journal of Adolescent Health Care, 9,* 105–113.

Troiden, R. R. (1989). The formation of homosexual identities. In G. Herdt (Ed.), *Gay and lesbian youth* (pp. 43–73). Binghamton, NY: Harrington Park Press.

Tuber, S., & Coates, S. (1985). Interpersonal phenomena in the Rorschachs of extremely feminine boys. *Psychoanalytic Psychology, 2,* 251–265.

Tuber, S., & Coates, S. (1989). Indices of psychopathology in the Rorschachs of boys with severe gender identity disorder: A comparison with normal control subjects. *Journal of Personality Assessment, 53,* 100–112.

Tuchman, W. W., & Lachman, J. H. (1964). An unusual perversion: The wearing of diapers and rubber pants in a 29-year-old male. *American Journal of Psychiatry, 120,* 1198–1199.

Tuckman, J., & Regan, R. A. (1966). Intactness of the home and behavioral problems in children. *Journal of Child Psychology and Psychiatry, 7,* 225–233.

Tully, B. (1992). *Accounting for transsexualism and transhomosexuality: The gender identity careers of over 200 men and women who have petitioned for surgical reassignment of their sexual identity.* London: Whiting & Birch.

Tuttle, G. E., & Pillard, R. C. (1991). Sexual orientation and cognitive abilities. *Archives of Sexual Behavior, 20,* 307–318.

Ulrichs, K. H. (1994). *The riddle of "man-manly" love: The pioneering work on male homosexuality* (2 vols, M. A. Lombardi-Nash, Trans.). Buffalo, NY: Prometheus Books. (Original work published 1864–1879)

Unger, R., & Crawford, M. (1992). *Women and gender: A feminist psychology.* New York: McGraw-Hill.

Unger, R. K. (1979). Toward a redefinition of sex and gender. *American Psychologist, 34,* 1085–1094.

Unger, R. K., & Crawford, M. (1993). The troubled relationship between terms and concepts. *Psychological Science, 4,* 122–124.

Van de Wiele, R. L., Bogumil, F., Dryenfurth, I., Ferin, M., Jewelewica, R., Warren, M., Rizkallah, J., & Mikhail, G. (1970). Mechanisms regulating the menstrual cycle in women. *Recent Progress in Hormone Research, 26,* 63–95.

Van den Aardweg, G. J. M. (1986). *On the origins and treatment of homosexuality: A psychoanalytic reinterpretation.* New York: Praeger.

Van den Brekel, E. J. G. (1986). Linkshandigheid [Left-handedness]. *Maandbericht Gezondheidsstatistiek, 5,* 5–9.

van den Wijngaard, M. (1991a). The acceptance of scientific theories and images of masculinity and femininity—1959±1985. *Journal of the History of Biology, 24,* 19–49.

van den Wijngaard, M. (1991b). *Reinventing the sexes: Feminism and biomedical construction of femininity and masculinity, 1959–1985.* Unpublished doctoral dissertation, University of Amsterdam.

Vasta, R., Lightfoot, C., & Cox, B. D. (1993). Understanding gender differences on the water-level problem: The role of spatial perception. *Merrill–Palmer Quarterly, 39,* 391–414.

Vecchio, T. J. (1966). Predictive value of a single diagnostic test in unselected populations. *New England Journal of Medicine, 274,* 1171–1173.

Verhulst, F. C., & Koot, H. M. (1992). *Child psychiatric epidemiology: Concepts, methods, findings.* Newbury Park, CA: Sage.

Verkauf, B. S., & Jones, H. W. (1970). Masculinization of the female genitalia in congenital adrenal hyperplasia: Relationship to the salt losing variety of the disease. *Southern Medical Journal, 63,* 634–638.

Voeller, B. (1990). Some uses and abuses of the Kinsey scale. In D. P. McWhirter, S. A. Sanders, & J. M. Reinisch (Eds.), *Homosexuality/heterosexuality: Concepts of sexual orientation* (pp. 32–38). New York: Oxford University Press.

Volkan, V. D. (1979). Transsexualism: As examined from the viewpoint of internalized object relations. In T. B. Karasu & C. W. Socarides (Eds.), *On sexuality: Psychoanalytic observations* (pp. 189–221). New York: International Universities Press.

Wachtel, S., Green, R., Simon, N. G., Reichart, A., Cahill, L., Hall, J., Nakamura, D., Wachtel, G., Futterweit, W., Biber, S. H., & Ihlenfeld, C. (1986). On the expression of H-Y antigen in transsexuals. *Archives of Sexual Behavior, 15,* 51–68.

Wakefield, J. C. (1992a). Disorder as harmful dysfunction: A conceptual critique of *DSM-III-R*'s definition of mental disorder. *Psychological Review, 99,* 232–247.

Wakefield, J. C. (1992b). The concept of mental disorder: On the boundary between biological facts and social values. *American Psychologist, 47,* 373–388.

Walinder, J. (1965). Transvestism: Definition and evidence in favor of occasional derivation from cerebral dysfunction. *International Journal of Neuropsychiatry, 1,* 567–573.

Walinder, J. (1967). *Transsexualism: A study of forty-three cases.* Göteborg, Sweden: Scandinavian University Books.

Wallach, H. D. (1961). Termination of treatment as a loss. *Psychoanalytic Study of the Child, 16,* 538–548.

Walters, W. A. W., & Ross, M. W. (Eds.). (1986). *Transsexualism and sex reassignment.* Oxford: Oxford University Press.

Ward, A. J. (1991). Prenatal stress and childhood psychopathology. *Child Psychiatry and Human Development, 22,* 97–110.

Ward, I. L. (1972). Prenatal stress feminizes and demasculinizes the behavior of males. *Science, 175,* 82–84.

Ward, I. L. (1984). The prenatal stress syndrome: Current status. *Psychoneuroendocrinology, 9,* 3–11.

Ward, I. L. (1992). Sexual behavior: The product of perinatal hormonal and prepubertal social factors. In A. A. Gerall, H. Moltz, & I. L. Ward (Eds.), *Handbook of behavioral neurobiology: Vol. 11. Sexual differentiation* (pp. 157–180). New York: Plenum Press.

Ward, I. L., Ward, O. B., Winn, R. J., & Bielawski, D. (1994). Male and female sexual behavior potential of male rats prenatally exposed to the influence of alcohol, stress, or both factors. *Behavioral Neuroscience, 108,* 1188–1195.

Ward, I. L., & Weisz, J. (1980). Maternal stress alters plasma testosterone in fetal males. *Science, 207,* 328–329.

Ward, I. L., & Weisz, J. (1984). Differential effects of maternal stress on circulating levels of corticosterone, progesterone, and testosterone in male and female rat fetuses and their mothers. *Endocrinology, 114,* 1635–1644.

Watabe, T., & Endo, A. (1994). Sexual orientation of male mouse offspring prenatally exposed to ethanol. *Neurotoxicology and Teratology, 16,* 25–29.

Watson, D. B. (1991). Laterality and handedness in adult transsexuals. *SIEC-CAN Journal, 6*(1), 22–26.

Watson, D. B., & Coren, S. (1992). Left-handedness in male-to-female transsexualism [Letter to the editor]. *Journal of the American Medical Association, 267,* 1342.

Weeks, J. (1985). *Sexuality and its discontents: Meanings, myths and modern sexualities.* London: Routledge & Kegan Paul.

Weeks, J. (1991). *Against nature: Essays on history, sexuality, and identity.* London: Rivers Oram Press.

Weiner, B. (1993). On sin versus sickness: A theory of perceived responsibility and social motivation. *American Psychologist, 48,* 957–965.

Weinrich, J. D. (1976). *Human reproductive strategy. I. Environmental predictability and reproductive strategy: Effects of social class and race. II. Homosexuality and nonreproduction: Some evolutionary models.* Unpublished doctoral dissertation, Harvard University.

Weinrich, J. D. (1980). Homosexual behavior in animals: A new review of observations from the wild, and their relationship to human homosexuality. In R. Forleo & W. Pasini (Eds.), *Medical sexology: The Third International Congress* (pp. 288–295). Littleton, MA: PSG.

Weinrich, J. D. (1985). Transsexuals, homosexuals, and sissy boys: On the mathematics of follow-up studies. *Journal of Sex Research, 21,* 322–328.

Weinrich, J. D. (1987). A new sociobiological theory of homosexuality applicable to societies with universal marriages. *Ethology and Sociobiology, 8,* 37–47.

Weisz, J. R., & Weiss, B. (1991). Studying the "referability" of child clinical problems. *Journal of Consulting and Clinical Psychology, 59,* 266–273.

Wellings, K., Field, J., Johnson, A. M., & Wadsworth, J. (1994). *Sexual behaviour in Britain: The National Survey of Sexual Attitudes and Lifestyles.* London: Penguin Books.

West, D. J. (1967). *Homosexuality.* Harmondsworth, England: Penguin Books.

Westhead, V. A., Olson, S. J., & Meyer, J. K. (1990). Gender identity disorders in adolescence. In M. Sugar (Ed.), *Adolescent sexuality* (pp. 87–107). New York: Norton.

Westney, L., Bruney, R., Ross, B., Clark, J. F. J., Rajguru, S., & Ahluwalia, B.

(1991). Evidence that gonadal hormone levels in amniotic fluid are decreased in males born to alcohol users in humans. *Alcohol and Alcoholism, 26,* 403–407.

Westphal, C. (1869). Die Konträre Sexualempfindung [The inverted sexual instinct]. *Archiven für Psychiatrie und Nervenkrankheiten, 2,* 73–108.

Weyl, N. (1987). Hormonal influences on sexual inversion: A dual inheritance model of Proust's homosexuality. *Journal of Social and Biological Structures, 10,* 385–390.

Whalen, R. E. (1993). Animal sexual differentiation: The early days and current questions. In M. Haug, R. E. Whalen, C. Aron, & K. L. Olsen (Eds.), *The development of sex differences and similarities in behavior* (pp. 77–86). Dordrecht, The Netherlands: Kluwer Academic.

Whalen, R. E., & Edwards, D. A. (1967). Hormonal determinants of the development of masculine and feminine behavior in male and female rats. *Anatomic Record, 157,* 173–180.

Whitam, F. L., Diamond, M., & Martin, J. (1993). Homosexual orientation in twins: A report on 61 pairs and three triplet sets. *Archives of Sexual Behavior, 22,* 187–206.

Whitam, F. L., & Mathy, R. M. (1986). *Male homosexuality in four societies: Brazil, Guatemala, the Philippines, and the United States.* New York: Praeger.

White, P. C., New, M. I., & Dupont, B. (1987). Congenital adrenal hyperplasia. *New England Journal of Medicine, 316,* 1519–1524, 1580–1586.

Whitehead, H. (1981). The bow and the burden strap: A new look at institutionalized homosexuality in native North America. In S. B. Ortner & H. Whitehead (Eds.), *Sexual meanings: The cultural construction of gender and sexuality* (pp. 80–115). Cambridge, England: Cambridge University Press.

Whiting, B. B., & Edwards, C. P. (1973). A cross-cultural analysis of sex differences in the behavior of children aged three through eleven. *Journal of Social Psychology, 91,* 171–188.

Widiger, T. A., Frances, A. J., Pincus, H. A., & Davis, W. W. (1990). DSM-IV literature reviews: Rationale, process, and limitations. *Journal of Psychopathology and Behavioral Assessment, 12,* 189–202.

Widiger, T. A., & Weissman, M. M. (1991). Epidemiology of borderline personality disorder. *Hospital and Community Psychiatry, 42,* 1015–1021.

Wiederman, M. W. (1993). Demographic and sexual characteristics of nonresponders to sexual experience items in a national survey. *Journal of Sex Research, 30,* 27–35.

Wiesen, M., & Futterweit, W. (1983). Normal plasma gonadotropin response to gonadotropin-releasing hormone after diethylstilbestrol priming in transsexual women. *Journal of Clinical Endocrinology and Metabolism, 57,* 197–199.

Wikan, U. (1977). Man becomes woman: Transsexualism in Oman as a key to gender roles. *Man, 12,* 304–319.

Wille, R., Borchers, D., & Schultz, W. (1987, June). *Prenatal distress: A dispo-*

sition for homosexuality? Paper presented at the meeting of the International Academy of Sex Research, Tutzing, Germany.

Willerman, L. (1973). Activity level and hyperactivity in twins. *Child Development, 44,* 288–293.

Williams, J. B. W., Gibbon, M., First, M. B., Spitzer, R. L., Davies, M., Borus, J., Howes, M. J., Kane, J., Pope, H. G., Rounsaville, B., & Wittchen, H. (1992). The Structured Clinical Interview for DSM-III-R (SCID): II. Multisite test–retest reliability. *Archives of General Psychiatry, 49,* 630–636.

Williams, K., Goodman, M., & Green, R. (1985). Parent–child factors in gender role socialization in girls. *Journal of the American Academy of Child Psychiatry, 26,* 720–731.

Williams, K., Green, R., & Goodman, M. (1979). Patterns of sexual identity development: A preliminary report on the "tomboy." *Research in Community and Mental Health, 1,* 103–123.

Williams, W. L. (1986). *The spirit and the flesh: Sexual diversity in American Indian culture.* Boston: Beacon Press.

Williamson, N. E. (1976). *Sons or daughters: A cross-cultural survey of parental preferences.* Beverly Hills, CA: Sage.

Williamson, N. E. (1983). Parental sex preferences and sex selection. In N. G. Bennett (Ed.), *Sex selection of children* (pp. 129–145). Orlando, FL: Academic Press.

Willmott, M. (1975). *Cognitive characteristics and sexual orientation: Observations based on three highly selected groups.* Unpublished master's thesis, University of Newcastle-upon-Tyne.

Willmott, M., & Brierley, H. (1984). Cognitive characteristics and homosexuality. *Archives of Sexual Behavior, 13,* 311–319.

Winkler, R. C. (1977). What types of sex-role behavior should behavior modifiers promote? *Journal of Applied Behavior Analysis, 10,* 549–552.

Wittig, M. A., & Petersen, A. C. (Eds.). (1979). *Sex-related differences in cognitive functioning.* New York: Academic Press.

Wolfe, B. E. (1979). Behavioral treatment of childhood gender disorders: A conceptual and empirical critique. *Behavior Modification, 3,* 550–575.

Wolfe, S. M. (1990). *Psychopathology and psychodynamics of parents of boys with a gender identity disorder of childhood.* Unpublished doctoral dissertation, City University of New York.

Wolfe, S. M. (1994, October). Case illustration of intervention strategies for boys with gender identity disorder and their families. In S. J. Bradley (Chair), *Gender identity disorder: Recent research and approaches to treatment.* Institute presented at the meeting of the American Academy of Child and Adolescent Psychiatry, New York.

Woodhouse, A. (1989). *Fantastic women: Sex, gender and transvestism.* New Brunswick, NJ: Rutgers University Press.

Woollett, A., White, D., & Lyon, L. (1982). Observations of fathers at birth. In N. Beail & J. McGuire (Eds.), *Fathers: Psychological perspectives* (pp. 71–91). London: Junction Books.

Wrate, R. M., & Gulens, V. (1986). A systems approach to child effeminacy and the prevention of adolescent transsexualism. *Journal of Adolescence, 9*, 215–229.

Young, W. C., Goy, R. W., & Phoenix, C. H. (1964). Hormones and sexual behavior. *Science, 143*, 212–218.

Yudkin, M. (1978). Transsexualism and women: A critical perspective. *Feminist Studies, 4*, 97–106.

Zaphiriou, M. (1978). David: The analysis of a latency boy with poor physical endowment. *Bulletin of the Hampstead Clinic, 1*, 17–30.

Zecca, G. M., Lertora, V., & Macchi, M. (1990). Trattamento dei disturbi dell'identita di genere nell'eta evolutiva: Primi risultati [Disorder of indentification of the sex during the growing ages: First results]. *Archivio Italiano di Urologia, 62*, 89–92.

Zera, D. (1992). Coming of age in a heterosexist world: The development of gay and lesbian adolescents. *Adolescence, 27*, 849–854.

Zimmerman, M., & Coryell, W. (1987). The Inventory to Diagnose Depression (IDD): A self-report scale to diagnose major depressive disorder. *Journal of Consulting and Clinical Psychology, 55*, 55–59.

Zucker, K. J. (1982). Childhood gender disturbance: Diagnostic issues. *Journal of the American Academy of Child Psychiatry, 21*, 274–280.

Zucker, K. J. (1984). [Review of *Growing up straight: What every family should know about homosexuality* and *Shaping your child's sexual identity*]. *Archives of Sexual Behavior, 13*, 387–390.

Zucker, K. J. (1985). Cross-gender-identified children. In B. W. Steiner (Ed.), *Gender dysphoria: Development, research, management* (pp. 75–174). New York: Plenum Press.

Zucker, K. J. (1988). Toward a developmental sexology [Review of *The "sissy boy syndrome" and the development of homosexuality*]. *Contemporary Psychology, 33*, 197–199.

Zucker, K. J. (1990a). Gender identity disorders in children: Clinical descriptions and natural history. In R. Blanchard & B. W. Steiner (Eds.), *Clinical management of gender identity disorders in children and adults* (pp. 1–23). Washington, DC: American Psychiatric Press.

Zucker, K. J. (1990b). Psychosocial and erotic development in cross-gender identified children. *Canadian Journal of Psychiatry, 35*, 487–495.

Zucker, K. J. (1990c). Treatment of gender identity disorders in children. In R. Blanchard & B. W. Steiner (Eds.), *Clinical management of gender identity disorders in children and adults.* (pp. 25–47). Washington, DC: American Psychiatric Press.

Zucker, K. J. (1992a). "It ain't the meat, it's the motion": Commentary on Rekers and Morey's (1989) "Sex-typed body movements as a function of severity of gender disturbance in boys." *Journal of Psychology and Human Sexuality, 5*, 69–73.

Zucker, K. J. (1992b). Gender identity disorder. In S. R. Hooper, G. W. Hynd, & R. E. Mattison (Eds.), *Child psychopathology: Diagnostic criteria and clinical assessment* (pp. 305–342). Hillsdale, NJ: Erlbaum.

Zucker, K. J. (1993, November). *Towards DSM-IV.* Paper presented at the XIII International Symposium on Gender Dysphoria, New York.

Zucker, K. J. (1994, July). Gender identity, sexual orientation, and sexual behavior in women with congenital adrenal hyperplasia. In K. J. Zucker (Chair), *Congenital adrenal hyperplasia: The nature and nurture of psychosexual differentiation.* Symposium presented at the meeting of the International Academy of Sex Research, Edinburgh.

Zucker, K. J., & Blanchard, R. (1994). Re-analysis of Bieber et al.'s 1962 data on sibling sex ratio and birth order in male homosexuals. *Journal of Nervous and Mental Disease, 182,* 528–530.

Zucker, K. J., Bradley, S. J., Corter, C. M., Doering, R. W., & Finegan, J. K. (1980). Cross-gender behaviour in very young boys: A normative study. In J. Sampson (Ed.), *Childhood and sexuality* (pp. 599–622). Montreal: Editions Etudes Vivantes.

Zucker, K. J., Bradley, S. J., Doering, R. W., & Lozinski, J. A. (1985). Sex-typed behavior in cross-gender-identified children: Stability and change at a one-year follow-up. *Journal of the American Academy of Child Psychiatry, 24,* 710–719.

Zucker, K. J., Bradley, S. J., & Hughes, H. E. (1987). Gender dysphoria in a child with true hermaphroditism. *Canadian Journal of Psychiatry, 32,* 602–609.

Zucker, K. J., Bradley, S. J., & Ipp, M. (1993). Delayed naming of a newborn boy: Relationship to the mother's wish for a girl and subsequent cross-gender identity in the child by the age of two. *Journal of Psychology and Human Sexuality, 6,* 57–68.

Zucker, K. J., Bradley, S. J., & Lowry Sullivan, C. B. (1992). Gender identity disorder in children. *Annual Review of Sex Research, 3,* 73–120.

Zucker, K. J., Bradley, S. J., Lowry Sullivan, C. B., Kuksis, M., Birkenfeld-Adams, A., & Mitchell, J. N. (1993). A gender identity interview for children. *Journal of Personality Assessment, 61,* 443–456.

Zucker, K. J., Bradley, S. J., Oliver, G., Hood, J. E., Blake, J., & Fleming, S. (1992, July). *Psychosexual assessment of women with congenital adrenal hyperplasia: Preliminary analyses.* Poster presented at the meeting of the International Academy of Sex Research, Prague.

Zucker, K. J., Doering, R. W., Bradley, S. J., Alon, N., & Lozinski, J. A. (1984, September). *Sex-typed fantasy play in cross-gender-identified children.* Poster presented at the meeting of the International Academy of Sex Research, Cambridge, England.

Zucker, K. J., Doering, R. W., Bradley, S. J., & Finegan, J. K. (1982). Sex-typed play in gender-disturbed children: A comparison to sibling and psychiatric controls. *Archives of Sexual Behavior, 11,* 309–321.

Zucker, K. J., Finegan, J. K., Doering, R. W., & Bradley, S. J. (1983). Human figure drawings of gender-problem children: A comparison to sibling, psychiatric, and normal controls. *Journal of Abnormal Child Psychology, 11,* 287–298.

Zucker, K. J., Finegan, J. K., Doering, R. W., & Bradley, S. J. (1984). Two subgroups of gender-problem children. *Archives of Sexual Behavior, 13,* 27–39.

Zucker, K. J., & Green, R. (1989). Gender identity disorder of childhood. In T. B. Karasu (Ed.), *Treatments of psychiatric disorders* (Vol. 1, pp. 661–670). Washington, D.C.: American Psychiatric Association.

Zucker, K. J., & Green, R. (1991). Gender identity disorders. In M. Lewis (Ed.), *Child and adolescent psychiatry: A comprehensive textbook* (pp. 604–613). Baltimore: Williams & Wilkins.

Zucker, K. J., & Green, R. (1992). Psychosexual disorders in children and adolescents. *Journal of Child Psychology and Psychiatry, 33,* 107–151.

Zucker, K. J., & Green, R. (1993). Psychological and familial aspects of gender identity disorder. *Child and Adolescent Psychiatric Clinics of North America, 2,* 513–542.

Zucker, K. J., Green, R., Bradley, S. J., Williams, K., Rebach, H. M., & Hood, J. E. (in press). Gender identity disorder of childhood: Diagnostic issues. In T. A. Widiger, A. J. Frances, H. A. Pincus, M. B. First, & W. W. Davis (Eds.), *DSM-IV sourcebook.* Washington, DC: American Psychiatric Association.

Zucker, K. J., Green, R., Garofano, C., Bradley, S. J., Williams, K., Rebach, H. M., & Lowry Sullivan, C. B. (1994). Prenatal gender preference of mothers of feminine and masculine boys: Relation to sibling sex composition and birth order. *Journal of Abnormal Child Psychology, 22,* 1–13.

Zucker, K. J., Kuksis, M., & Bradley, S. J. (1988, August). *Gender constancy judgments in cross-gender-identified children.* Poster presented at the meeting of the International Academy of Sex Research, Minneapolis.

Zucker, K. J., Lozinski, J. A., Bradley, S. J., & Doering, R. W. (1992). Sex-typed responses in the Rorschach protocols of children with gender identity disorder. *Journal of Personality Assessment, 58,* 295–310.

Zucker, K. J., Wild, J., Bradley, S. J., & Lowry, C. B. (1993). Physical attractiveness of boys with gender identity disorder. *Archives of Sexual Behavior, 22,* 23–34.

Zucker, K. J., Wilson, D. N., Kurita, J. A., & Stern, A. (1995). *Children's appraisals of sex-typed behavior in their peers.* Manuscript submitted for publication.

Zucker, K. J., & Yoannidis, T. (1983, April). *The relation between gender labeling and gender constancy in preschool children.* Poster presented at the meeting of the Society for Research in Child Development, Detroit.

Zuger, B. (1966). Effeminate behavior present in boys from early childhood: I. The clinical syndrome and follow-up studies. *Journal of Pediatrics, 69,* 1098–1107.

Zuger, B. (1970a). Gender role determination: A critical review of the evidence from hermaphroditism. *Psychosomatic Medicine, 32,* 449–463.

Zuger, B. (1970b). The role of familial factors in persistent effeminate behaviors in boys. *American Journal of Psychiatry, 126,* 1167–1170.

Zuger, B. (1974). Effeminate behavior in boys: Parental age and other factors. *Archives of General Psychiatry, 30,* 173–177.

Zuger, B. (1976). Monozygotic twins discordant for homosexuality: Report of a pair and significance of the phenomenon. *Comprehensive Psychiatry, 17,* 661–669.

Zuger, B. (1978). Effeminate behavior present in boys from childhood: Ten additional years of follow-up. *Comprehensive Psychiatry, 19,* 363–369.

Zuger, B. (1980). Homosexuality and parental guilt. *British Journal of Psychiatry, 137,* 55–57.

Zuger, B. (1984). Early effeminate behavior in boys: Outcome and significance for homosexuality. *Journal of Nervous and Mental Disease, 172,* 90–97.

Zuger, B. (1988). Is early effeminate behavior in boys early homosexuality? *Comprehensive Psychiatry, 29,* 509–519.

Zuger, B. (1989). Homosexuality in families of boys with early effeminate behavior: An epidemiological study. *Archives of Sexual Behavior, 18,* 155–166.

Zuger, B., & Taylor, P. (1969). Effeminate behavior present in boys from early childhood: II. Comparison with similar symptoms in non-effeminate boys. *Pediatrics, 44,* 375–380.

Index